EXPERIMENTAL LEUKEMOGENESIS

Japanese Cancer Association

GANN Monographs on Cancer Research

GANN Monographs on Cancer Research are intended for the publication of the proceedings of international conferences and symposia dealing with cancer or closely related research fields, and series of papers on specific subjects of importance to cancer research. Publication of each individual monograph is to be decided by the Editorial Board of the Japanese Cancer Association with the final approval of the Board of Directors of the said Association. It is hoped that series of GANN Monographs on Cancer Research will serve as an important source of international information in cancer research.

Tomizo Yoshida, M. D.

JAPANESE CANCER ASSOCIATION
GANN Monograph on Cancer Research No. 12

EXPERIMENTAL LEUKEMOGENESIS

Edited by TADASHI YAMAMOTO
HARUO SUGANO

UNIVERSITY PARK PRESS

UNIVERSITY PARK PRESS
Baltimore • London • Tokyo
Library of Congress Cataloging in Publication Data

Japanese Cancer Association Symposium on Experimental Leukemia Research in Japan, Tokyo, 1970. Experimental leukemogenesis.
(GANN monograph on cancer research, no. 12)
1. Leukemia, Experimental—Congresses. I. Yamamoto, Tadashi, 1917– ed. II. Sugano, Haruo, ed. III. Title. IV. Nippon Gan Gakkai. V. Series.
RC643.J36 1970 616.1'55'071 72-2137
ISBN 0-8391-0650-5

UTP No. 3047-67656-5149
Printed in Japan.

Originally published by
UNIVERSITY OF TOKYO PRESS

PREFACE

This volume presents in greater detail papers from the Japanese Cancer Association Symposium on Experimental Leukemia Research in Japan held in Tokyo on November 13 and 14, 1970. In contemplating a theme for this volume, the Association's first thought was to consider the ever-increasing viral leukemia research, particularly studies concerning oncornavirus-induced leukemia, as a result of the discovery of a very high, early incidence of myelogenous leukemia in rats, which was not proved to be of viral nature, after oral administration of butyl-nitrosourea. As the symposium organizers, we both felt that although an appropriate motif could be the possible synergistic relation of chemical or physical origins to viral leukemogenesis as a target of current research it would be premature to assume that all the leukemia and allied diseases require a virus. It seemed more fitting to give investigators in Japan interested in this field of research an opportunity to reveal their data. This volume, therefore, is somewhat like a resume of the current studies on experimental leukemia and allied diseases in Japan.

At this time, a brief survey of the history of tumor virus research in Japan would be suitable. In the well-known book "Experimental Leukemia" (1968) edited by Dr. Marvin A. Rich, Dr. Jacob Furth, in his article of a historical sketch of experimental leukemia, refers to Akira Fujinami's summary (1930) of his contributions in which Fujinami stressed the biologic aspects of transplantable avian tumors and did not consider the evidence for a causative filtrable agent to be conclusive. Even Professor Fujinami, who also discovered the Fujinami chicken sarcoma virus, an inducible sarcoma, independent of Peyton Rous's Rous sarcoma virus, was confused by theories of so-called filtrable minute cells. (At present, however, the discovery of viral agents can be adequately accomplished on the basis of his data on inducing sarcomas in ducks and silky fowl as well as alternately in domestic fowl.) It was rather clear that the firmly traditional concept of malignancy as an autonomous growth without any additional growth hindered the development of tumor virus research. Professor Fukuzo Oshima, in summarizing his contributions at a general assembly of the Japanese Pathologist Society in 1951, identified the virus tumor as an intermediate between inflamation and neoplasia. Professor Shigeyasu Amano was the first to introduce a modern virologic aspect into recent cancer research based on his electron-microscopic observations on mouse mammary tumor virus and mouse leukemia virus, particularly the studies on the tissue-cultured Amano virus-induced leukemia cell line. In 1962, after two years of successive joint discussion meetings of virologists and oncologists, he established a new research group on tumor viruses aided by a grant from the Ministry of Education of Japan.

On November 30, 1963, Professor Amano introduced to researchers in the field, young Dr. Masakazu Hatanaka, who showed the base composition of RNA of the Amano virus and even the positive hybridization results of viral RNA with the virus-producing cultured cell DNA just a year before Dr. Howard M. Temin proposed his provirus theory. Because of the sudden death of Professor Amano on March 30, 1964, the results were mentioned only in *Nippon Rinsho*, **22**, 1203 (1964). Curiously enough, at that time, many molecular biologists were sceptical of his results. As a suddenly appointed successor to Professor Amano, one of the editors (Tadashi Yamamoto) had to tackle first the problem of autonomous growth without additional growth employing a series of mouse ascites sarcomas induced by Schmidt-Ruppin strain of Rous sarcoma virus. As yet, the basis of leukemia and allied diseases, particularly of virus-induced leukemia, has not been fully acertained. Further studies on the analysis of cellular and host factors, as well as of the virus itself, are expected. An ancient Zen saying in Chinese states 喫茶去 (chi cha chui; after drinking tea let us go on or after drinking tea let us get back); at this stage it would be preferable for us to go on.

The editors are indebted to all of the contributors of this volume, and especially to Dr. Takeshi Odaka and Dr. Yoji Ikawa for their excellent assistance.

Tadashi Yamamoto
Haruo Sugano

CONTENTS

VIRAL LEUKEMOGENESIS

GANN Monograph on Cancer Research 12, 1972

NATURAL TRANSMISSION OF AVIAN LEUKOSIS VIRUSES AMONG CHICKENS

Takehiko SHIMIZU
*National Institute of Animal Health**

Avian leukosis viruses are widespread among the chicken population in Japan. The infection is due mainly to subgroup A viruses and only occasionally to subgroup B viruses. In practice, infection by subgroups C and D, if present, seems to have been overlooked in Japan. The difference between the incidence of infection with subgroup A and B viruses may be explained by the genetic susceptibility of the commercial chicken population. The viruses are transmitted from parent to offspring *via* the egg and from bird to bird after hatching in rearing units. The vertical as well as horizontal transmission results in the widespread infection and perpetuation of the viruses.

Avian leukosis virus problems have been relatively refractory to investigation because the techniques for assaying the causative viruses have been unsatisfactory. Through painstaking investigations over a period of 20 years, Burmester and his co-workers (*1*, *2*) first demonstrated by chick inoculation tests that the viruses were in some cases transmitted through the egg and in other cases transmitted by contact between infected and noninfected chickens. Then, Rubin *et al.* (*12–14*) developed an *in vitro* assay technique for the viruses and confirmed the above facts in some detail. In recent years the avian leukosis viruses have been classified into 4 subgroups, A, B, C, and D, on the basis of their envelope properties, such as antigenicity, host range, and interference pattern (*6*). Therefore, it is important to understand how each subgroup of the viruses is involved in natural transmission. From the practical point of view, however, it seems unlikely that subgroup C and D viruses play important roles in the field, because no viruses of these subgroups have been isolated from field cases, although a number of attempts have been made. Thus, our studies (*8*, *9*) have been concerned mainly with the transmission of subgroup A and B viruses among chickens. In this paper, the mode of natural transmission of avian leukosis viruses will be discussed in the light of our findings as well as evidence provided by others.

Incidence of Infection of Avian Leukosis Viruses

Although considerable data (*11*, *15*) have been presented to suggest that avian leukosis viruses may exist in virtually every commercial flock of chickens, there has

* Josuihoncho 1500, Kodaira, Tokyo 187 (清水武彦).

been little definite information on the incidence of infection with each subgroup of the viruses. An attempt was made to obtain serological evidence of infection with each subgroup of the viruses. A total of 514 chicken sera were collected from eight localities, from northern to southern Japan, irrespective of breeds and ages. The sera were tested for neutralizing antibodies for both subgroups A and B using RSV(RAV-1)* and RSV(RAV-2) as indicators for subgroups A and B, respectively. As shown in Table I, there were no significant differences by localities in positive incidence of antibodies for either subgroup. However, the antibody incidence for subgroup A, ranging from 36.9 to 52.0%, was considerably higher than that for subgroup B, ranging from 3.2 to 16.9%, indicating that subgroup A viruses play a

TABLE I. Incidence of Neutralizing Antibodies for Avian Leukosis Viruses among Chickens in Various Localities

Locality	No. tested	Subgroup A		Subgroup B	
		No. pos.	% pos.	No. pos.	% pos.
Miyagi	63	24	38.1	3	4.8
Saitama	62	28	45.1	2	3.2
Shizuoka	68	28	41.2	3	4.4
Gifu	65	24	36.9	6	9.2
Nara	65	30	46.2	7	10.8
Shimane	63	30	47.6	4	6.3
Ehime	63	30	47.6	5	7.9
Kumamoto	65	34	52.3	11	16.9
Totals	514	228	(44.4)	41	(8.0)

TABLE II. Incidence of Virus Isolation from Apparently Abnormal Chickens

Group No.	Age (days)	No. tested	No. positive	
			Subgroup A	Subgroup B
1	60–90	18	4	3(3)†
2	94	10	3	1(1)
3	200	8	0	0
4	200–270	10	5	1(1)
5	70	5	1	0
6	90	6	4	0
7	100	5	4	0
	138	23	13	1
	219	5	1	0
8	70	36	10	0
9	160–270	15	5	2(1)
Totals (%)		141	50 (34.5)	8 (5.7)

† Parentheses indicate the number of specimens coinfected with subgroup A and B viruses.

* Abbreviations used: RSV, Rous sarcoma virus; RAV, Rous associated virus; RIF, resistant inducing factor; FFU, focus forming unit.

more important role in natural transmission among chickens. The results of virus isolation from chickens of various ages also indicated that the subgroup A viruses were much more prevalent than the subgroup B viruses. A total of 141 specimens were submitted to our laboratory for diagnosis, and most of them were judged to be affected with Marek's disease on the basis of histopathological findings. They were tested for RIF-active viruses by inoculating a C/O-type chick embryo cell culture with a 20% suspension of the liver. The materials were also inoculated into the nonproducing (NP) cells derived from a C/O-type cell culture originally infected with Bryan's high titer strain of RSV and tested for the inducing ability of infectious RSV. The results are shown in Table II. The RIF-active viruses were isolated from 52 specimens, among which 44 were infected with subgroup A, 8 coinfected with subgroups A and B, and 2 infected with subgroup B. The results agreed essentially with those obtained in another way, through the NP cell-activation method. These findings indicate that the incidence of infection with subgroup A is roughly 5 to 6 times higher than that of subgroup B and that there are few or no cases of infection with viruses other than subgroups A and B in Japan.

Horizontal Transmission after Hatching

Widespread infection was observed among chickens with avian leukosis viruses, especially with subgroup A viruses. In order to discover when and how chickens are infected after hatching, an experimental flock of chicken, most of which were susceptible to infection with subgroup A viruses, was examined for infection with subgroup A viruses by testing the development of antibodies. A chicken flock was pedigree-hatched and reared in intimate contact for at least the first 3 months of life. They contained some congenitally infected chicks (Nos. 32, 33, and 35) out of a total of 43 chicks. As indicated in Table III, at 1 week after hatching, 70% of the chicks had maternal antibodies, which became undetectable at 2 months of age. At 3 months of age, 20% of the chicks developed antibodies again. Antibody-positive incidence increased to 56% at 5 months of age and thereafter remained almost unchanged. These results indicate that a few weeks before 3 months of age chickens begin to be infected and most of the susceptible chickens are infected before 5 months of age, suggesting that the spread of infection proceeds rather slowly, compared with other acute viral diseases, although the efficiency of contact transmission may be affected by many factors.

Congenital Transmission and Genetic Susceptibility of Chickens

Rubin *et al.* (*13*, *14*) have indicated that egg infection is of primary importance in the dissemination of avian leukosis viruses. However, most of available data are concerned only with the transmission of subgroup A viruses in a few commercial chicken flocks. Information on subgroup B virus infection is scanty, especially on the incidence of egg infection. In addition, it is known that the susceptibility of chickens to infection with any subgroup of the viruses is specific (*16*) and is controlled by a single pair of autosomal dominant genes (*4*, *15*). Phenotype distribution of susceptibility in the chicken population is one of the important

TABLE III. Development of Neutralizing Antibodies in Chickens after Hatching†

Dam No.	Progeny chick No.	Antibody status					
		1 wk.	2 mos.	3 mos.	5 mos.	7 mos.	17 mos.
771	1	⧻	−	−	⧺	+	⧺
	2	⧻	−	−	⧺	+	
	41	⧺		−	⧺	⧺	
	43	⧺	−	⧺	⧺	⧻	
	9	⧻	−	−	−	−	−
	44	⧻	−	±	⧺	⧺	
	45	⧺	−	−	−		−
784	47	⧻	−	±	⧻	⧻	
	48	⧻	−	±	⧺	⧻	
	50	⧻	−	⧺	⧺	⧻	
802	10	⧻	−	±	⧻	⧻	
	57	⧺	−	−	⧻	⧻	⧻
817	14	−	−	−	⧺	⧺	⧻
	59	−	−	+	±	−	−
	19	⧻	−	±	⧻	⧻	⧻
	21	⧻	±	±	±	−	−
861	22	⧻	−	−			
	62	⧻	±	±	+	−	
	64	⧺	±	−			
	65	⧻	−	±	−	−	−
	28	⧻		⧻	⧻	⧻	⧻
	74	⧺	−	−	−	−	−
	75	⧻	±	⧻	⧻	⧻	
957	76	⧻	±	+	⧺	+	
	77	⧻	−	−	−	−	
	78		−	−	−	−	−
	79	⧻	−	−	−	−	−
	30	⧻	−	⧺			
965	31	⧻	−	−	−	−	
	80	⧻	−	−	⧺	⧺	
	81	⧺	−				
	32	−	−	−	−	−	
967	33	−	−	−	−	−	−
	35	−	−	−	−	−	
	39	±	−	−	⧺	+	⧺
	40	−	−	−	+	⧺	⧻
	85	−	−	−	−	−	−
976	86	±	−		⧻	⧻	⧻
	87	−	−	−	−	−	−
	88	±	−	−	−	−	−
	90	±	±	⧻	⧻	⧻	
No. pos./No. tested		28/40	0/39	8/39	21/37	20/36	8/20
	(%)	(70.0)	(0)	(20.5)	(56.7)	(55.5)	(40.0)

† Neutralizing antibodies were tested as follows: A mixture of equal volumes of a 1 : 5 dilution of serum and RSV (RAV-1) containing 2,000 FFU/0.1 ml was incubated at 37° for 40 min and assayed for surviving RSV by focus formation. The degree of neutralization is expressed as −, ±, +, ⧺, and ⧻, which correspond to surviving fractions >0.5, 0.2–0.49, 0.1–0.19, 0.01–0.09, and <0.01, respectively.

factors responsible for the natural transmission of the viruses. Thus, an attempt was made to determine the incidence of egg infection and the phenotype distribution in some chicken flocks.

A total of 240 fertile eggs were collected from various flocks, 91 from breeding lines of chickens and 149 from 3 commercial flocks. They were incubated at 38° for 10 days. The cultures were prepared individually from the chick embryos, transferred 3 times at 3–4 day intervals and tested for RSV foci by inoculating both RSV(RAV-1) and RSV(RAV-2). Those that developed the expected number of foci were considered susceptible and free of leukosis viruses of that subgroup. Resistant cultures were further tested to determine whether the resistance was genetic or due to leukosis virus infection. For this, the supernatant fluid from the cultures, which remained without challenge with RSV, was tested for the virus in known susceptible C/O-type cell cultures. The results are shown in Table IV. No viruses of either subgroup were recovered from 91 eggs from purebred lines tested, whereas RIF-active viruses were detected in 6 out of 149 eggs from commercial flocks. Of 6 isolates, 5 belonged to subgroup A and only 1 to subgroup B, indicating that in egg infection as well subgroup A viruses have a higher incidence than subgroup B viruses. This situation seems to be comparable to that of some chicken flocks in the United States as reported by Calnek(*3*). Some differences were also observed in phenotype distribution between purebred lines and commercial flocks. The majority of embryos from all purebred lines were resistant to either or both subgroups A and B, *i.e.*, resistance to subgroup A (C/A and C/AB) and subgroup B (C/B and C/AB) was found in 66.1% and 73.5%, respectively. On the other hand, nearly 70.5% of the embryos from commercial flocks were susceptible

TABLE IV. Incidence of Virus Infection and Genetic Resistance to Subgroup A and B Viruses in Chick Embryos from Various Flocks

a. Purebred lines

Flock code	No. tested	Virus isolation (No. pos.)		Phenotype classification			
		Subgroup A	Subgroup B	C/O	C/A	C/B	C/AB
B–1	12	0	0	6	3	3	0
B–2	13	0	0	4	8	1	0
B–3	24	0	0	0	1	0	23
B–4	18	0	0	0	2	2	14
B–5	14	0	0	0	0	5	9
B–6	10	0	0	0	0	10	0
Totals (%)	91	0 (0)	0 (0)	10 (10.9)	14 (15.6)	21 (23.0)	46 (50.5)

b. Commercial flocks

Flock code	No. tested	Subgroup A	Subgroup B	C/O	C/A	C/B	C/AB
C–1	30	1	0	23	0	7	0
C–2	40	1	0	22	0	18	0
C–3	79	3	1	58	3	18	0
Totals (%)	149	5 (3.4)	1 (0.7)	103 (69.1)	3 (2.0)	43 (28.8)	0 (0)

to both subgroups and the remaining 30% of these embryos were resistant to one of the subgroups of the viruses. It is noteworthy that the majority of chickens from commercial flocks were susceptible to subgroup A viruses, which were most prevalent in the field.

DISCUSSION

The present results of the antibody survey as well as virus isolation not only confirmed the earlier finding (*11*) that avian leukosis viruses are widely disseminated among chickens but also revealed that most of the infections are due to subgroup A viruses, while infection with subgroup B viruses is extremely limited. The great difference in the rate of infection with each of these subgroups may be due in part to the difference in the incidence of genetic resistance to each virus subgroup in chickens.

The failure to isolate viruses other than those in subgroups A and B from the field cases, even by the NP cell-activation method, suggests that subgroups C and D may play little or no role in Japan. To confirm this, further studies, such as antibody surveys, must be made.

It is important for the perpetuation and dissemination of the viruses that congenital infection of chicken embryos was demonstrated even at low incidence, because the majority of congenitally infected embryo develop into viremic chickens, which may be a major source of horizontal infection among chickens (*14*). In fact, when a flock containing congenitally infected chickens was reared in intimate contact, evidence was obtained that horizontal infection effectively occurred by the fifth month of life. Together, these findings provide possible explanations for the widespread dissemination of avian leukosis viruses among chickens.

Recently, however, ample evidence (*5*, *7*, *10*, *17*) seems to support the hypothesis that the repressed or defective genome of avian leukoviruses is widely distributed among chickens and transferred to their offspring through the egg as a single dominant autosomal gene. The function of such a viral genome in chickens is not known in detail. It is conceivable, however, that the interaction between such a viral genome and infectious virus such as phenotypic mixing or recombination may occur frequently (*7*), because both forms of avian leukoviruses have ubiquitous distribution among chickens. If this is the case, the natural history of avian leukosis viruses would prove to be more complicated, and further studies will be required on this problem.

REFERENCES

1. Burmester, B. R., and Gentry, R. F. The transmission of avian lymphomatosis by contact. *Cancer Res.*, **14**, 34 (1954).
2. Burmester, B. R., and Waters, N. F. The role of the infected egg in the transmission of visceral lymphomatosis. *Poult. Sci.*, **34**, 1415 (1955).
3. Calnek, B. W. Lymphoid leukosis virus: A survey of commercial breeding flocks for genetic cellular resistance and incidence of embryo infection. *Avian Dis.*, **12**, 104 (1968).

4. Crittenden, L. B., Stone, H. A., Reamer, R. H., and Okazaki, W. Two loci controlling genetic cellular resistance to avian leukosis-sarcoma viruses. *J. Virol.*, **5**, 898 (1967).
5. Dougherty, R. H., and Di Stefano, H. S. Lack of relationship between infection with avian leukosis virus and the presence of COFAL antigen in chick embryos. *Virology*, **29**, 586 (1966).
6. Duff, R. G., and Vogt, P. K. Characteristics of two new avian tumor virus subgroups. *Virology*, **39**, 18 (1969).
7. Hanafusa, H., Miyamoto, T., and Hanafusa, T. A cell-associated factor essential for formation of an infectious form of Rous sarcoma virus. *Proc. Natl. Acad. Sci. U.S.*, **66**, 314 (1970).
8. Hihara, H., Ishizaki, R., Mizuno, and Y. Shimizu, T. Serological properties of avian leukosis viruses isolated from field cases (in Japanese). *Kachikueiseishikenjo Kenkyuhokoku* (*Bull. Natl. Inst. Anim. Health*), **61**, 1 (1970).
9. Mizuno, Y., Yuasa, N., Hihara, H., Ishizaki, R., and Shimizu, T. Neutralizing antibodies against avian leukosis viruses in abnormal chicken sera (in Japanese). *Kachikueiseishikenjo Kenkyuhokoku* (*Bull. Natl. Inst. Anim. Health*), **60**, 1 (1970).
10. Payne, L. N., and Chubb, R. C. Studies on the nature and genetic control of an antigen in normal chick embryo which reacts in the COFAL test. *J. Gen. Virol.*, **3**, 379 (1968).
11. Purchase, H. G. The epizootiology of the avian leukosis complex. *In* "Comparative Leukemia Research," ed. by M. Wennergren, Pergamon Press, Oxford and New York, p. 209 (1966).
12. Rubin, H. A virus in chick embryos which induces resistance *in vitro* to infection with Rous sarcoma virus. *Proc. Natl. Acad. Sci. U.S.*, **46**, 1105 (1960).
13. Rubin, H., Cornelius, A., and Fanshier, L. The pattern of congenital transmission of avian leukosis virus. *Proc. Natl. Acad. Sci. U.S.*, **47**, 1058 (1961).
14. Rubin, H., Fanshier, L., Cornelius, A., and Hughes, W. F. Tolerance and immunity in chickens following congenital and contact infection with avian leukosis virus. *Virology*, **17**, 143 (1962).
15. Shimizu, T., Ishizaki, R., Hihara, H., Mizuno, Y., Sazawa, H., and Sugimori, T. The development of an experimental chicken flock free of avian leukosis virus (in Japanese). *Kachikueiseishikenjo Kenkyuhokoku* (*Bull. Natl. Inst. Anim. Health*), **57**, 9 (1968).
16. Vogt, P. K., and Ishizaki, R. Reciprocal patterns of genetic resistance to avian tumor viruses in two lines of chickens. *Virology*, **26**, 664 (1965).
17. Weiss, R. A. Host range of Bryan strain Rous sarcoma virus synthesized in the absence of helper virus. *J. Gen. Virol.*, **5**, 511 (1969).

GANN Monograph on Cancer Research 12, 1972

VERTICAL TRANSMISSION OF MLV-MOLONEY AND MSV-MOLONEY, AND RELATED PROBLEMS

Noriaki IDA, Kayata OGAWA, Yasuhiro OHBA, Michiko TAKADA, Etsuko YOKOGI, and Yoji IKAWA
Toyo Kogyo Hospital and Cancer Institute***

1) Vertical transmission of Moloney leukemia virus and Moloney sarcoma virus in various strains of mice are described, with emphasis on placental transmission of these viruses. 2) The virus prepared from congenital sarcoma thus induced (MSV-CS-Moloney substrain) showed a high potency in induction of brain tumors (gliomas or hemangioendotheliomas) in rats and mice. 3) A tissue culture line of oligodendroglial cells was established from one of the MSV-CS-induced brain tumors in the rat.

The results reported here represent extensions of a study designed to gain some information on the congenital transmission, that is, from parents to offspring, of the Moloney leukemia virus (MLV) and Moloney sarcoma virus (MSV) in mice.

Most congenital sarcomas were found in offspring whose mothers had been dually infected with MSV and MLV. The cell-free extracts prepared from the congenital sarcoma thus induced seemed to have had higher oncogenicity toward the production of brain tumors in rats or mice. For this reason, the data included information on brain tumors in rats induced by the MSV-CS-Moloney substrain prepared from the congenital sarcoma in mice.

It is also reported that the tissue culture line of oligodendroglial cells was established from one of the brain tumors in the rats infected with this virus.

Vertical Transmission of MLV-Moloney in Various Strains of Mice

Gross (*13*) observed that filtrates of embryos from AK mice, as well as filtrates of ovaries and testes of AK mice (*14*), induced leukemia when inoculated into C3H mice at birth. From these results this investigator reasoned that leukemia in mice was an " egg-borne virus disease " and that the effective agent could be transmitted from one generation to the next through the embryos. Thus, the possibility of " vertical transmission " of a leukemia virus was suggested. Similar studies on the avian leukosis virus have been reported by Cottral *et al.* (*5*).

Early studies (*1*, *10*, *39*) indicated that leukemia in mice was not transmissible through the mother's milk. However, more recently it has been shown that cer-

* Huchu-cho 5621, Aki-gun, Hiroshima 730 (井田憲明, 小川加弥太, 大場康寛, 高田美智子, 横木悦子).
** Kami-Ikebukuro 1-37-1, Toshima-ku, Tokyo 170 (井川洋二).

tain leukemia viruses are transmissible through the milk of viremic or leukemic mice (*16, 33, 36*). Dmochowski *et al.* (*6*) recently demonstrated the presence of mature leukemia virus particles in the spleen and thymus of these animals. Previously, the Passage A virus, a more active line of the Gross agent, was shown to be transferred through the maternal line of mice, more particularly through the milk of infected mothers (*8, 15, 16*).

The ova transfer method was used by Fekete and Otis (*7*) to investigate the possibility of the uterine environment affecting the natural transmission of a leukemia agent. They concluded that extrinsic factors, such as the influence of nursing by foster mothers from a low-leukemia strain and the combined influence of such nursing and uterine environment in low-leukemia strain mothers, do not alter the incidence of leukemia and the expression of genetic tendencies.

1. Embryonal transmission of virus in A/LN and BALB/c strain mice

The experiments we reported previously (*27*) were, therefore, undertaken to investigate the possible natural modes of transmission of the Moloney leukemia agent in A/LN and BALB/c strains of mice. This study included the following: a) embryonal transmission of leukemia virus in A/LN strain mice, b) embryonal transmission of leukemia virus in BALB/c strain mice, c) embryonal transmission of leukemia virus at the 12th day of gestation in BALB/c strain mice, and d) reciprocal foster-nursing of offspring between virus-injected BALB/c mothers and normal intact BALB/c mothers.

Evidence was obtained for the transfer of murine leukemia virus across extraembryonic membranes. Pregnant A/LN and BALB/c mice were inoculated intravenously with a mouse-derived Moloney leukemia virus preparation. The periods of inoculation ranged from the 1st through the 18th day of gestation, based on time of detection of the vaginal plug. Immediately after birth the offspring of the viremic mothers were given to normal, untreated BALB/c or Swiss female mice for nursing. These animals were then observed for the development of leukemia. The results obtained indicate that the virus will cross the placental barrier and infect the fetus. It is interesting that several of the mothers remained free of the disease through the period of observation, whereas their offspring died with the virus-induced neoplasm.

2. Reciprocal foster-nursing: transmission of the virus through mother's milk in BALB/c mice

To determine additional routes of transmission of the virus from mother to offspring, reciprocal foster-nursing was carried out. Mothers receiving the virus at the 12th day of gestation foster-nursed a number of mice obtained from normal BALB/c mothers. Of the offspring surviving until the first observation of leukemia, the disease developed in 20.8% at an average age of 39.5 weeks. These results confirm and extend previous findings (*15, 36*) that the leukemia virus can be transmitted to successive generations through the milk of viremic mothers.

Many others (*2, 17, 23, 28, 31, 34, 35, 40–42, 46*) have investigated the vertical transmission from parent to offspring of various murine leukemia viruses.

Generally, the milk of virus-infected mothers is the most effective route in low-leukemia mouse strains, but there seems to be a different situation in the high-leukemia strains such as AK and C58 (*1*, *7*, *10*, *17*, *39*). Friend virus showed a low degree of transmission through mother's milk and a rather high degree of transmission of immunity against the same virus (*41–43*).

Recently, Huebner (*20*) and Huebner and Todaro (*22*) announced on the basis of sero-epidemiological and cell culture studies that the C-type RNA virus genome in mice was transmitted vertically as part of the genetic inheritance of most if not all cells. Except in certain strains of mice which have inherent genetic susceptibilities for expression of the viral particle and the viral *gs* antigen and frequently also susceptibility to early tumor expression, the virus is generally transmitted in a repressed or " switched-off " state. Physical and chemical inducers and old age result in cancers that are correlated with the frequent " switch-on " of large amounts of *gs* antigen and frequently also with fully infectious virus. Thus, it was suggested that the vertically transmitted C-type RNA virus genome is a major determinant of both natural and induced oncogenesis in mice.

The above investigators suggested that " an understanding of how normal cells and normal animals prevent expression of endogenous viral information would appear to offer one of the best hopes for the control of naturally occurring cancers." Thus, vertical transmission of the C-type RNA virus appears to be an important subject regarding the etiology of these neoplasms.

Vertical Transmission of MSV-Moloney in Swiss ICR Mice

As described previously, Ida *et al.* (*23*, *27*, *28*) reported that leukemia virus will cross the placental barrier and infect the fetus. Recently, Moloney (*45*) reported, from the passage line of the Moloney leukemia virus, the isolation of agents that are sarcomatogenic for mice, rats, and hamsters. Perk *et al.* (*47*) and Ikawa and Sugano (*29*) studied the pathogenesis of a rhabdomyosarcoma virus isolate. They reported that the growth of the tumor was very rapid in the muscle tissue, and that regardless of the route of inoculation, the neoplasms arose from muscle tissue by attaching to and penetrating adjacent organs. The titration pattern of some stocks of MSV indicated that the infection of mouse cells was defective and required simultanous infection with a murine leukemia virus for production of infectious progeny MSV (*18*).

As was reported before (*25*, *26*) experiments were undertaken to investigate the possible natural modes of transmission of the Moloney sarcoma agent in Swiss ICR mice. We studied the embryonal transmission of MSV in Swiss mice and also the effect of reciprocal foster-nursing of offspring between virus-infected Swiss mothers and normal intact mothers.

1. Animals, sarcoma, and leukemia virus

Swiss ICR mice were derived from the colonies of Cent. Lab. Exp. Anim. Japan, Inc., Tokyo. Both sarcoma and leukemia viruses (Moloney) were propagated and prepared as described previously (*44*). The dose of the virus injected was 0.1 ml each time, and its concentration was a standard (1 g equiv./ml) virus concentration.

2. *Injection of MSV in pregnant mice*

Pregnant mice were injected intraperitoneally with 0.1 ml doses MSV repeatedly to see if MSV is transmitted to the embryos across the placental barrier. In order to avoid mortality among the embryos and yet achieve adequate dose, we selected the method of repeated injections of the virus at certain periods during pregnancy. The virus was injected three times daily or every other day, with some exceptions. Various groups were set up as follows: injection of MSV was initiated 1) before placenta was established, 2) after placenta was established, 3) at a critical period of fetal growth, 4) at an early period in more advanced pregnancy, and 5) at a later stage of gestation. In addition, dual injection of MSV and MLV was also performed to take advantage of any possible synergism between MLV and MSV. The day of gestation was estimated from the time of first detection of the vaginal plug.

At birth, the offspring were given to normal Swiss ICR foster mothers to avoid possible transmission of either a virus or its antibody through the mother's milk. Our tentative objective in these experiments was detection of " MSV-vertical transmission " through the placenta. When sarcoma developed in the offspring, several studies, including histology and other biological examinations, were conducted.

3. *Embryonic transmission of murine sarcoma virus in Swiss mice*

As indicated above, MSV was injected into pregnant Swiss mice at various

TABLE I. Vertical Transmission of Sarcoma Virus through the Placental Barrier

No.	Experimental group			No. of mother mice injected	No. positive/ No. of offspring obtained	Age at tumor-detection (days)
	Time of injection	Days of gestation	Virus			
1	Before placenta	4, 5, 6	MSV	5	0/51	
	is established		MSV plus MLV	14	0/156	
2	After placenta	7, 9, 11	MSV	14	0/147	
	is established		MSV plus MLV	8	0/87	
3	At a critical	9, 11, 13	MSV	6	0/56	
	period of fetal		MSV plus MLV	7	0/68	
	growth	(11–19)[a]	MSV plus MLV	(3)	1/(25)	7
4	At an early period	13, 15, 18	MSV	15	1/83	19
	in later stage of		MSV plus MLV	15	(1)[b], 2/73	(43), 47, 38
	pregnancy					
5	At a later stage of	15, 17, 18	MSV	6	0/27	
	pregnancy (1)		MSV plus MLV	11	2/66	15, 15
6	At a later stage of	15, 16, 17,	MSV	9	1/77	14
	pregnancy (2)	18, 19	MSV plus MLV	13	2/125	13, 8

[a] Sarcoma developed at the thigh lesion in 7-day-old offspring from the mother injected with MSV and MLV during the period from the 11th to the 19th day of gestation every day, successively. This additional group consisted of 25 offspring obtained from 3 litters.

[b] Sarcoma developed in suckling mice when inoculated at birth with the cultured fluid of the lung tissue of the offspring who showed dyspnea at 43 days of age.

TABLE II. Virus-induced Congenital Sarcomas, Their Tissue Cultures and Transplantations

Sarcoma induced				Tissue culture			Transplantation	
Identification of sarcoma	Experimental group (No. of mother)	Location of tumor	LP (days)	T-C (days of culture)	No. positive/ No. of animals inoc. with supernatant	MLP (days)	No. positive/ No. of animals transplanted	MLP (days)
Sa-1	MSV. MLV (11) No. 2F	Thigh	7	5 (+)	10/10	10	(1) 12/12 (+)	3
				9 (+)	4/9	16	(2) 11/11 (+)	3
				16 (+)	3/12	32	(3) 11/11 (+)	5
				29 (−)	0/10	—		
Sa-2	MSV (13) No. 2F	Pectoral, thoracic cavity, back	19	3 (+)	12/12	15	—	—
				8 (+)	12/12	9		
Sa-3	MSV. MLV (13) No. 7F	Lung tissue	43	4 (−)	0/10	—		
				7 (+)	1/10	20[a]	(1) 10/10 (+)	5
		Thigh	20[a]	15 (+)	10/10	15	(2) 13/13 (+)	3
				10 (+)	4/10	33	(3) 18/18 (+)	5
				13 (+)	2/9	50		
				20 (−)	0/12	—		
				33 (−)	0/10	—		
Sa-4	MSV. MLV (13) No. 2F	Pectoral	47	—	—	—	(1) 5/5 (+)	5
							(2) 8/8 (+)	5
							(3) 10/10 (+)	5
Sa-5	MSV. MLV (13) No. 8F	Pectoral, thoracic cavity	38	3 (+)	10/10	10	(1) 8/8 (+)	5
				12 (+)	17/17	12	(2) 10/10 (+)	5
Sa-6	MSV. MLV (15) No. 4F	Pectoral	15	2 (+)	6/6	12	(1) 3/3 (+)	5
				5 (+)	15/15	12	(2) 25/25 (+)	6
				8 (+)	12/12	9	(3) 35/35 (+)	5
Sa-7	MSV. MLV (15) No. 1F	Submental	15	3 (−)	0/9	—	(1) 2/10 (+)	10
				4 (+)	6/10	10	(2) 20/20 (+)	5
				8 (+)	7/12	6	(3) 10/10 (+)	5
				10 (+)	8/14	23	(4) — (15)[b]	
				11 (+)	5/11	44	169/169	3-5
				18 (+)	4/10	78		
Sa-8	MSV (15) No. 1F	Diaphragm, thoracic cavity, abdominal wall, left leg	14	4 (+)	10/10	10	(1) 35/35 (+)	5
							(2) 28/28 (+)	5
							(3) 10/10 (+)	4
Sa-9	MSV. MLV (15) No. 4F	Dorsal	13	5 (+)	12/12	7	(1) 13/13 (+)	6
				10 (+)	10/10	15	(2) 13/13 (+)	3
				15 (+)	10/10	14	(3) 15/15 (+)	5
				19 (+)	8/8	15		
				26 (+)	2/14	22		
				39 (+)	3/10	35		
Sa-10	MSV. MLV (15) No. 14F	Abdominal wall, hemorrhagic ascites	8	3 (+)	10/10	9	(1) 10/10 (+)	3
				8 (+)	10/10	14	(2) 11/11 (+)	3
				12 (+)	3/9	36	(3) 14/14 (+)	5
				19 (+)	3/13	9		

[a] Sarcoma developed in 1 of 10 mice inoculated at birth with the cultured fluid of the lung tissue of an offspring showing dyspnea at 43 days of age.

[b] Serial transplantations were conducted up to the 15th passages, and all mice were positive.

stages of gestation. Sarcomas were found in some offspring extremely early in life, and in several animals leukemias were also found later in life.

As shown in Tables I and II, sarcomas developed in 9 offspring in the group in which the virus was injected at a later stage of pregnancy. The location of these tumors was the pectoral muscle, abdominal wall, thoracic wall, submental region, dorsal muscle, thigh and legs (Photos 1 and 2). The time of tumor detection or obtaining a positive result was 7, 8, 13, 14, 15, 15, 19, 38, 43, and 47 days of age.

The age at tumor development was extremely young. Most of the tumor masses were histologically identical with malignant rhabdomyoblastoma. Besides these experiments, one of the offspring of the 13th day group using MSV and MLV showed dyspnea at 43 days of age. The mouse was killed and the lung tissue was cultured. When cell-free supernatant of the culture fluid was inoculated into newborn mice, rhabdomyosarcoma developed at the site of inoculation with a mean latent period of 20 days. Thus, sarcomas developed in the offspring exposed to the MSV-M in their uterine life. The term " congenital sarcoma " is applicable to these cases because of extremely early onset of sarcoma and the manner of induction.

4. *Histology of the sarcoma tissue*

In most of the cases, the sarcoma tissue was more or less associated with striated muscle tissue which remained thin and ran in the same direction. Most of the tumor masses were histologically identical to the thigh tumor primarily induced by direct injection of newborn mice with Moloney MSV, and more closely resembled myogenic sarcoma than fibrosarcoma. Large spindle-shaped cells with abundant pale blue cytoplasm, large, relatively clear nuclei, and prominent nucleoli occupied the greater part of the tumor tissue in the Hematoxylin-Eosin stained section. These occasionally contained round giant cells such as are frequently seen in human rhabdomyosarcomas. Thus, the overall findings were consistent with malignant rhabdomyoblastoma (see Photos 3–7).

5. *Electron-microscopic study*

Electron-microscopic findings on the tumors were, generally, identical to those observed in the primary tumors induced in the thighs of newborn or suckling mice. The tumor cells were spindle-shaped and contained an elongated nucleus. The cisternae of the endoplasmic reticulum contained a moderately electron-dense precipitate. Mitochondrial profiles were usually circular or oval. Numerous fibrils were in the cytoplasmic matrix of these cells and in some cases were very prominent. The matured C type often was present on the surface of the tumor cell, and a particle budding from the plasma membrane was also seen at the surface of the tumor cell in some areas (Photos 8 and 9).

6. *Inoculation of tissue-culture fluid of congenital sarcomas*

Tissue-culture of 8 sarcomas and a lung tissue were successfully accomplished. Ten fragments of tumor tissue were implanted in Eagle's minimum essential medium with 20% fetal bovine serum. Cell-free supernatant of the tissue-culture fluid harvested on a certain culture day (2–29 days) was inoculated into newborn Swiss mice intramuscularly. As shown in Table II, most of the animals developed sarcoma at the site of inoculation.

7. *Transplantation of the primary congenital sarcoma*

Eight sarcomas were transplanted into suckling mice of the same strain. Most of the recipients developed sarcomas at the site of injection within 3–5 days. The second and third cell transfers were also 100% successful (see Table II). Thus, evidence was obtained from the results of mouse sarcoma culture, tumor transplantation, as well as electron-microscopic study, that these tumors contained MSV.

8. *Isolation of leukemogenic virus from congenital sarcoma*

As described previously, 8 sarcomas and a lung tissue of the congenitally infected offspring were cultured. When the supernatant of the tissue culture fluids of these tumors was inoculated intramuscularly into newborn mice, sarcoma

TABLE III. Isolation of Leukemogenic Virus from Congenital Sarcoma

Identification of sarcoma			Tissue culture				
			T-C (days)	No. of sarcomas/ No. of animals inoculated	MLP (days)	No. of leukemias/ No. of animals inoculated	MLP (days)
Sa-1	MSV. MLV (11)	Thigh	5 (+)	10/10	10	—	
			9 (+)	4/9	16	3/9	133
			16 (+)	3/12	32	1/12	141
			29 (−)	0/10	—	5/10	132 (113–161)
Sa-3	MSV. MLV (13)	Lung-thigh	5 (+)	10/10	15	—	
			10 (+)	4/10	33	2/10	161 (137–185)
			13 (+)	2/9	50	3/9	133
Sa-7	MSV. MLV (15)	Submental	3 (+)	0/9	—	0/9	
			4 (+)	6/10	10	0/10	
			8 (+)	7/12	6	0/12	
			10 (+)	8/14	23	1/14	119
			11 (+)	5/11	44	0/11	
			18 (+)	4/10	78	3/10	161 (146–192)
Sa-9	MSV. MLV (15)	Dorsal	5 (+)	12/12	7	—	
			10 (+)	10/10	15	—	
			15 (+)	10/10	14	—	
			19 (+)	8/8	15	—	
			26 (+)	2/14	22	3/14	155 (141–174)
			39 (+)	3/10	35	2/10	113
Sa-10	MSV. MLV (15)	Abdominal wall	3 (+)	10/10	9	—	
			8 (+)	10/10	14	—	
			12 (+)	3/9	36	3/9	148
			19 (+)	3/13	9	0/13	

developed in the recipients and all tissues used showed positive results. In addition, lymphocytic leukemias developed in some recipient mice that did not show early sarcomas. That is, leukemia was found in 26 (16%) of 162 animals inoculated with T-C fluids from five different sources of sarcoma (Table III). Their latent period ranged from 113 to 192 days. Thus, isolation of a leukemogenic virus from MSV-M-induced sarcoma was achieved by the tissue culture method. It seems likely that leukemia virus could be transmitted in association with MSV-M during vertical transmission.

According to Snell (*58*), in young mice spontaneous rhabdomyosarcomas were sometimes observed, probably arising from embryonic rests in striated muscle. This was observed in dba females and dba/C57 black stock hybrids. The earliest case occurred in a 2.5-month-old dba female. Since the natural occurrence of this type of tumor is extremely rare in mice, the results obtained in our experiment seem to constitute clear evidence of vertical transmission of the oncogenic virus.

Most of the tumors developed in the offspring obtained from mothers infected at a later stage of pregnancy, and not in the offspring from mothers infected early in gestation. Altered immune response of the host animals could be responsible for this.

In general, the latent period for MSV-induced tumor in suckling mice is as short as 5 days. Therefore, malignant transformation must be initiated sometime during fetal life. The fetuses exposed to the virus at an early stage may be protected by passive transfer of maternal antibodies against MSV-M; and the fetuses exposed later in pregnancy may escape from such passive immunization. In addition, immunological mechanisms are so poorly developed during the neonatal period that virus multiplication and the growth of transformed neoplastic cells are facilitated to quite an extent in newborn mice. Therefore, a state of specific immunological tolerance to viral antigens occurs as a consequence of fetal infection (*4*).

It appears that the potency of the vertically transmitted MSV-M increases with the help of MLV and leads to the induction of congenital sarcoma. Since the leukemogenic component was separated from the sarcomas by tissue culture, it can be speculated that MLV was also transmitted vertically together with MSV-M. Harvey and East (*19*) demonstrated that leukemogenic agents of MSV-H were separated by vertical transmission from infected female mice.

Dilution of MSV seems to be a main factor in these phenomena. However, it should be borne in mind that sarcoma virus can, in some way, accelerate leukemia virus growth in a system less susceptible to leukemia. This represents a functional synergistic relationship between RNA viruses (*9*). Thus, leukemia virus growth might be accelerated by MSV-M in congenital sarcomas. The complexity of sarcoma-leukemia interaction during intrauterine infection is under further investigation.

Brain Tumor in Rats Induced with MSV-CS-Moloney Substrain

1. The origin of MSV-CS-Moloney substrain

As has been reported previously (*25, 26*), sarcomas developed after an extremely short latent period in several offspring whose mothers were injected intraperitoneally with both MSV and MLV. The tumor thus induced could be called a "congenital sarcoma (CS)." The virus was prepared from the transplanted tumors of congenital sarcomas according to Moloney's method (*44*). This virus seemed to have much higher oncogenicity, as judged from the incidence and onset of brain tumors in rats and mice (*24*). Enhancement of murine sarcoma virus oncogenicity in mice might occur through coinfection with MLV in the fetal tissue, as was suggested in other experiments (*61*). The new sarcoma virus obtained in our laboratory was tentatively called the MSV-CS-Moloney substrain.

2. Brain tumor induction with MSV-CS-Moloney

When MSV-CS-Moloney was inoculated intraperitoneally into newborn Sprague-Dawley rats, sarcomas and bone tumors developed in the recipients. In

TABLE IV. Incidence of Intracranial Tumors of Sprague-Dawley Rats Inoculated with MSV-CS-Moloney Substrain[a] or MSV-Moloney Intracerebrally

Virus	Age at inoculation (days)	No. of rats bearing brain tumor/No. inoculated	%	ALP (days)	Other tumor
MSV-CS-Moloney substrain	1–3	23/24	95.8	16	
MSV-Moloney	1–3	2/11	18.2	75	1[b]
Control	1–3	0/25	0.0	—	

[a] MSV-CS-Moloney substrain: MSV originated from virus-induced congenital sarcoma.
[b] Leukemia developed in 1 of 11 animals at 84 days of age.

TABLE V. Induction of Sarcomas in Rats and Mice after Intramuscular Injection of Whole Cell Suspensions of Rat Brain Tumor

Brain tumor used for transplantation	Rats			Mice		
	No. of "takes"/ No. injected	%	ALP (days)	No. of induction/ No. injected	%	ALP (days)
No. 6	6/9	67	15			
10	15/15	100	11	16/16	100	4
11				15/15	100	5
12				15/15	100	5
13				15/15	100	6
14				13/13	100	4
15				16/16	100	4
16	11/11	100	14	13/13	100	5
Totals	32/35	91.4	13	118/118	100	5

TABLE VI. Development of Sarcoma and Bone Tumor in Rats after Transplantation of Rat Brain Tumor in the Left Thigh Region

Rats		Induction of tumor			
		Sarcoma		Bone tumor	
No.	Sex	Location	ALP (days)	Location	ALP (days)
35	22 F	Left thigh (32)	13	L. femur (24)	37
	13M			L. leg (17)	38
				R. leg (1)	65
				L. foot (2)	44
				R. foot (4)	37
				L. arm (3)	43
				R. arm (1)	59
				L. tibia (1)	41

TABLE VII. Development of Sarcoma and Leukemia in Swiss ICR Mice Inoculated with Cell-free Supernatant of Tissue Culture Fluid of Rat Brain Tumor

ID No. of rat	No. of mice inoculated	No. of sarcomas (incidence)	ALP (days)	Range	No. of leukemias (incidence)	ALP (days)	Range
6. RBT_1	19	15	21	(10–93)	2	159	(136–181)
7. RBT_2	13	0	—	—	3	112	(108–121)
9. RBT_3	10	6	28	(18–77)	2	110	(108–112)
10. RBT_4	10	1	148	(148)	0	—	—
12. RBT_5	13	13	50	(29–90)	1	52	(52)
13. RBT_6	9	6	33	(9–68)	0	—	—
14. RBT_7	10	3	33	(15–68)	0	—	—
15. RBT_8	10	1	9	(9)	4	117	(87–137)
16. RBT_9	5	5	50	(31–65)	1	65	(65)
Total RBT_{1-9}	99	50 (50.5%)	35	(9–148)	13 (13.3%)	112	(52–181)

addition, when MSV-CS-Moloney substrain was injected intracerebrally into the newborn rats in a dose of 0.04 ml of 1.0 g equiv./ml virus concentration, 95.8% of 24 animals developed brain tumor (Table IV). Intramuscular injection of whole-cell suspensions of these rat brain tumors into either suckling rats or mice produced sarcomas at the site of injection. Their incidence was 91.4% and 100%, respectively (Table V). Bone tumors were also found in the rats thus treated (Table VI).

Histological study of the brain tumors of the rats and mice showed endotheliomas and gliomas, and some classified as gemistocytic astrocytomas (Photo 10). Following intramuscular inoculation of mice with cell-free supernatants of tissue culture fluids of the rat brain tumors, myogenic sarcoma developed early and leukemia at a later time (Table VII).

Oncogenicity of MSV-Moloney has previously been documented in mice

(*45*), rats (*48*), and hamsters (*21*). In general, tumor production rarely occurs in rats inoculated intramuscularly with MSV-Moloney virus (*47*, *60*). Only thymectomized newborn rats are susceptible to the virus, and tumors thus induced can be transplanted to the syngeneic host (*60*).

It has been well established that several organs, such as the brain, anterior chamber of eyes, testes, and cheek pouch, in hamster represent immunologically weak sites. The Moloney strain of MSV was shown to be capable of inducing hemangioendotheliomas, meningiomas, and gliomas in newborn rats inoculated intracerebrally (*56*). The formation of hemangioendotheliomas in the brain of rats appears to suggest that potent virus is able to bring about a malignant transformation of the mesenchymal cell system. Since the discovery of murine sarcoma virus, it has been thought that the oncogenic effect on this agent was confined to tissues of mesenchymal origin. The induction of gliomas in rats shows the oncogenic effect of this virus on ectodermally derived tissue such as neuroglia.

Oncogenic viruses produced various types of brain tumor in animals when inoculated intracerebrally. Polyoma virus (*54*) and SV40 (*11*, *30*, *55*) produced sarcomas and ependymomas, respectively, in hamsters and in *Mastomys natalensis*. Meningeal sarcomas were induced in chickens and turkeys (*59*, *62*) by Rous sarcoma virus. Several strains of Rous sarcoma virus induced meningiomas and gliomas in hamsters (*49*, *51*, *52*), rabbits (*53*), and dogs (*50*). Mouse brain tumor was also induced by the same virus (*32*). It was observed that hemangioendotheliomas, meningiomas, and gliomas developed in rats when MSV-Moloney was inoculated intracerebrally at birth (*56*, *57*).

It has already been pointed out (*49*, *52*, *53*) that high doses of RSV are needed to produce oncogenesis in the brain of the hamster and rabbit. Mammals such as the hamster are genetically somewhat resistant to infection by the avian sarcoma virus (*52*). In our experiment, only a small dose of MSV-CS-Moloney substrain was needed to induce intracranial tumor in the rats. As was suggested by Rabotti *et al.* (*53*), the choice of the brain as a target organ may be of some importance.

Rabson *et al.* (*55*) were unable to isolate the virus from the SV40-induced brain tumor in mastomys. Many other investigators (*12*, *63*) have had similar difficulties in recovering DNA viruses, such as SV40 and polyoma virus, from the virus-induced tumors. In addition, RSV does not seem to replicate in the hamster brain, although this virus grew in the chicken (*52*) and other fowl (*59*).

However, MSV-CS-Moloney replicated rather efficiently in the brain of inoculated rats. Intramuscular injection of whole-cell suspension of rat brain tumor into suckling rats produced myogenic sarcomas and bone tumors at the site of injection. Also, intramuscular inoculation of cell-free supernatants of tissue culture fluids of rat brain tumor caused multiple sarcomas in mice. Thus, it was evident that the MSV-CS-induced rat brain tumor does, indeed, contain MSV.

Tissue Culture Line of Oligodendroglial Cells Originating from MSV-CS-Moloney-Induced Rat Brain Tumors

As was described previously in this paper, brain tumors developed in Sprague-Dawley rats when the MSV-CS-Moloney substrain was inoculated intracerebrally into suckling rats. The results reported herein concern the tissue culture line of the oligodendroglial cells that originated from MSV-CS-Moloney induced brain tumors of rat.

1. Tissue culture of MSV-CS-Moloney-induced rat brain tumor and morphology of the cultured cells

A solid brain tumor was found in a 3-month-old rat inoculated with MSV-CS-Moloney substrain intracerebrally at birth with a dose of 0.06 ml of 1.0 g equiv./ml virus concentration (Photo 11). This brain tumor was cultured in Eagle's minimum essential medium containing 20% unheated fetal calf serum, 10% triptose phosphate broth, and 0.5% lactalbumin with kanamycin (6 mg/100 ml). In the culture media, tumor cells proliferated rapidly within 24 hr and progressed for several days, after which they showed " conspicuous clumping." An end-to-end arrangement in long strings was noted for most of the cells (Photos 12–13). These cells were globose or pearlike with a variable number of short but slender protoplasmic processes arising sharply from perikarya (Photos 13–15). These processes were seen to branch once or twice dichotomously, and they formed attachments with processes from similar cells. This dichotomous branching may be represented by a short flat ribbonlike expansion at the extremity of the branches (Photo 14). The cell outlines showed bright refractility which seems characteristic of this type of cell (Photos 12–15). These vigorously growing tumor cells showed round nuclei eccentrically located in rather small cells with numerous delicate processes. These cultured cells were passed through culture media successively and continued to proliferate until the 23rd passage, reached at the time of this writing. Thus, a monoclonous oligodendroglial cell line in tissue culture was established.

2. Transplantation and metastasis of the oligodendroglial cells in rats

These cells are transplantable successively into suckling rats intracerebrally,

TABLE VIII. Intracerebral Injection of the Cultured Oligodendroglial Cells in Rats

Tissue culture passage	No. of "takes"/ No. of rats injected	%	Interval between transplantation and death (days)
4th	10/10	100	12
	13/13	100	12
7th	17/17	100	7
20th	8/8	100	8

TABLE IX. Intracerebral Transplantation of Oligodendroglial Cell-transplanted Brain Tumor in Rats

Transplantation generation	No. of "takes"/ No. of rats transplanted	%	Interval between transplantation and death (days)
1st	16/16	100	9
	17/17	100	7
2nd	8/8	100	7

TABLE X. Subcutaneous Transplantation of Oligodendroglial Cell Brain Tumor in Rats

Transplantation generation	No. of "takes"/ No. of rats transplanted	%	Interval between transplantation and death (days)
1st	15/15	100	12
2nd	14/14	100	21
3rd	14/15	93	10

subcutaneously, or intramuscularly. The young rats bearing the transplanted subcutaneous tumor showed metastases to various organs such as lungs, liver, spleen, kidneys, regional lymph nodes, peritoneum, and, occasionally, thymus. Ascitic forms of these cells were also observed in the adult rat with subcutaneous transplanted tumors. It was noted, by the tissue culture method, that these transplanted brain tumors, subcutaneous tumors, and metastatic lesions consisted of the same type of cells, that is, oligodendroglial cells (Tables VIII, IX, and X).

3. Induction of brain tumors in rats and sarcomas in mice with the cell-free extracts of oligodendroglial cells or transplanted brain tumors

Cell-free extracts of cultured cells and transplanted brain tumors had the potency to induce brain tumors in rats or sarcomas in mice, when inoculated at birth, intracerebrally, or intramuscularly (Table XI). Thus, the monoclonous cultured oligodendroglial cells appeared to be malignant brain tumor cells, judging from their origin, transplantability, and inductivity.

TABLE XI. Induction of Brain Tumor in Rats and Sarcoma in Mice with Cell-free Extracts of Oligodendroglial Cells or Oligodendroglial Cell-transplanted Brain Tumor

Source	Animal	Route (dose)	No. of animals injected	Brain tumors	Myogenic sarcomas	%	ALP (days)
Oligodendroglial cell extracts	Mice	im (0.1)	5		5	100	10
Oligodendroglial cell transplanted brain tumor extracts	Mice	im (0.1)	21		21	100	7
	Rats	ic (0.06)	8	8		100	27

When MSV-CS-Moloney substrain, prepared from congenital sarcoma, was inoculated intracerebrally into newborn rats, brain tumors developed in the recipients, as was reported previously (*24*). Similar results were demonstrated by Ribacchi and Giraldo (*56*). One of the cultured rat brain tumors thus induced showed oligodendroglial cells, the characteristics of which were described in this paper.

Canti *et al.* (*3*) reported the appearances of living oligodendroglial cells of the human glioma group *in vitro*. Lumsden and Pomerat (*38*) demonstrated normal oligodendrocytes in tissue culture, originating from the corpus callosum of the rat. The characteristic features of these cells, as described by these authors (*37*), were similar to those of the cultured cell line established in our laboratory.

It should be noted that these cultured oligodendroglial cells can be transplanted not only intracerebrally but also subcutaneously into young rats. As was described previously, subcutaneous oligodendroglial cell tumors grew to 5 cm^3 in size and were very soft and rather demarcated from the surrounding tissues. Metastasis of these cells was observed in various organs, such as lungs, liver, spleen, kidneys, lumbar and axillary lymph nodes, and, infrequently, thymus. When the tumors and metastatic lesions of these organs were tissue cultured, typical oligodendroglial cells were noted as early as several hours after commencing the tissue culture.

Since it is extremely interesting to know if these oligodendroglial cells contain MSV, cell-free extract from these cells or the oligodendroglial cell-transplanted brain tumor was inoculated into newborn rats intracerebrally and into mice intramuscularly. Both cases were positive, namely, brain tumors developed in rats and myogenic sarcomas in mice, as shown in Table XI. The newly induced rat brain tumors were cultured and the resultant cells were no longer the same type as the original.

Thus, the oligodendroglial cells cultured monoclonously *in vitro* appeared to be malignant brain tumor cells, judging from various characteristics such as origin, transplantability, and inductivity. The establishment of a MSV-induced ectodermal tumor cell line appears unusual. These oligodendroglial cells in tissue culture will be used for the study of the interaction between RNA oncogenic virus and host cells.

REFERENCES

1. Barnes, W. A., and Cole, R. K. The effect of nursing on the incidence of spontaneous leukemia and tumors in mice. *Cancer Res.*, **1**, 99 (1941).
2. Buffett, R. F., Grace, J. T. Jr., DiBerardino, L. A., and Mirand, E. A. Vertical transmission of murine leukemia virus. *Cancer Res.*, **29**, 588 (1969).
3. Canti, R. G., Bland, J. O. W., and Russell, D. S. Tissue culture of gliomata. *Res. Pub. Assoc. Nerv. Mental. Dis.*, **16**, 1 (1937).
4. Chieco-Bianchi, L., Tridente, G., Pennelli, N., and Fiore Donati, L. Role of immunological tolerance in viral leukemogenesis of the mouse. *Bibl. Haematol.*, **31**, 40 (1968).
5. Cottral, G. P., Burmester, B. R., and Water, N. F. Egg transmission of avian lymphomatosis. *Poult. Sci.*, **33**, 1174 (1954).
6. Dmochowski, L., Grey, C. E., Padgett, F., and Sykes, J. A. Studies on the structure of the mammary tymor-inducing virus (Bittner) and of leukemia virus (Gross). *In* "Viruses, Nucleic Acids and Cancer (Proc. 17th Annual Symposium on Fundamental Cancer Research)," University of Texas, M. D. Anderson Hospital and Tumor Institute, Williams and Wilkins Co., Baltimore, p. 85 (1963).
7. Fekete, E., and Otis, H. K. Observations on leukemia in AKR mice born from transferred ova and nursed by low leukemic mothers. *Cancer Res.*, **14**, 445 (1954).
8. Feldman, D. G., Gross, L., and Dreyfuss, Y. Electron microscopic study of the Passage A mouse leukemia virus in mammary glands of pregnant, virus-injected, C3H(f) mice. *Cancer Res.*, **23**, 1604 (1963).
9. Fischinger, P. J., Moore, C. O., and O'Connor, T. E. Isolation and identification

of a helper virus found in the Moloney sarcoma-leukemia virus complex. *J. Natl. Cancer Inst.*, **42**, 605 (1969).

10. Furth, J., Cole, R. K., and Boon, M. C. The effect of maternal influence upon spontaneous leukemia of mice. *Cancer Res.*, **2**, 280 (1942).
11. Gerber, P., and Kirschstein, R. L. SV40-induced ependymomas in newborn hamsters. 1. Virus-induced relationships. *Virology*, **18**, 582 (1962).
12. Girardi, A. J., Sweet, B. H., Slotnick, V. B., and Hilleman, M. R. Development of tumors in hamsters inoculated in the neonatal period with vacuolating virus, SV40. *Proc. Soc. Exp. Biol. Med.*, **109**, 649 (1962).
13. Gross, L. Presence of leukemic agent in normal testes and ovaries of young mice of AK line. *Acta Haematol.*, **10**, 18 (1953).
14. Gross, L. Mouse leukemia: An egg-borne virus disease; with a note on mouse salivary gland carcinoma. *Acta Haematol.*, **13**, 13 (1955).
15. Gross, L. Vertical transmission of passage A leukemia virus from inoculated C3H mice to their untreated offspring. *Proc. Soc. Exp. Biol. Med.*, **107**, 90 (1961).
16. Gross, L. Transmission of mouse leukemia virus through milk of virus-injected C3H female mice. *Proc. Soc. Exp. Biol. Med.*, **109**, 830 (1962).
17. Gross, L., and Dreyfuss, Y. How is the mouse leukemia virus transmitted from host to host under natural conditions? *In* "Carcinogenesis: A Broad Critique (Proc. 20th Annual Symposium on Fundamental Cancer Research)," University of Texas, M. D. Anderson Hospital and Tumor Institute, Williams and Wilkins Co., Baltimore, pp. 9–21 (1967).
18. Hartley, J. W., and Rowe, W. P. Production of altered cell foci in tissue culture by defective Moloney sarcoma virus particles. *Proc. Natl. Acad. Sci. U.S.*, **55**, 780 (1966).
19. Harvey, J. J., and East, J. Biological activity and separation of a leukemogenic virus from murine sarcoma virus-Harvey (MSV-H). *Int. J. Cancer*, **4**, 655 (1969).
20. Huebner, R. J. Identification of leukemogenic viruses: Specifications for vertically transmitted, mostly " Switched Off " RNA tumor viruses as determinants of the generality of cancer. *Bibl. Haematol.*, **36**, 22 (1970).
21. Huebner, R. J., Hartley, J. W., Rowe, W. P., Lane, W. T., and Capps, W. I. Rescue of the defective genome of Moloney sarcoma virus from a noninfectious hamster tumor and the production of pseudotype sarcoma viruses with various murine leukemia viruses. *Proc. Natl. Acad. Sci. U.S.*, **56**, 1164 (1966).
22. Huebner, R. J., and Todaro, G. J. Oncogenes of RNA tumor viruses as determinants of cancer. *Proc. Natl. Acad. Sci. U.S.*, **64**, 1087 (1969).
23. Ida, N., Fukuhara, A., and Ohba, Y. Several aspects of vertical transmission of Moloney virus. *Natl. Cancer Inst. Monograph*, **22**, 287 (1966).
24. Ida, N., Ikawa, Y., Ogawa, K., Takada, M., and Yokogi, E. Intracranial tumors in rats and mice produced by MSV-CS-Moloney substrain. *Proc. Japan. Cancer Assoc. (29th Annual Meeting)*, 97 (1970).
25. Ida, N., Ikawa, Y., and Ohba, Y. Studies on hypodiploid and hyperdiploid virus-induced mouse leukemias and the vertical transmission of MSV-Moloney. *Bibl. Haematol.*, **36**, 221 (1970).
26. Ida, N., Ikawa, Y., Ohba, Y., and Yamada, S. Vertical transmission of MSV-Moloney in Swiss ICR mice. *Abstr. Papers (10th Int. Cancer Congr.)*, 163 (1970).
27. Ida, N., Moloney, J. B., and Taylor, H. G. Vertical transmission of Moloney leukemia virus in A/LN and BALB/c strains of mice. *GANN*, **56**, 239 (1965).

28. Ida, N., Moloney, J. B., Taylor, H. G., and Trentin, J. J. Placental transmission of Sarcoma 37 leukemia virus. *In* "Res. Report M 11/P 11, Houston," University of Texas, M. D. Anderson Hospital and Tumor Institute, p. 226 (1961).
29. Ikawa, Y., and Sugano, H. Histogenesis of ICR/Swiss mice-adapted-MSV-induced thigh tumors (in Japanese). *Nippon Byōri Gakkai Kaishi* (*Trans. Japan. Pathol. Soc.*), **58**, 101 (1969).
30. Kirschstein, R. L., and Gerber, P. Ependymomas produced after intracerebral inoculation of SV40 into newborn hamsters. *Nature*, **195**, 299 (1962).
31. Krischke, W., and Graffi, A. The transmission of the virus of myeloid leukemia of mice by the milk. *Acta Unio Int. Contra Cancrum*, **19**, 360 (1963).
32. Kumanishi, T. Brain tumors induced with Rous sarcoma virus, Schmidt-Ruppin strain. 1. Induction of brain tumors in adult mice with Rous chicken sarcoma cells. *Japan. J. Exp. Med.*, **37**, 461 (1967).
33. Law, L. W. Influence of foster-nursing on virus induced and spontaneous leukemia in mice. *Proc. Soc. Exp. Biol. Med.*, **111**, 615 (1962).
34. Law, L. W. Studies of experimental transmission of leukemogenic virus infection in mice. *J. Natl. Cancer Inst.*, **34**, 543 (1965).
35. Law, L. W. Transmission studies of a leukemogenic virus, MLV, in mice. *Natl. Cancer Inst. Monograph*, **22**, 267 (1966).
36. Law, L. W., and Moloney, J. B. Studies of congenital transmission of a leukemia virus in mice. *Proc. Soc. Exp. Biol. Med.*, **108**, 715 (1961).
37. Lumsden, C. E. *In* "Pathology of Tumors of the Nervous System," ed. by D. S. Russell, L. J. Rubinstein, and C. R. Lumsden, Edward Arnold Ltd., London, pp. 281–335 (1963).
38. Lumsden, C. E., and Pomerat, C. M. Normal oligodendrocytes in tissue culture: A preliminary report on the pulsatile glial cells in tissue cultures from the corpus callosum of the normal adult rat brain. *Exp. Cell Res.*, **2**, 103 (1951).
39. MacDowell, E. C., and Richter, M. N. Mouse leukemia IX: The role of heredity in spontaneous cases. *Arch. Pathol.*, **20**, 709 (1935).
40. Mirand, E. A. *In* "Transmission of Viruses by the Water Route," ed. by G. Gerg, John Wiley & Sons, New York, pp. 269–285 (1967).
41. Mirand, E. A., Buffett, R. F., and Grace, J. T., Jr. Mode of transmission of Friend virus disease. *Proc. Soc. Exp. Biol. Med.*, **121**, 970 (1966).
42. Mirand, E. A., and Grace, J. T., Jr. Transmission of Friend virus disease from infected mothers to offspring. *Virology*, **16**, 344 (1962).
43. Mirand, E. A., Grace, J. T. Jr., and Buffett, R. F. Passive and active immunity to Friend virus disease. *Nature*, **209**, 696 (1966).
44. Moloney, J. B. Biological studies on a lymphoid-leukemia virus extracted from sarcoma 37. I. Origin and introductory investigations. *J. Natl. Cancer Inst.*, **24**, 933 (1960).
45. Moloney, J. B. A virus-induced rhabdomyosarcoma of mice. *Natl. Cancer Inst. Monograph*, **22**, 139 (1966).
46. Nakakuki, K., Shisa, H., and Nishizuka, Y. Possible transmission of leukemia virus in AKR mice through milk. *GANN*, **57**, 427 (1966).
47. Perk, K., Moloney, J. B., and Jenkins, E. G. Further studies on the relationship of a rhabdomyosarcoma virus to muscle tissue. *Int. J. Cancer*, **2**, 43 (1967).
48. Perk, K., Shacht, D. A., and Moloney, J. B. Pathogenesis of a rhabdomyosarcoma (undifferentiated type) in rats induced by a murine sarcoma virus (Moloney). *Cancer Res.*, **28**, 1197 (1968).
49. Rabotti, G. F., Anderson, W. R., and Sellers, R. L. Oncogenic activity of Mill

Hill (Harris) strain of Rous virus for hamsters. *Nature*, **206**, 946 (1965).
50. Rabotti, G. F., Grove, A. S. Jr., Sellers, R. L., and Anderson, W. R. Induction of multiple brain tumours (gliomata and leptomeningeal sarcomata) in dogs by Rous sarcoma virus. *Nature*, **209**, 884 (1966).
51. Rabotti, G. F., and Raine, W. A. Brain tumors induced in hamsters inoculated intracerebrally at birth with Rous sarcoma virus. *Nature*, **204**, 898 (1964).
52. Rabotti, G. P., Raine, W. A., and Sellers, R. L. Brain tumors (glioma) induced in hamsters by Bryan's strain of Rous sarcoma virus. *Science*, **147**, 504 (1965).
53. Rabotti, G. P., Sellers, R. L., and Anderson, W. A. Leptomeningeal sarcomata and gliomata induced in rabbits by Rous sarcoma virus. *Nature*, **209**, 524 (1966).
54. Rabson, A. S., and Kirschstein, R. L. Intracranial sarcomas produced by polyoma virus in Syrian hamsters. *Arch. Pathol.*, **69**, 663 (1960).
55. Rabson, A. S., O'Conor, G. T., Kirschstein, R. L., and Braniyan, W. J. Papillary ependymomas produced in Rattus (Mastomys) natalensis inoculated with vacuolating virus (SV40). *J. Natl. Cancer Inst.*, **29**, 765 (1962).
56. Ribacchi, R., and Giraldo, G. Intracranial tumors in rats injected intracerebrally with murine sarcoma virus (MSV), Moloney's strain, Preliminary report. *Lav. Anat. Pat. Perugia*, **26**, 141 (1966a).
57. Ribacchi, R., and Giraldo, G. Plasmacytomas occurring in the bones of rats injected intracerebrally with murine sarcoma virus (MSV), Moloney's strain, Preliminary report. *Lav. Anat. Pat. Perugia*, **26**, 149 (1966b).
58. Snell, G. D. *In* " Biology of the Laboratory Mouse," ed. by G. D. Snell, Dover Publications, New York, pp. 194 and 206 (1961).
59. Spencer, H. J., and Groupé, V. Pathogenesis of virus-induced Rous sarcoma. I. Distribution of virus and tumor foci in chicks and turkeys. *J. Natl. Cancer Inst.*, **29**, 397 (1962).
60. Ting, R. C. Tumor induction in thymectomized rats by murine sarcoma virus (Moloney) and properties of the induced virus-free tumor cells. *Proc. Soc. Exptl. Biol. Med.*, **126**, 778 (1967).
61. Turner, W., and Chirigos, M. A. Enhancement of murine sarcoma virus (Moloney) oncogenicity in mice by coinfection with Rauscher leukemia virus. *Proc. Am. Assoc. Cancer Res.*, **9**, 72 (1968).
62. Vigier, P. Passage intracérébral du virus de sarcoma de Rous chez la poussin nouveau-né. *Bull. Cancer*, **44**, 409 (1957).
63. Vogt, M., and Duibecco, R. Studies on cells rendered neoplastic by polyoma virus: The problem of the presence of virus-related materials. *Virology*, **16**, 41 (1962).

EXPLANATION OF PHOTOS

PHOTO 1. Swiss ICR mouse (Sa-5, female) bearing sarcoma in the pectoral muscle.
This sarcoma was detected in an offspring whose mother was dually infected with MSV and MLV during pregnancy. The mouse was killed at 38 days of age.

PHOTO 2. Swiss ICR mouse (Sa-1, female) bearing sarcoma in the thigh lesion.
This sarcoma was detected at 7 days of age in an offspring whose mother was infected with MSV and MLV during pregnancy. The mouse was killed at 15 days of age.

PHOTO 3. Malignant rhabdomyosarcoma (Sa-5, pectoral lesion; see Photo 1). This view of a congenital sarcoma shows both large elongated cells and a few short, small spindle cells, as well as some mononuclear round cells. Hematoxylin and Eosin.

PHOTO 4. Malignant rhabdoblastoma, showing rather round cells, oriented in various directions

in bundles or whorls with relatively large cytoplasm and centrally placed nuclei.
Sa-1, thigh lesion; see Photo 2. Hematoxylin and Eosin. ×1,000

PHOTO 5. A large elongated tumor cell with multiple nuclei possessing several distinct nucleoli.
Sa-5, pectoral lesion. Hematoxylin and Eosin. ×1,000

PHOTO 6. Mononuclear round tumor cell with lightly stained large nucleus.
Sa-5, pectoral lesion. Hematoxylin and Eosin. ×1,000

PHOTO 7. Tumor cell imprint colored with Wright's stain. Large, rather round cells with curled endings possessing 1 or 2 round nuclei in which many large distinct nucleoli and clumps of chromatin can be seen. Sa-8. ×1,000

PHOTO 8. A spindle-shaped tumor cell. The elongated nucleus, mitochondria with mostly circular or oval profiles, and ergastoplasm showing an orientation along the long axis of the cell are evident. Part of the cytoplasm of the tumor cell shows a flocculent, granular precipitate in the cisternae of the endoplasmic reticulum. ×11,000

PHOTO 9. Virus particles are seen on the surface of the tumor cell and a particle budding from the plasma membrane. Fibrils are in the cytoplasmic matrix. ×25,000

PHOTO 10. Gemistocytic astrocytoma induced in Swiss ICR mouse with MSV-CS-Moloney substrain.

PHOTO 11. Large or small round cells with numerous slender short processes are observed in the solid brain tumor of a 3-month-old Sprague-Dawley rat which was inoculated intracerebrally at birth with MSV-CS-Moloney substrain. These cells show a rather large spherical nucleus often laterally located.

PHOTO 12. Clusters of cultured oligodendroglial cells at the 20th passage, photographed using an interference-phase attachment. The outlines of most of the cells show bright refractility. ×200

PHOTO 13. Cultured oligodendroglial cells at the 20th passage. Polyhedral cells forming attachment with short processes from other similar type of cells are observed.

PHOTOS 14 and 15. Same cells as above. Bipolar or tripolar cells with dichotomous branching, having various types of expansion, are seen at the extremity of the processes.

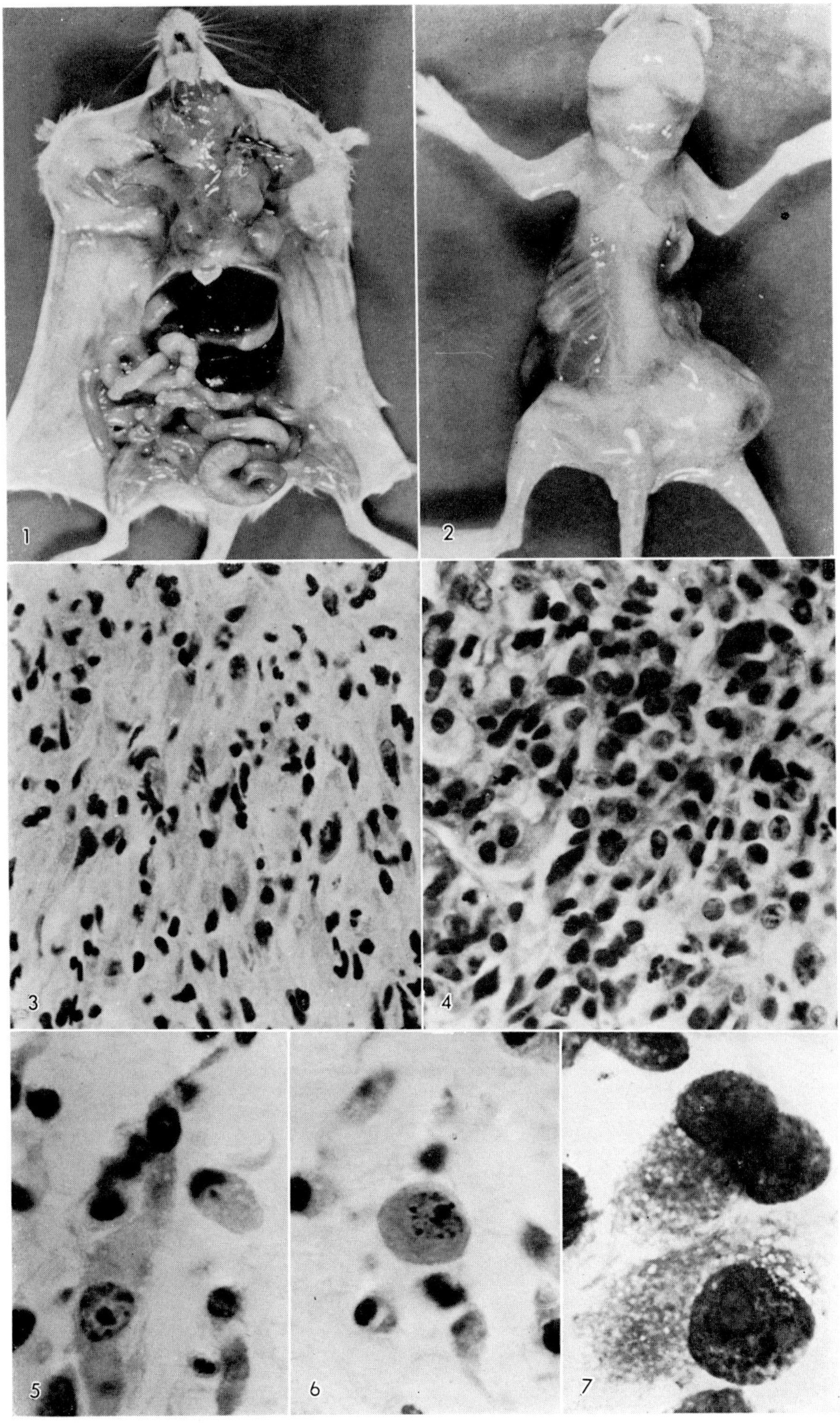
1
2
3
4
5
6
7

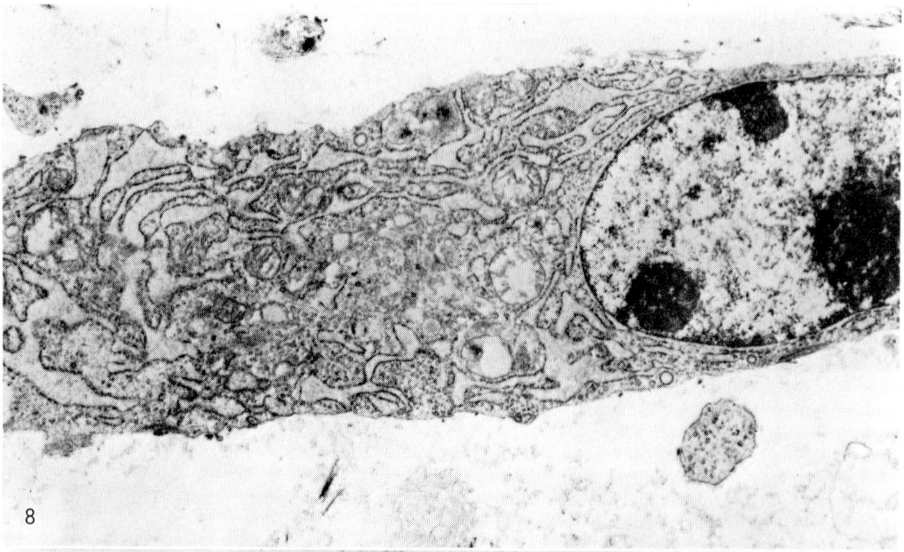
8

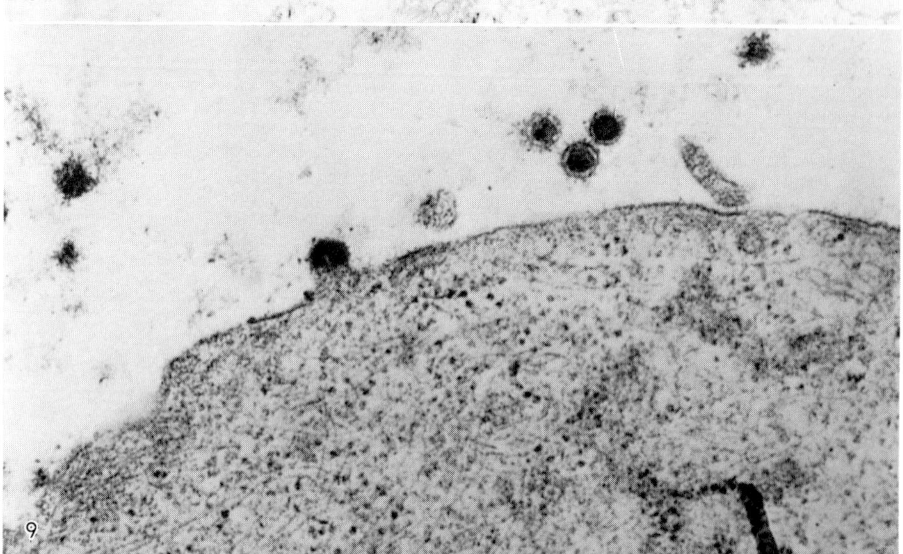
9

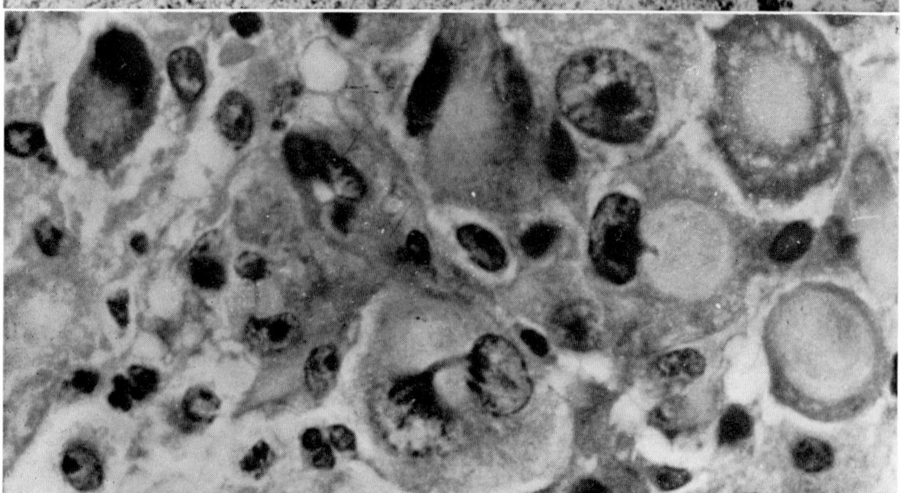
10

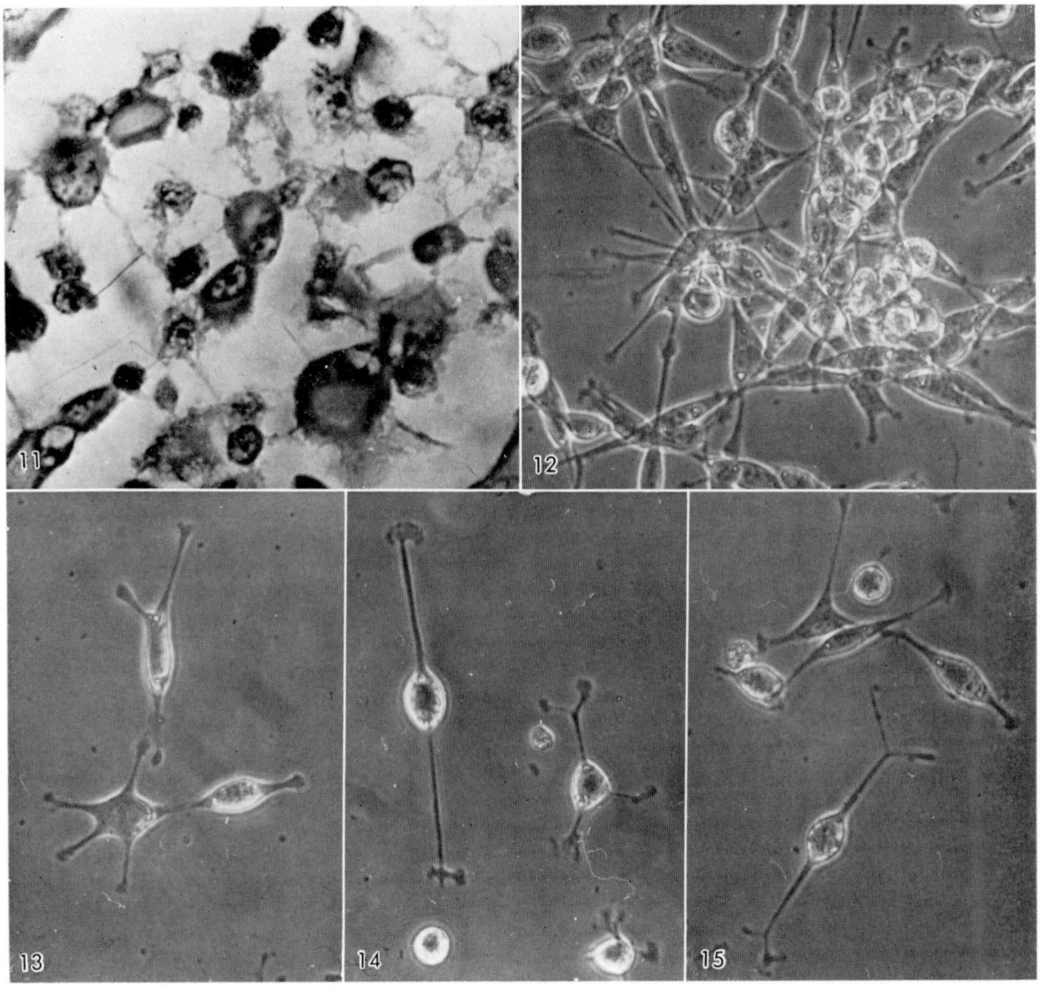
11
12
13
14
15

PATHOGENESIS OF FRIEND VIRUS-INDUCED LEUKEMIA IN MICE*

Yoji IKAWA,† Haruo SUGANO, and Mitsuru FURUSAWA

*Department of Pathology, Cancer Institute** and Laboratory of Embryology, Faculty of Science, Osaka City University****

Leukemic disease induced in DDD mice by infection with Friend virus maintained at the Cancer Institute, Tokyo, since 1960, was shown to be malignant erythroblastosis because the cell membrane of the proliferating cells had the same antigens as the erythrocytes.

The cells of the transplantable Friend tumors were lacking in these antigens, suggesting that they were selected by transplantation from the reactively proliferating cells of early lesions of Friend disease. The role of Friend virus in the appearance of the truly neoplastic cells among the early splenic lesions awaits future study although the virus does induce an incomplete maturation arrest of proerythroblasts resulting in fatal erythroblastosis.

Historical Review of Friend Virus

In 1957, Friend described the recovery of a virus from the enlarged spleen of a Swiss mouse which had been inoculated with a cell-free extract of Ehrlich ascites tumor cells (*10*). The rationale of this experiment was based on Selby's electron-microscopic studies of Ehrlich ascites tumor cells and the finding of intracytoplasmic virus particles which, however, were later identified as reovirus particles (*38*). The electron micrographs of Friend virus particles shown by de Harven in 1958 (*4*, *5*) were consistent with classical type C particles, round, 100 nm in diameter, with dense nucleoids.

Friend virus, routinely prepared as 10% homogenates of the virus-infected enlarged mouse spleens, induces splenomegaly in susceptible mice approximately 1 week after intraperitoneal inoculation. This lesion is followed by the appearance of blastic cells in the peripheral blood, and diffuse infiltration of the blastic cells into the liver causing fatal hemorrhage.

The oncogenic activity of the virus inducing the leukemic state, described as Friend disease, varies among the different host strains of mice. Rats are resistant to the virus. When inoculated into resistant mice (*30*, *31*) or rats (*6*, *26*) im-

* Supported in part by a Grant-in-Aid for Scientific Research from the Ministry of Education of Japan.

† Present address: Viral Leukemia and Lymphoma Branch, National Cancer Institute, NIH, Bethesda, Maryland 20014, U.S.A.

** Kami-Ikebukuro 1-37-1, Toshima-ku, Tokyo 170 (井川洋二, 菅野晴夫).

*** Sugimoto-cho, Higashisumiyoshi-ku, Osaka 5 (古沢　満).

mediately after birth, the virus induces lymphocytic lymphoma after a latent period of several months.

Lymphoma-inducing viruses associated with Friend disease are considered as helper agents in the defective Friend virus system (*9*). The attenuated Friend virus (*41*) obtained from long-term *in vitro* cultures may also be in the same category.

In comparing the relation between Moloney sarcoma virus and Moloney leukemia virus, the virus causing classical Friend disease should be considered the " Friend erythroblastosis virus," and the lymphoma-inducing virus isolated from the same system should be considered the " Friend leukemia virus," or " Friend associated virus." The Friend virus described herein is accordingly " Friend erythroblastosis virus " in association with " Friend leukemia virus."

The Friend virus was kindly supplied by Dr. C. Friend in 1960. The agent was passed through ddOM mice until 1965 and then through DDD mice at the Cancer Institute, Tokyo, by routine intraperitoneal injection.

Friend Disease: Reticulum Cell Sarcoma or Erythroblastosis?

Friend virus in DDD mice causes splenomegaly within 2 weeks after inoculation. These DDD mice constitute an inbred albino strain established at the Institute of Medical Science, University of Tokyo. Subsequently the blastic cell count in the peripheral blood increases to 500,000/mm^3 in association with an increase in the erythroblast count.

The description of the above disease is detailed in previous reports by Friend (*10*), Metcalf *et al.* (*27*), and Kasuga and Oota (*23*). In fact, the enlarged spleens consisted of spindle or polygonal cells, and since hepatomegaly occurred in splenectomized mice, the disease was interpreted as an undifferentiated reticulum cell sarcoma associated with erythroblastosis.

The nature of Friend virus-induced disease as an undifferentiated reticulum cell sarcoma is also supported by the morphological character of the transplantable tumors derived from the splenic or hepatic lesions of Friend disease (*3*, *11*, *28*). Since the establishment of the transplantable tumors, histological studies have been concerned primarily with them, and hence many classical pathologists have raised questions regarding the neoplastic character of the virus-induced disease.

Kobayashi described the relation between the presence of virus and the maintenance of the neoplastic character in a minimal virus-producing transplantable Friend tumor (*25*), and Maruyama and Oboshi made over 100 clones of a Friend tumor cell line but was unable to establish a nonproducing cell line (*29*). Fieldsteel was the first to establish a nonproducing cell line of the Friend tumor (*8*).

Friend *et al.* in 1965 obtained a cell line that differentiated along the erythrocytic line (*12*, *13*, *32*, *36*). Prior to this, erythrocytic differentiation was also demonstrated by Soule *et al.* in a Stansly leukemia cell line (*39*).

Rauscher in 1962 described a murine leukemia virus which simulates the activity of Friend virus (*35*). In Rauscher disease, the primary lesions were the principal materials available for the study of its histogenesis. In 1966, Yokoro and Thorell (*40*) employing microspectrophotometry determined hemoglobin concentrations on impression smears of blastic cells from the hepatic lesions of Rauscher disease. Dunn and Green (*7*) described the disease as reactive proliferation of erythroid and myeloid cells, insisting on its involving only hematopoietic organs.

Friend Disease as Malignant Erythroblastosis

Ikawa *et al.* reported in 1965 (at the 24th Annual Meeting of the Japanese Cancer Association) on the early focal splenic lesions of Friend disease induced by inoculation with diluted virus material (*22*).

Prior to this, Axelrad and Steeves (*2*), and Pulznik and Sachs (*33*) described spleen focus assays for Friend virus and Rauscher virus, respectively. The number of splenic foci was proportionate to the quantity of virus inoculated.

Microscopic spleen foci of Friend disease in DDD mice were recognized as early as 2 days after inoculation with the virus and can be described as a uniform accumulation of polygonal cells along the trabeculae in the red splenic pulp (*22*).

Electron-microscopic studies of early spleen foci of Friend disease revealed 2 types of blastic cells, one simulating proerythroblasts, and the other, basophilic erythroblasts, both shedding virus (*19*). The resemblance of spleen focus cells to erythroblasts was first suggested by Sugano. Budding of virus particles was also observed in cells morphologically corresponding to normoblasts.

In 1967, Ikawa and Sugano observed early lesions of Friend disease in the bone marrow of splenectomized mice and concluded that the hepatomegaly in splenectomized mice was secondary to the bone marrow lesions (*17*). Thus, the hypothesis that Friend disease was malignant erythroblastosis was established (*18*).

Pulse labeling of the spleen focus cells with ^{3}H-thymidine showed a labeling index higher than 75% (Photos la and 1b, Table I), suggesting a short generation time comparable to that of erythroblasts (*20*), thus allowing the early lesions of Friend disease to replace the entire spleens, which resulted in spleens weighing over 2.0 g.

TABLE I. Tritiated Thymidine Pulse Labeling of the Cells of Spleen Foci of Friend Virus-induced Leukemia

	No. of SF checked	No. of cells checked	No. of cells labeled	Labeling index(%)
Cells of SF, 3–5 days p.i.	20	2288	2484	86.1
Cells of SF, 7–11 days p.i.	7	8651	6660	76.9

SF : spleen foci. p.i. : post infection.

Impression smears of spleen foci of Friend disease stained with Giemsa solution revealed classical proerythroblasts with occasional small normoblasts.

In 1966, Ikawa and Sugano established 6 transplantable Friend tumor strains after hundreds of experiments of transplanting 7- to 12-day spleen foci to syngenic mice (*15, 16*). The subcutaneously transplanted tumors were called SFST-1 to -6 (Spleen Focus-derived Solid Tumor -1 to -6). All of them were converted to ascites forms, SFAT-1 to -6. SFAT-1, -2, -4, and -5 cytologically showed uniform monocytoid cells, whereas SFAT-3 and -6 consisted of erythroid cells at different stages (Photos 2a and 2b).

Sassa *et al.* demonstrated a high heme synthesis in SFAT-3 and SFAT-6 cells (*37*). Kasuga, employing an immunofluorescence technique, showed the presence of globin in SFAT-3 cells (*24*).

Conclusive Evidence of Erythroid Origin

Recently, we obtained conclusive evidence that the cells neoplastically proliferating in Friend disease were of an erythroid origin. Adachi and Furusawa purified normal erythrocyte membranes and obtained an erythrocyte membrane-specific antibody by immunizing guinea pigs (*1*). This specific antibody reacts only to erythrocytic series of any strain of mice from proerythroblasts to mature erythrocytes (*14*).

When the spleen focus cells of Friend disease were stained with the same fluorescein-labeled antibody, all of them fluoresced (Photo 3), and the cells of the spleen in the advanced stage of Friend disease also reacted to the antibody. The results indicate that the cell membrances of these proliferating cells in Friend disease have the same proteins as normal erythrocytes.

Precursors of Proliferating Cells Which Comprise Friend Disease

The proliferating cells in the spleen following infection with Friend virus are erythroid. The question arises, which cells in the red splenic pulp were forced to proliferate and cause fatal erythroblastosis: stem cells or proerythroblasts? This question was also raised by Pluznik *et al.* (*34*).

Repeated syngenic red blood cell transfusion resulted in polycythemia and a decrease in the population of erythroblasts in the spleen (Photo 4a). An intraperitoneal injection of 6 cobalt units of erythropoietin (supplied through the courtesy of Dr. T. Asano, Teikokuzoki Pharmaceutical Co., Tokyo) induced synchronous production of proerythroblasts along the splenic trabeculae and arterioles in the red splenic pulp 24 hr after inoculation (Photo 4b). This was followed by the appearance of small erythroblasts surrounding the large proerythroblasts at 48 hr.

Seventy-two hours after injection of erythropoietin into the polycythemic mice, the erythropoietic state becomes almost normal. If erythropoietin is injected into normal mice, the population of erythroblasts in the spleen increases, resulting in a moderately enlarged spleen of around 0.45 g (normal weight, about 0.12 g).

When Friend virus was injected into mice with different degrees of erythropoiesis, splenomegaly paralleled the quantity of proerythroblasts at the time of infection, which suggests that the erythropoietin-induced proerythroblasts are one of the target cells of Friend virus.

The proerythroblasts synchronously induced by erythropoietin in the spleens of DDD mice were labeled with tritiated thymidine and were observed autoradiographically with and without Friend virus. Approximately 90% of the spleen focus cells, 24 hr and 48 hr after Friend virus infection, showed silver

TABLE II. Autoradiographic Study of ^{3}H-Thymidine-labeled, Erythropoietin (Ep)-induced Procrythroblasts with or without Friend Virus Infection

Spleens (post infection)	Materials	No. of cells checked	No. of cells labeled (over 5 grains)	Labeling index
Ep only	Proerythroblasts	228	210	92.1
	Other cells in red splenic pulp	586	24	4.1
FV after labeling (24 hr)	FV-induced SF cells	351	302	86.3
	Other cells in red splenic pulp	1012	68	6.7
FV after labeling (48 hr)	FV-induced SF cells	311	283	91.0
	Other cells in red splenic pulp	982	83	8.5

FV: Friend virus. SF: Spleen foci.

grains (Photos 5a and 5b) and were proven to be formed by the proliferation of the labeled proerythroblasts (Table II). Without Friend virus, the labeled proerythroblasts differentiated into smaller erythroblasts which were positive for silver grains autoradiographically (Photo 6).

Arrest of Maturation of Proerythroblasts by Friend Virus

Approximately 70% of erythropoietin-induced proerythroblasts differentiate into smaller erythroblasts, while 30% remain as reserve cells, some of which remain undifferentiated 1 week after stimulation by erythropoietin. When infected with Friend virus in high titer, approximately 90% of erythropoietin-induced proerythroblasts remained undifferentiated (Table III).

The maturation arrest of erythropoietin-induced proerythroblasts by infection with Friend virus was less in BALB/c mice (Table III) (*21*), which might explain the unsuccessful transplantation of splenic lesions of Friend disease in BALB/c mice. In Rauscher disease, anisocytosis is more conspicuous than in Friend disease. This finding suggests the remarkable tendency of Rauscher virus-induced erythroblastoid cells to differentiate into erythrocytes.

TABLE III. 48-Hour Friend Virus-induced Spleen Foci in Polycythemic Mice with Pulse-labeled, Erythropoietin-induced Proerythroblasts

Mouse strain	No. of foci checked	Large proerythroblastoid cells†		Small erythroblasts†	
		No. of cells checked	No. of cells labeled	No. of cells checked	No. of cells labeled
DDD	46	2622	2361	111	104
BALB/c	17	796	653	393	325

† In a section of the spleen material.

Are Primary Friend Cells Reactively Proliferating?

Both the reactivity of primary Friend cells to an erythrocyte membrane-specific antibody and their differentiating potentiality support the suggestion that the cells are reactively proliferating and that Friend disease is not in the category of a true neoplasm.

However, the survival times of DDD mice intraperitoneally inoculated with 10^6 cells of SFAT-1 to -6 were 18 to 25 days. At autopsy, up to 15 to 20 ml of ascites fluid accumulated, including 3 to 6×10^8 cells, mesenterial infiltration was conspicuous, and paratracheal and axillary lymph node metastases were observed. In this respect, the neoplastic character of the transplantable Friend tumors may be comparable to those of Ehrlich ascites tumors or Yoshida ascites tumor. Chromosomes of SFAT-1 and SFAT-3 cells were analyzed, and they revealed, respectively, 2 and 3 large metacentric chromosomes among 42 chromosomes. In a preliminary study the chromosomes of spleen focus cells were mostly normal, including several cells with 41 chromosomes.

Since these findings suggested that the transplantable tumor cells were rarely selected out of the spleen focus cells and were comparable to truly neoplastic cells, the cell membrane was checked by the previously described erythrocyte membrane-specific antibody procedure. The cells of all the transplantable Friend tumors and Friend cell lines were negative for erythrocyte membrane-specific antigens.

Do Spleen Focus Cells Provide a Key to Viral Leukemogenesis?

The cells of primary lesions of Friend disease are antigenically different from those of the transplantable tumors. Since the 7- to 12-day spleen foci were used in establishing SFAT-1 to -6 strains, the early splenic foci of Friend disease may provide truly neoplastic cells among the other reactively proliferating cells. An understanding of leukemogenesis by type C viruses may be found in a more complete study of these reactively proliferating erythroid cells.

A substrain of Friend virus maintained in Rosewell Park Memorial Institute, Buffalo, New York, causes anemia in susceptible mice. If this anemia is due to the complete maturation arrest of proerythroblasts, the transplantability of the primary lesions of Friend disease induced by the substrain may be higher, and the early lesions may provide more frequent truly neoplastic cells. The substrain was kindly supplied by Dr. R. Steeves, and pathogenesis of the virus-induced lesion is now under investigation.

Acknowledgments

We would like to thank Dr. John B. Moloney for reading the manuscript, and Dr. Thelma B. Dunn for her advice.

REFERENCES

1. Adachi, H., and Furusawa, M. Immunological analysis of the structural molecules of erythrocyte membrane in mice. I. Analysis of the aqueous phase molecules obtained by butanol fraction of erythrocyte membrane. *Exp. Cell Res.*, **50**, 490 (1968).
2. Axelrad, A. A., and Steeves, R. A. Assay for Friend leukemia virus in rapid

quantitative method based on enumeration of macroscopic spleen foci in mice. *Virology*, **24**, 513 (1964).

3. Buffet, R. F., and Furth, J. A transplantable reticulum-cell sarcoma variant of Friend's viral leukemia. *Cancer Res.*, **19**, 1063 (1959).
4. de Harven, E., and Friend, C. Electron microscopic study of a cell-free induced leukemia of the mouse. A preliminary report. *J. Biophys. Biochem. Cytol.*, **4**, 151 (1958).
5. de Harven, E., and Friend, C. Further electron microscope studies of a mouse leukemia induced by cell-free filtrates. *J. Biophys. Biochem. Cytol.*, **7**, 747 (1960).
6. Dawson, P. J., and Fieldsteel, A. H. Lymphatic leukemia in rats and mice inoculated with Friend virus. *Brit. J. Cancer*, **20**, 114 (1966).
7. Dunn, T. B., and Green, A. W. Morphology of BALB/c mice inoculated with Rauscher virus. *J. Natl. Cancer Inst.*, **36**, 987 (1966).
8. Fieldsteel, A. H., Dawson, P. J., and Scholler, J. Virus-free Friend virus-induced tumor, *in vivo* and *in vitro* characteristics. *J. Natl. Cancer Inst.*, **36**, 71 (1966).
9. Fieldsteel, A. H., Kurahara, C., and Dawson, P. J. Moloney leukemia virus as a helper in retrieving Friend virus from a non-infectious reticulum cell sarcoma. *Nature*, **223**, 1274 (1969).
10. Friend, C. Cell-free transmission in adult Swiss mice of a disease having the character of a leukemia. *J. Exp. Med.*, **105**, 307 (1957).
11. Friend, C., and Haddad, J. R. Tumor formation with transplants of liver from mice with virus-induced leukemia. *J. Natl. Cancer Inst.*, **25**, 1279 (1960).
12. Friend, C., Patuleia, M. C., and de Harven, E. Erythrocytic maturation *in vitro* of murine (Friend) virus-induced leukemic cells. *Natl. Cancer Inst. Monograph*, **22**, 505 (1966).
13. Friend, C., Scher, W., Holland, J. G., and Sato, T. Hemoglobin synthesis in murine virus-induced leukemic cells *in vitro*: Stimulation of erythroid differentiation by dimethyl sulfoxide. *Proc. Natl. Acad. Sci. U.S.*, **68**, 378 (1971).
14. Furusawa, M., and Adachi, H. Immunological analysis of the structural molecules of erythrocyte membrane in mice. II. Staining of erythroid cells with labelled antibody. *Exp. Cell Res.*, **50**, 497 (1968).
15. Ikawa, Y., and Sugano, H. An ascites tumor derived from early splenic lesion of Friend's disease. *GANN*, **57**, 641 (1966).
16. Ikawa, Y., and Sugano, H. Transplantation of spleen foci of Friend disease (in Japanese). *Nippon Byōri Gakkai Kaishi* (*Trans. Soc. Pathol. Japan*), **55**, 139 (1966).
17. Ikawa, Y., and Sugano, H. Focal lesions of Friend's disease in bone marrow. *GANN*, **58**, 305 (1967a).
18. Ikawa, Y., and Sugano, H. Histogenesis of Friend virus-induced leukemia (malignant erythroblastosis) and its short latency (in Japanese). *Ann. Rept. Co-op. Res.* (*Cancer*), 317 (1967b).
19. Ikawa, Y., and Sugano, H. Spleen focus of Friend's disease. An electron microscopic study. *GANN*, **58**, 155 (1967c).
20. Ikawa, Y., and Sugano, H. Target cell analysis of Friend virus by using erythropoietin (in Japanese). *Proc. Japan. Cancer Assoc.* (*26th Ann. Meeting*), 224 (1967d).
21. Ikawa, Y., and Sugano, H. Maturation arrest of erythropoietin-induced proerythroblasts in DDD mice caused by infection with Friend leukemia virus. *Abstr. Papers, 10th Int. Cancer Congr.*, **155**, (1970).

22. Ikawa, Y., Sugano, H., and Oota, K. Spleen focus of Friend's disease. A histological study. *GANN*, **58**, 61 (1967).
23. Kasuga, T., and Oota, K. Pathological characteristics of Friend disease (in Japanese). *Gan no Rinsho* (*Japan. J. Cancer Clin.*), **8**, 251 (1962).
24. Kasuga, T. Presence of globin in Friend ascites tumor cells: An immunofluorescence study (in Japanese). *Proc. Japan. Cancer Assoc.* (*26th Ann. Meeting*), 223 (1966).
25. Kobayashi, H. Immunopathological studies on the Friend virus-induced ascitic tumor (in Japanese). *Acta Pathol. Japon.*, **16**, 79 (1966).
26. Kobayashi, H., Hosokawa, M., Takeishi, N., Sendo, F., and Kodama, T. Transplantable Friend virus-induced tumors in rats. *Cancer Res.*, **29**, 1385 (1969).
27. Metcalf, D., Furth, J., and Buffet, R. F. Pathogenesis of mouse leukemia caused by Friend virus. *Cancer Res.*, **19**, 52 (1959).
28. Oboshi, S., Aoki, K., Sato, R., and Baba, T. Friend virus ascites sarcoma: A transplantable ascites tumor variant induced from Friend's viral leukemia. *GANN*, **55**, 73 (1964).
29. Oboshi, S., and Maruyama, K. Electron microscopic analysis of converting process of Friend ascites tumor cells into nonproducer. *In* " Electron Microscopy," ed. by R. Uyeda, Maruzen Co. Ltd., Tokyo, Vol. II, p. 217 (1966).
30. Odaka, T., and Ikawa, Y. Friend virus-induced transplantable tumors of C57BL/6 origin containing unusually minute amounts of infectious virus. *Int. J. Cancer*, **3**, 211 (1968).
31. Odaka, T., Ikawa, Y., and Takizawa, K. Disappearance of infectious virus from Friend virus-induced C57BL/6 tumors. *Int. J. Cancer*, **4**, 403 (1969).
32. Patuleia, M., and Friend, C. Tissue culture studies on murine virus-induced leukemia cells: Isolation of single cells in agar-liquid medium. *Cancer Res.*, **27**, 726 (1967).
33. Pluznik, D. H., and Sachs, L. Quantitation of a murine leukemia virus with a spleen colony assay. *J. Natl. Cancer Inst.*, **33**, 535 (1964).
34. Pluznik, D. H., Sachs, L., and Resnitzky, P. The mechanism of leukemogenesis by the Rauscher leukemia virus. *Natl. Cancer Inst. Monograph*, **22**, 3 (1966).
35. Rauscher, F. J. A virus-induced disease of mice characterized by erythrocytopoiesis and lymphoid leukemia. *J. Natl. Cancer Inst.*, **29**, 515 (1962).
36. Rossi, G. B., and Friend, C. Erythropoietic activity in spleen colonies resulting from the inoculation of virus (Friend) induced leukemic cells in mice. *Proc. Natl. Acad. Sci. U.S.*, **58**, 1373 (1967).
37. Sassa, S., Takaku, F., Nakao, K., Ikawa, Y., and Sugano, H. Heme synthesis in Friend ascites tumor cells. *Proc. Soc. Exp. Biol. Med.*, **127**, 527 (1968).
38. Selby, C. C., Grey, C. E., Lichtenberg, S., Friend, C., Moore, A. E., and Biesele, J. J. Submicroscopic cytoplasmic particles occasionally found in the Ehrlich mouse ascites tumor. *Cancer Res.*, **14**, 790 (1954).
39. Soule, H. D., Albert, S., Wolf, P. L., and Stansly, P. G. Erythropoietic differentiation of stable cell lines derived from hematopoietic organs of mice with virus-induced leukemia. *Exp. Cell Res.*, **42**, 380 (1966).
40. Yokoro, K., and Thorell, B. Cytology and pathogenesis of Rauscher virus disease in spleenectomized mice. *Cancer Res.*, **26**, 536 (1966).
41. Yoshikura, H., Hirokawa, Y., Ikawa, Y., and Sugano, H. Infectious but nonleukemogenic Friend leukemia virus obtained after prolonged cultivation *in vitro*. *Int. J. Cancer*, **4**, 636 (1969).

EXPLANATION OF PHOTOS

PHOTO 1a. A spleen focus of FLV-induced leukemia, 3 days after the virus infection.

PHOTO 1b. An autoradiographic picture of the same spleen focus by pulse tritium-labeling.

PHOTO 2a. Friend ascites tumor (SFAT-1) consisting of uniform cells.

PHOTO 2b. Friend ascites tumor (SFAT-3) consisting of various types of erythroid cells.

PHOTO 3. Impression smear of a spleen focus stained with FITC-labeled mouse erythrocyte membrane-specific antibody.

PHOTO 4a. Spleen of a polycythemic mouse lacking in erythroblasts.

PHOTO 4b. Spleen with synchronous production of proerythroblasts after erythropoietin injection.

PHOTO 5a. A spleen focus of FLV-induced leukemia 48 hr after FLV infection following synchronous production of proerythroblasts by injection with erythropoietin to transfusion polycythemic mice.

PHOTO 5b. An autographic picture of the same focus. Silver grains which had specifically been present in erythropoietin-induced proerythroblasts can be seen immigrating in the focus cells.

PHOTO 6. An autoradiographic picture of erythropoietin-induced proerythroblasts 48 hr after synchronous induction and labeling. Silver grains seen in dark, small erythroblasts.

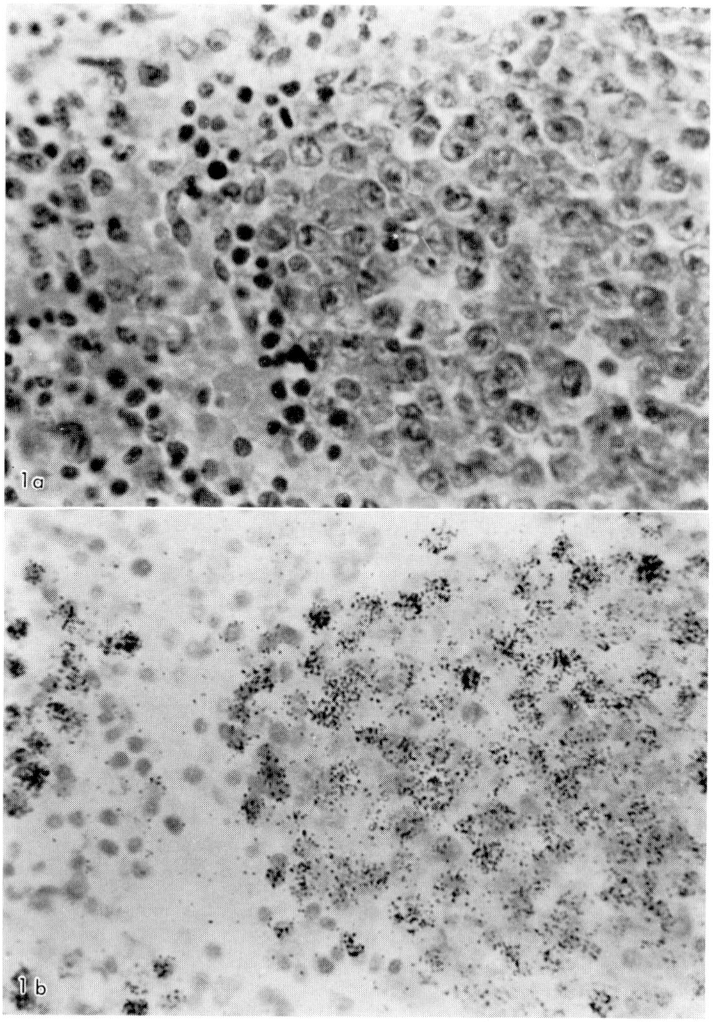
1a
1b

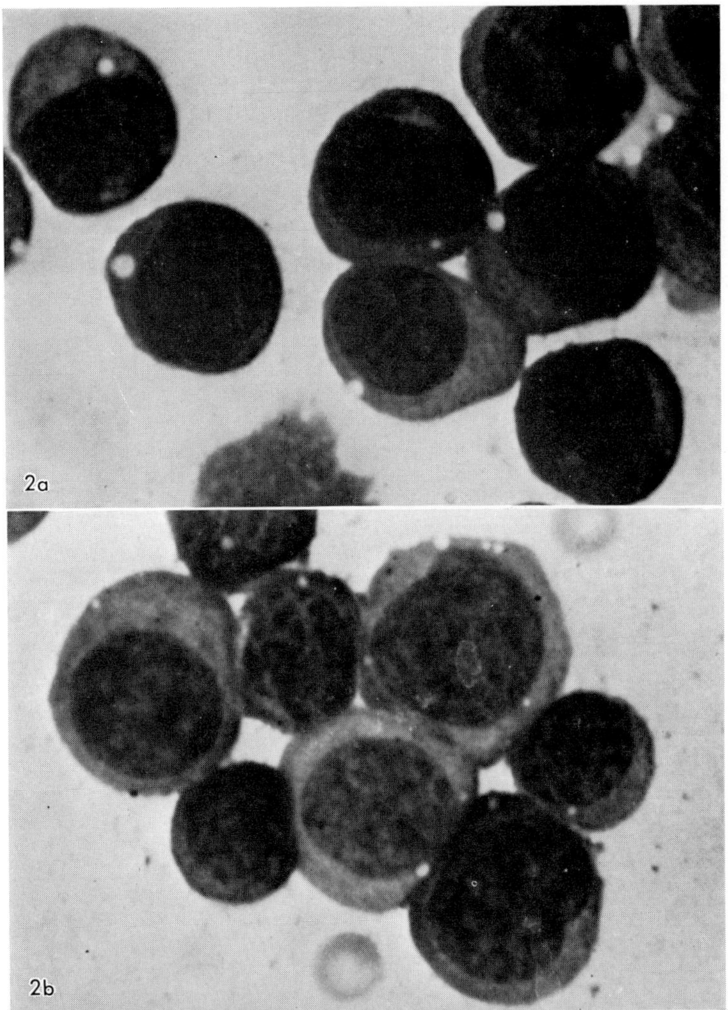
2a
2b

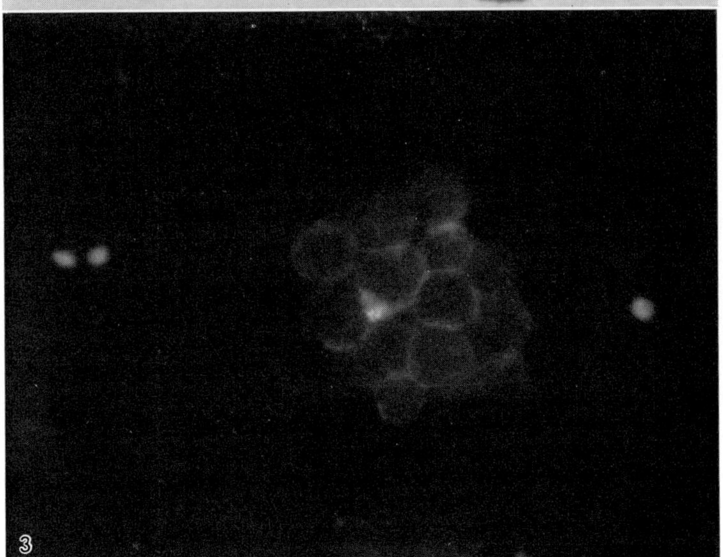
3

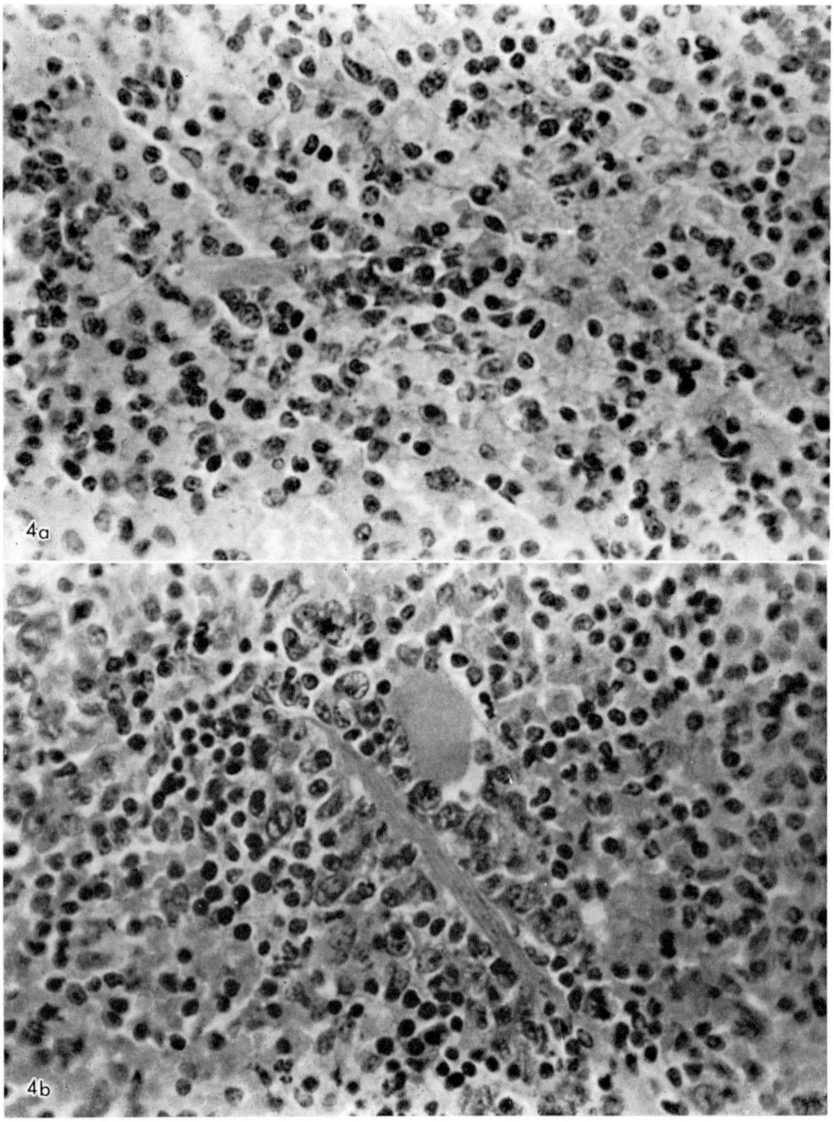
4a
4b

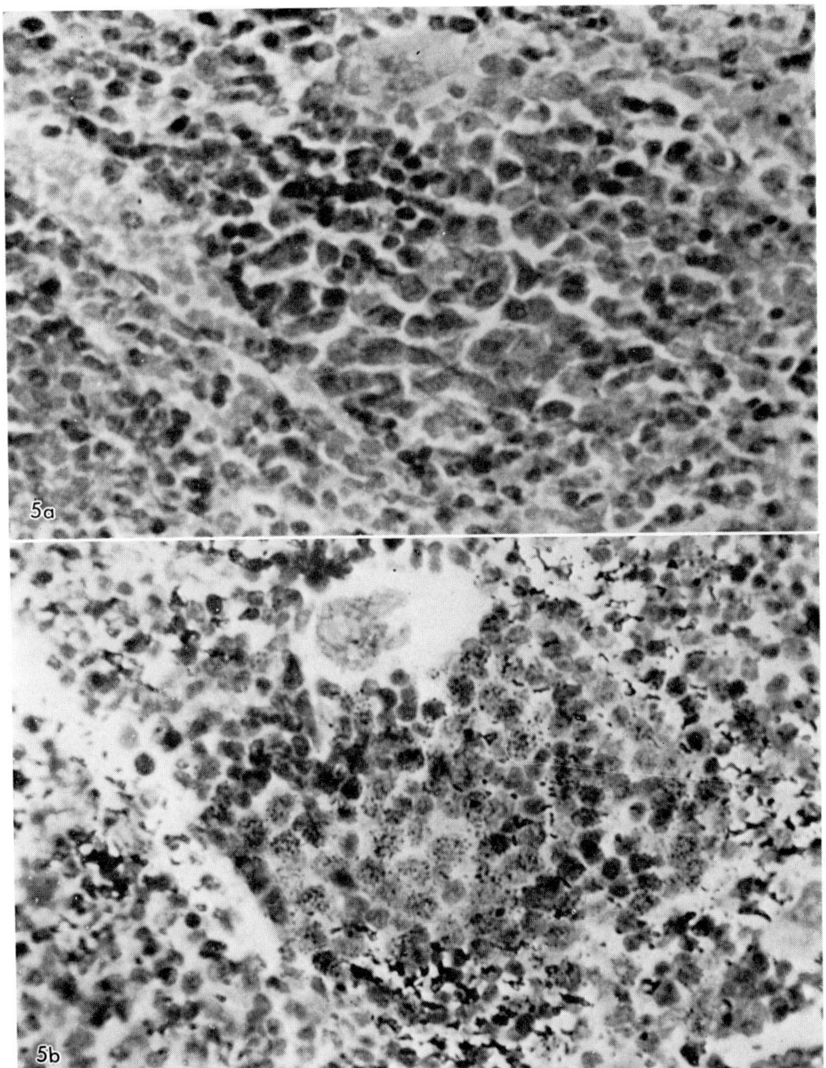
5a
5b

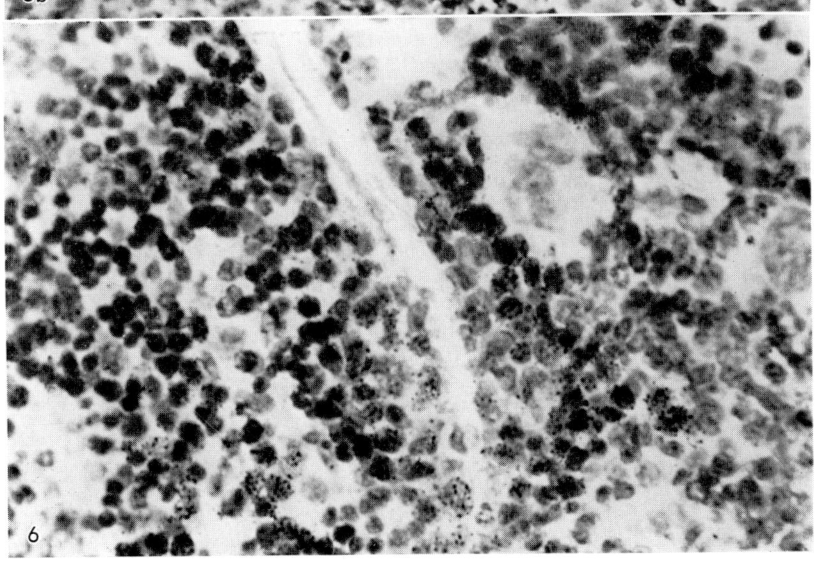
6

GANN Monograph on Cancer Research 12, 1972

LEUKEMOGENESIS BY RAUSCHER VIRUS IN MICE

Shozo IRINO, Isao MIYOSHI, Tatsuo SEZAKI, Tadami NAGAO, Hirokuni TAGUCHI, Koichi HARA, and Kiyoshi HIRAKI

*Department of Internal Medicine, Okayama University Medical School**

This paper presents the results of our experiments on the histogenesis and target cells of Rauscher leukemia, virus-target cell interaction, the role of hemolytic anemia, and the pathophysiology of iron, protein, hemoglobin, vitamin B_{12}, and folic acid in Rauscher leukemia. From these findings we conclude that Rauscher disease is a neoplastic process involving an erythroid cell series, and we believe that the elucidation of this disease may lead to the solution of the problem of the interrelationships among virus, host, and leukemia.

Rauscher virus is a potent leukemogenic virus isolated by Rauscher (*11*) in 1962, which induces erythroleukemia after a short latency in various strains of susceptible mice. Rauscher disease is characterized by marked hepatosplenomegaly and the presence of erythroblasts in the peripheral blood. The nature of this disease is considered by Rauscher (*11*) to be erythrocytopoiesis followed by lymphoid leukemia, but it has also been reported that erythroleukemia is followed by myeloblastic leukemia (*1*). There is still a controversy over whether erythroid proliferation in Rauscher disease is reactive hyperplasia or a neoplastic process (*2–5*, *10*, *13*, *15*). The present paper is concerned with hematological and cytohistological aspects of Rauscher disease and virus-target cell interaction *in vivo* and *in vitro*. Furthermore, results are presented on the role of hemolytic anemia, ferrokinetics, protein, hemoglobin, vitamin B_{12}, and folic acid in Rauscher disease.

Hematological and Cytohistological Analysis

Young adult BALB/c mice were injected with Rauscher virus. Nearly all of them developed leukemia and died with marked hepatosplenomegaly an average period of 90 days after virus inoculation. One week after virus inoculation, scattered foci of reticulum cells and erythroblasts were already noted under the capsule and around the lymph follicles of the spleen and in the sinusoids of the liver. The cellular infiltration became conspicuous with the progression of the disease, involving other organs, like the lungs and kidneys. In the bone marrow an increase of erythroblasts and reticulum cells also occurred, though to a lesser degree. In the splenectomized, Rauscher virus-inoculated mice, the tumorous infiltration of

* Shikata-cho 2-5-1, Okayama 700 (入野昭三, 三好勇夫, 瀬崎達雄, 長尾忠美, 田口博国, 原功一, 平木　潔).

these cells was more pronounced in the bone marrow and liver. The peripheral blood picture showed a transient decrease of red cells, white cells, and thrombocytes in 1 week, and an increase of nucleated cells, reticulocytes, erythroblasts, and smudge cells in about 2 weeks after virus inoculation, and a few Rauscher cells (*5*), characteristic of Rauscher leukemia, appeared 3 to 4 weeks after virus inoculation. Rauscher leukemia, therefore, may be defined as an erythroleukemia or an erythroreticulum cell leukemia, originating in the spleen and bone marrow.

Target Cell and Virus Cell Interaction in vivo *and* in vitro

A 3-month-old BALB/c mouse with Rauscher leukemia was sacrificed and the enlarged spleen was aseptically minced in an RPMI-1640 medium. The resulting cell suspension in the RPMI-1640 medium supplemented with 20% calf serum was kept stationary in tubes and bottles at 37°. The cultured cells (OUMS-1) were composed of a mixture of fibroblastoid and round cells (*7*). May-Grünwald-Giemsa stained preparations showed immature cells resembling reticulum cells and erythroblasts in various stages of maturity (Photo 1). When the cells were grown in medium with ^{59}Fe added, cellular incorporation of the isotope was demonstrated by a well-type scintillation counter. Microspectrophotometry disclosed a significant absorption at a Soret band of 406 nm in the mature erythroblast-like cells, suggesting the presence of hemoglobin (Fig. 1). The cellular ultrastructures were compatible with those of undifferentiated reticulum cells, proerythroblasts, and their precursors. Thin-section electron microscopy of the cultured cells revealed many type C virus particles in the intercellular spaces and intracytoplasmic vacuoles, and also a small number of doughnut-shaped immature and budding particles (Photo 2). Bioassay of the supernatant fluid was positive (*8*).

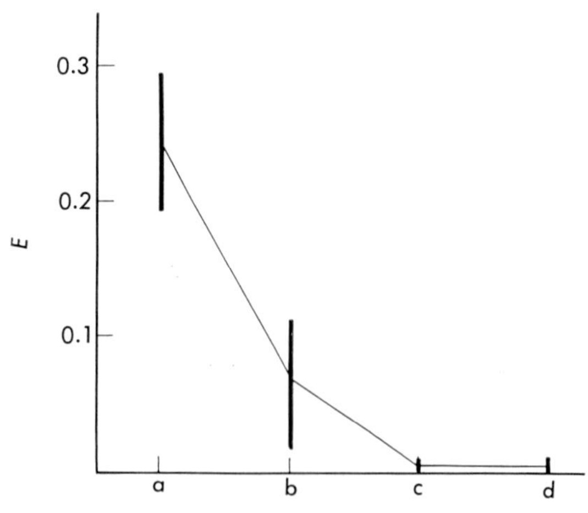

FIG. 1. Microspectrophotometry of the OUMS-1 cells at a Soret band of 406 nm

a: erythrocytes; b: mature erythroblast-like cells; c: large round cells; d: fibroblast-like cells.

These findings indicated an erythroid nature of the cell line derived from the leukemic spleen, which corresponds well to the *in vivo* state of Rauscher leukemic mice

In order to clarify the mode of virus-target cell interaction, electron microscopy was carried out on the localization and morphology of virus particles in the spleen of mice with various stages of Rauscher disease following inoculation. No virus particles were seen 2 to 4 days after virus inoculation; after 1 week a few virus particles budding from the membranes of megakaryocytes (Photo 3) and in the intercellular spaces were occasionally observed. These virus particles measured approximately 120 nm in diameter and were mature type C particles. Until 4 to 6 weeks after virus inoculation, multiplication of virus particles in the megakaryocytes continued to be active and this appeared to be a primary site of virus replication. However, after 10 weeks, when the disease process was fully advanced, virus particles in the megakaryocytes were significantly reduced, with many virus particles in the intercellular spaces. At this stage budding of virus particles from the cell membrane of presumably leukemic cells was observed (Photo 4). Rauscher and Allen (*12*) reported the eclipse phase to be 1 to 4 days after virus inoculation on the basis of bioassay studies, and Silvestre *et al.* (*14*) observed virus budding by electron microscopy 4 days after inoculation. These findings were confirmed by our experiments, as follows. Fetus of Swiss mouse was trypsinized and cultured in YLE medium with 10% calf serum at 37° and the cultured cells were inoculated with 3 ml of 10% Rauscher leukemic spleen extract. Its infectivity titer was $10^{4.5}ID_{50}$ per 0.2 ml. Absorption time was 2 hr at 37°. Leukemogenic activity became manifest 6 days after virus inoculation and reached a titer of $10^{3.0}$ ID_{50}/ml 7 days after virus inoculation. Immediately after virus absorption, the inoculated virus particles were seen attached to the cell surface and appeared to be engulfed into the cytoplasm by phagocytosis. No formation of new virus particles could yet be recognized 3 days after virus absorption, but a fair number of virus particles were seen 7 days after virus absorption. Budding virus particles were still contiguous with the plasma membrane.

It is thought that the inoculated virus particles, which first attach to the cell surface, enter the cell by phagocytosis and that after an eclipse period of 6 to 7 days they are extruded extracellularly by budding. This period of virus eclipse is estimated to be about 6 days, longer than that of other infectious viruses, which may be a characteristic of leukemia virus replication (*9*).

Hemolytic Anemia, Ferrokinetics, Protein, Hemoglobin, Vitamin B_{12}, and Folic Acid

On the basis of the findings described above, Rauscher leukemia is considered an erythroleukemia or erythroreticulum cell leukemia, originating in splenic erythroid cells. Therefore, the role of hemolytic anemia, ferrokinetics, protein, hemoglobin, vitamin B_{12}, and folic acid in Rauscher leukemia was investigated.

A broad distribution curve of erythrocyte diameter was obtained from stained smears of leukemic peripheral blood. The diameter ranged in size from 3 to 9 μ during the development of leukemia, as compared to the normal size of 4 to 7 μ.

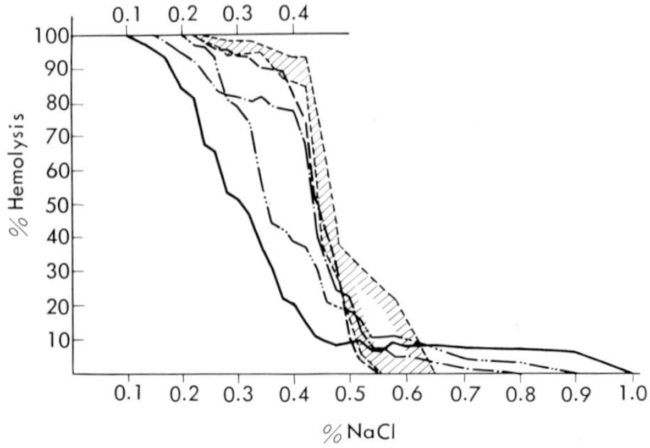

FIG. 2. Osmotic fragility curve of erythrocytes in Rauscher virus leukemia ////// normal range; — — — 1 week; — · — 4 weeks; — ·· — 8 weeks; ——— 12 weeks.

Characteristic osmotic fragility curves were obtained in leukemic mice by controlled salt concentration, with some cells showing increased fragility and some cells showing decreased fragility. These increased as well as decreased fragilities became more evident in the advanced stage of leukemia (Fig. 2); at 12 weeks after inoculation, hemolysis was observed in salt concentrations of 0.9 to 0.1%. The leukemic serum showed a slightly icteric color, and bilirubin was detected by the Hijman Van den Bergh method. Quantification of serum bilirubin was performed by a modification of Michaelson's original method. The direct and indirect bilirubin values were increased in the initial stage of leukemia and further increased in the advanced stage. In the leukemic serum, the total bilirubin was 1.2 mg/dl and direct bilirubin was 0.9 mg/dl, compared with means of 0.2 mg/dl and 0 mg/dl respectively in normal serum. The mean serum iron level in leukemic mice was 311 μg/dl, compared with the mean of 227 μg/dl in normal mice. Decreased haptoglobin, estimated by hemoglobin binding capacity using agar gel electrophoresis, indicated that hemolysis occurred in the leukemic mice. Excessive iron deposits were clearly demonstrated histologically in the leukemic liver and spleen, and especially in the kidneys, by the Berlin Blue staining method. Morphologically, stamp preparations of leukemic liver and spleen stained with May-Grünwald-Giemsa stain revealed a number of phagocytized red cells in the large reticulum cells (Photo 5).

Determination of red blood cell (RBC) survival was performed by noncohort labeling (^{51}Cr) techniques; ^{51}Cr-labeled RBC obtained from leukemic mice showed a shortened survival time in normal mice and became further shortened in leukemic mice, compared with that of labeled RBC from normal mice. The survival time of labeled RBC from normal mice was also shortened when injected into the leukemic mice (Fig. 3). These results suggested that shortened RBC survival time in leukemic mice was induced by both intracorpuscular and extracorpuscular causes resulting in a hemolytic anemia. Both direct and indirect Coombs tests with anti-mouse-globulin rabbit serum were positive in a few mice with advanced

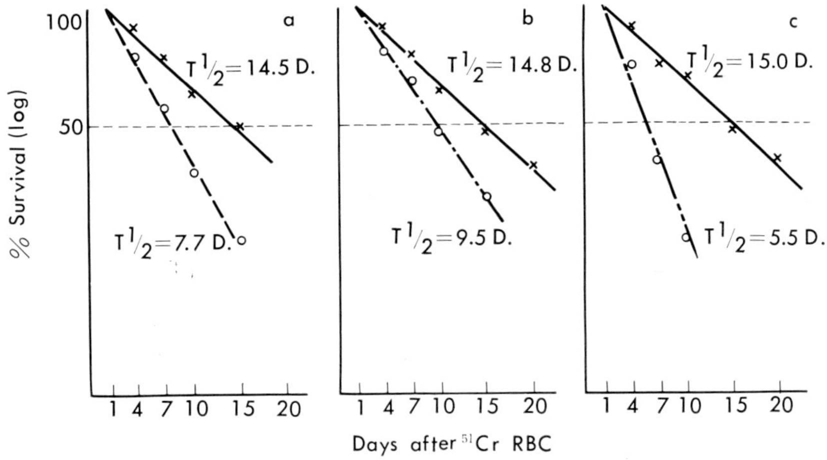

FIG. 3. Survival time of ^{51}Cr-labeled red blood cells in normal and Rauscher leukemia mice

a : ——— normal RBC, — — — leukemia RBC } in nor. mice; b : ——— nor. RBC in nor. mice, — - — nor. RBC in leuk. mice; c : ——— nor. RBC in nor. mice, ----- leuk. RBC in leuk. mice.

Rauscher leukemia (Photo 6). It may be interesting in this connection to note that, among AKR mice developing Rauscher leukemia after inoculation with cell-free filtrate of the supernatant culture fluids of our established mouse cell line, 63% showed a peculiar renal glomerular hyalinization and 50% showed hematoxylin bodies in the capillaries and small vessels of the lung and kidneys (Photo 7). The hematoxylin bodies were Feulgen-positive and presumably derived from the nuclear material (*6*). It remains to be seen whether an autoimmune mechanism is involved in the pathogenesis of these pathological features–glomerulopathy and hematoxylin bodies–in Rauscher viral leukemia, and it will likely be very important to elucidate how hemolytic anemia, and peculiar renal and pulmonary alterations are interrelated with the neoplastic proliferations of erythroid cells and with the host conditions.

In the study of ferrokinetics, individual mice were given intravenous injections of 1.0 μCi of ^{59}Fe in 0.25 ml of the physiological saline solution. Changes in plasma iron, mean radioiron clearance time (^{59}Fe T 1/2) and the reappearance rate (%) of ^{59}Fe in RBC were studied. In addition, the percentage uptake of injected ^{59}Fe and the percentage uptake of ^{59}Fe/g by the spleen, liver, and bone marrow were determined at 6, 24, or 48 hr after injection of ^{59}Fe (Fig. 4, Tables I and II). One week after infection, prior to the significant enlargement of the spleen, elevated plasma iron and shortened ^{59}Fe T 1/2 were noticed. The percentage uptake by the spleen and percentage uptake / g of spleen were increased, with a depressed ^{59}Fe reappearance rate. From 4 to 7 weeks, plasma iron levels became lower but they were still higher than normal, and ^{59}Fe T 1/2 was below normal. However, the reappearance rate gradually increased with the lapse of time since infection, and at 7 weeks after infection the 24-hr reappearance rate was over 100%.

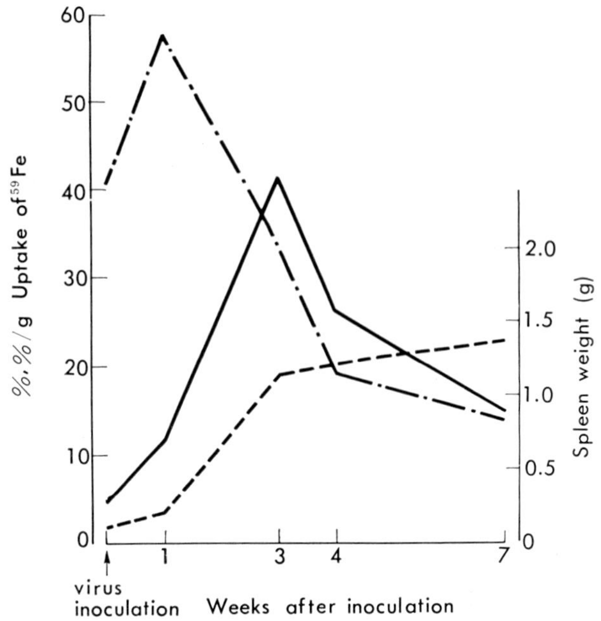

FIG. 4. Twenty-four hours uptake of ^{59}Fe in spleen and spleen weight following inoculation with Rauscher virus
— - — %/g; ——— %; - - - - spleen weight.

TABLE I. Uptake of ^{59}Fe in Femur and Tibia in Mice after Infection with Rauscher Virus

Time after inoculation (wk)	6	24	48 (hr)
Control	1.9	1.2	0.6
1	1.8	1.0	0.6
3	0.7	1.0	—
4	0.4	0.4	0.3
7	0.3	0.3	0.2

TABLE II. Plasma Fe, Blood Clearance, and Reappearance of ^{59}Fe in Mice Infected with Rauscher Leukemia Virus

Time after inoculation (wk)	Plasma Fe (μg %)	^{59}Fe T½ (min)	^{59}Fe reappearance (%)	
			24	48 (hr)
Control	229.6	62.6	69.2	97.3
1	559.8	39.0	28.2	29.3
4	466.0	51.8	59.7	67.0
7	311.7	45.0	102.2	87.9

The percentage uptake/g of spleen decreased sharply, accompanied by an increase in the splenic weight, while the total uptake by the spleen increased for 1 to 3 weeks after infection; thereafter both decreased, but they were still higher than normal levels. In the liver, the slight increase in the percentage uptake and decrease in the percentage uptake/g were not so significant, compared with those of the spleen. Bone marrow showed a decreased percentage uptake during the development of leukemia. These ferrokinetics data indicate that shortened ^{59}Fe T 1/2, decreased reappearance rate, and increased uptake by the spleen at the initial stage of leukemia, which constitute evidence of ineffective erythropoiesis, are related to the malignant proliferation of the erythroid cells. The shortened ^{59}Fe T 1/2, increased reappearance rate, and increased uptake of spleen at the advanced stage indicate that the maturation of erythroid cells is accelerated.

Observations on the serum protein and hemoglobin during the progression of Rauscher leukemia are considered most useful for the interpretation of host-virus or -tumor interactions and were sequentially pursued in parallel with the histological and hematological studies.

Two to three weeks after virus inoculation, we observed a decrease of γ- and α-globulins, especially, α_1-globulin, and a marked increase of β-globulin; 4 to 6 weeks after virus inoculation there was a slight increase of γ-globulin; and 12 to 16 weeks after virus inoculation, γ- and α_1-globulins were markedly reduced, despite the persisting elevation of β-globulin in comparison with the control. Of particular interest was the emergence of an abnormal fraction (mean: 1.02 g/dl) between α_2- and β-globulins about 4 weeks after virus inoculation. This abnormal fraction, which rapidly increased up to the advanced leukemic stage (Fig. 5, Photo 8), was never observed in the control, in mice with other reticular tissue neoplasms. It was not related to serum hemoglobin, haptoglobin, or glucoprotein but appeared to be related to the lipoprotein. Electrophoretically, this lipoprotein was due to retarded mobility of normal lipoprotein (Photos 9 and 10). Immunoelectrophoresis showed an increase of IgG in the initial and middle stages, and a decrease of IgG and an increase of transferrin in the advanced stage (Photo 11).

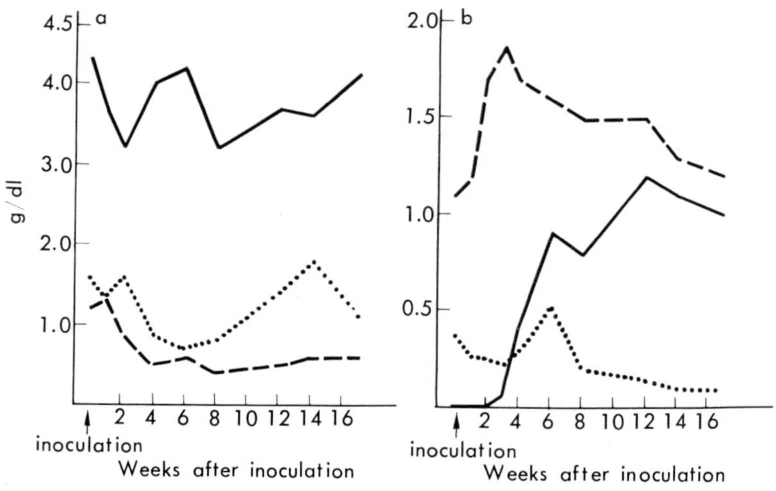

FIG. 5. Changes in each serum protein fraction in Rauscher leukemia

a: ——— albumin; — — — α_1-globulin; ········ α_2-globulin.

b: ——— abnormal; — — — β-globulin; ········ γ-globulin.

After sequential time intervals following Rauscher virus inoculation, hemolysates prepared from peripheral blood were analyzed by cellulose acetate membrane, agar, and starch gel electrophoresis. No abnormal hemoglobin was detectable in mice with Rauscher leukemia. Hemolysates from both normal and leukemic mice exhibited identical absorption curves with the α-band at 576 nm and the β-band at 541 nm. By starch gel electrophoresis, hemoglobin was separated into six fractions using hemolysates prepared from peripheral blood of normal and leukemic mice. These six fractions were denoted as I to VI, from anode to cathode (Photo 12). A decrease of fraction I+II, and fraction IV and an increase of fraction III were observed in leukemic mice (Fig. 6). This tendency was more evident in hemolysates prepared from the spleen. Fractions III and IV were 67.1% and 13.5% in the advanced stage of Rauscher disease, 49.6% and 42.6% in normal mice, respectively (Table III). The same pattern of fractions as in Rauscher leukemic mice was observed in fetal and newborn mice, but the abnormal fraction which appeared in the early stage of fetuses was not observed in Rauscher leukemic mice. The difference between the electrophoretic pattern of fractions

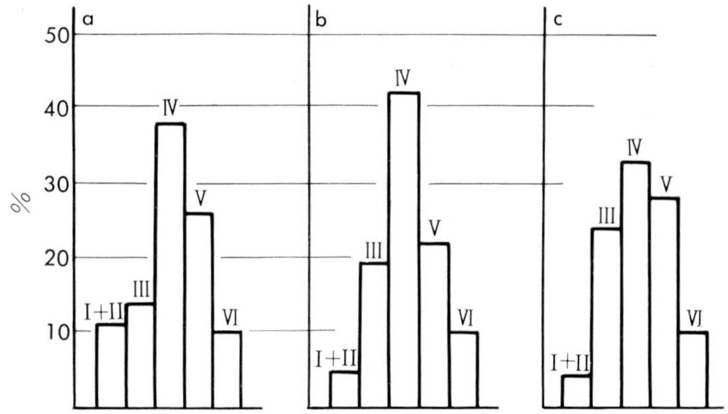

FIG. 6. Changes in the relative ratio of the hemoglobin subcomponents during the development of leukemia
a: normal; b: stage I (0–10 wk); c: stage II (10–20 wk).
( ): weeks after inoculation.

TABLE III. Relative Ratio of Hemoglobin Subcomponents in the Spleen of Leukemic Mouse

Leukemic mouse No.	Spleen weight (g)	Subcomponent (%) I	II	III	IV
1	1.4	2.9	18.1	47.4	31.6
2	2.5	2.4	16.6	56.4	24.6
3	2.5	0.5	12.5	60.6	26.4
4	3.0	0.9	18.4	67.1	13.5
Mean		1.7	16.4	57.9	24.0
Normal mouse	0.09	1.0	6.9	49.6	42.6

in normal and phenylhydrazine-induced anemic mice was not observed. The Betke staining, which is used for the demonstration of Hb F and is positive in almost all red cells from newborn mice, showed an average of 31.6% positive red cells from leukemic mice in contrast to an average of 8.6% positive cells from normal mice (Photo 13). It was found that the number of Betke-positive cells increases with the progression of Rauscher leukemia, suggesting abnormalities in hemoglobin synthesis.

From these findings, hemoglobin synthesis in Rauscher leukemia is considered to be similar to that of fetuses in relation to the neoplastic proliferation of erythroid cells.

Figure 7 shows a comparison of the vitamin B_{12} content in normal and in Rauscher leukemic mice as determined by the method used by the committee for the assay of vitamin B_{12} of the Japan Vitamin Society. There was no significant difference in serum vitamin B_{12} levels, but the vitamin B_{12} content in the liver and spleen was lower in leukemic mice than in normal mice, suggesting an increased metabolic demand by the tumor cells.

The folic acid content was likewise determined using *Lactobacillus casei* according to the Water and Morine method. In Rauscher leukemic mice the folic acid content in the serum and liver was low, while that in the spleen was high in comparison with those of normal mice (Fig. 8). The decrease in the serum and liver was considered to be due to an increased demand, and the rise in the spleen was ascribed to an increased number of immature erythroblasts. It is known that immature erythroblasts contain several times as much folic acid as mature erythroblasts. It is conceivable that this phenomenon holds true for the splenic erythroblasts in Rauscher leukemia.

Folic acid, 40 μg/kg, was injected intravenously into Rauscher leukemic and normal mice. The serum folic acid level 15 min after injection was lower in Rauscher leukemic mice than in normal mice (Fig. 9), suggesting an increased demand for folic acid in affected mice.

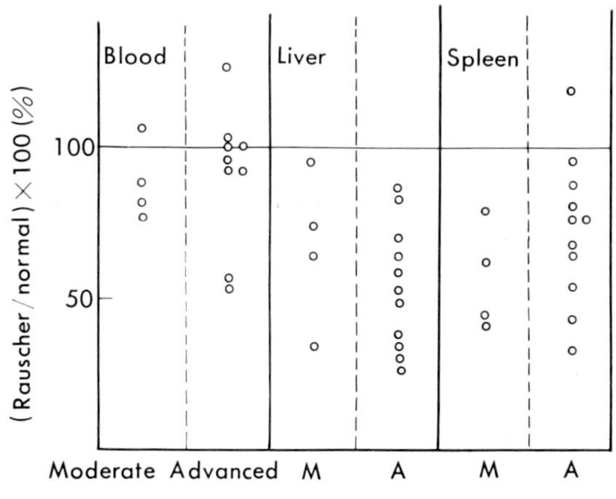

FIG. 7. Vitamin B_{12} of Rauscher leukemic mice
Moderate: spleen weight 500–930 mg.
Advanced: spleen weight 1150–2700 mg.

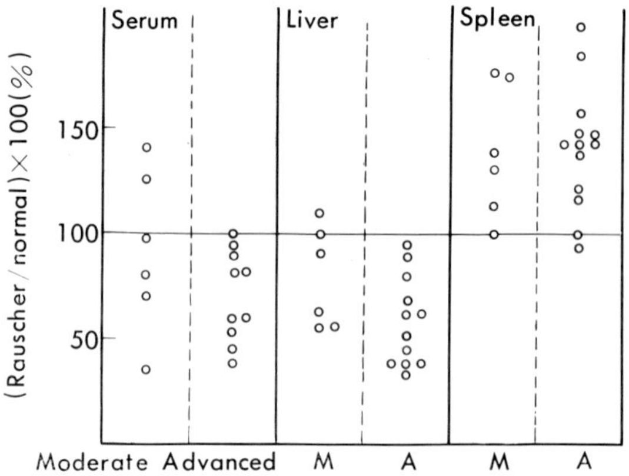

FIG. 8. Folic acid of Rauscher leukemic mice
Moderate: spleen weight 500–930 mg.
Advanced: spleen weight 1150–2700 mg.

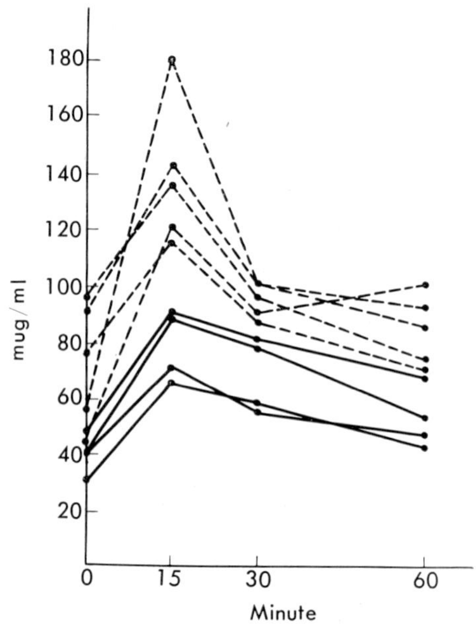

FIG. 9. Folic acid clearance test in Rauscher leukemic mice
– – – – normal mouse; ——— Rauscher mouse. (40 μg/kg i.v.).

REFERENCES

1. Boiron, M., Levy, J. P., Lasneret, J., Oppenheim, S., and Bernard, J. Pathogenesis of Rauscher leukemia. *J. Natl. Cancer Inst.*, **35**, 865–884 (1965).
2. Brodsky, I., Kahn, S. B., Ross, E. M., Petkov, G., and Braverman, S. D. Prelymphoid leukemia phase of Rauscher virus infection. *J. Natl. Cancer Inst.*, **38**, 779–787 (1967).
3. Dunn, T. B., and Green, A. W. Morphology of BALB/c mice inoculated with Rauscher virus. *J. Natl. Cancer Inst.*, **36**, 987–1001 (1966).

4. Irino, S. Studies on the pathogenesis of Rauscher disease (erythroleukemia) induced by Rauscher virus (in Japanese). *Acta Haematol. Japon.*, **28**, 877–881 (1965).
5. Irino, S., Osato, H., Dabasaki, H., and Hiraki, K. Rauscher virus and Rauscher disease. I. Peripheral blood picture with special reference to the occurrence of Rauscher cells (in Japanese). *Igaku to Seibutsugaku* (*Medicine and Biology*), **72**, 305–309 (1966).
6. Miyoshi, I., Osato, Y., Dabasaki, H., Irino, S., and Hiraki, K. Glomerulopathy and hematoxylin bodies in Rauscher murine leukemia. *GANN*, **58**, 85–87 (1967).
7. Miyoshi, I., Tsubota, T., Irino, S., and Hiraki, K. Establishment of erythroblastic cell lines from the spleen of mice with Rauscher leukemia. *GANN*, **59**, 439–441 (1968).
8. Miyoshi, I., Tsubota, T., Nagao, T., Takata, H., Irino, S., and Hiraki, K. Continuous viral multiplication and neoplastic transformation in cell lines established from spleen of mice with Rauscher leukemia. *GANN*, **60**, 583–590 (1969).
9. Ota, Z., Suzuki, S., Muguruma, M., Nagao, T., and Hiraki, K. An electron microscopic study of the development of Rauscher leukemia virus in cultured Swiss mouse embryo cells (in Japanese). *Igaku to Seibutsugaku* (*Medicine and Biology*), **76**, 48–50 (1968).
10. Pluznik, D. H., Sachs, L., and Resnitzky, P. The mechanism of leukemogenesis by the Rauscher leukemia virus. *Natl. Cancer Inst. Monograph*, **22**, 3–12 (1966).
11. Rauscher, F. J. A virus-induced disease of mice characterized by erythrocytopoiesis and lymphoid leukemia. *J. Natl. Cancer Inst.*, **29**, 515–543 (1962).
12. Rauscher, F. J., and Allen, B. V. Growth curve of a murine leukemia virus in mice. *J. Natl. Cancer Inst.*, **32**, 269–275 (1964).
13. Siegel, B. V., Weaver, W. J., and Koler, R. D. Mouse erythroleukemia of viral etiology. *Nature*, **201**, 1042–1043 (1964).
14. Silvestre, D., Levy, J.-P., Leclerc, J.-C., and Boiron, M. Ultrastructural study of the Rauscher virus in the mouse. *Pathol. Biol.*, **14**, 559–564 (1966).
15. Yokoro, K., and Thorell, B. Cytology and pathogenesis of Rauscher virus disease in splenectomized mice. *Cancer Res.*, **26**, 536–543 (1966).

EXPLANATION OF PHOTOS

PHOTO 1. The established cell line (OUMS-1) composed of a mixture of fibroblastoid and round cells. A few intermingled mature erythroblast-like cells can be seen. After 306 days *in vitro*, 76th passage. May-Grünwald-Giemsa. ×270

PHOTO 2. Numerous type C virus particles observed between two OUMS-1 cells. They are mostly mature particles with electron-dense nucleoids; a few immature doughnut-shaped particles are also present. After 253 days *in vitro*, 50th passage.

PHOTO 3. Virus particles budding from the megakaryocyte of the mouse 1 week after virus inoculation.

PHOTO 4. Virus particles budding from the leukemic cells of the mouse 10 weeks after virus inoculation.

PHOTO 5. Stamp preparations of leukemic liver and spleen stained with May-Grünwald-Geimsa stain showing a number of phagocytized red cells in the large reticulum cells.

PHOTO 6. Direct Coombs test with anti-mouse-globulin rabbit serum. Left: red blood cells of a normal mouse. Right: red blood cells of an advanced Rauscher leukemic mouse.

PHOTO 7. Diffuse deposition of homogeneous, eosinophilic material in all the glomeruli, some of which are, in addition, infiltrated with leukemic cells. Hematoxylin and Eosin. ×100

PHOTO 8. Electrophoretic serum protein changes in Rauscher leukemia.

PHOTO 9. Lipoprotein in the serum of Rauscher leukemia (Sudan Black B staining).

PHOTO 10. Migration of lipoprotein on paper electrophoresis in relation to serum protein changes in Rauscher leukemia. In each group: upper-ponseau, middle-sudan black, lower-ponseau and sudan black double staining

PHOTO 11. Immunoelectrophoresis of the Rauscher leukemic mouse serum.

Upper: advanced stage of Rauscher leukemia. Middle: initial stage of Rauscher leukemia. Lower: control (normal mouse serum). Tr.: transferrin. Transferrin increases in the advanced stage of Rauscher leukemia (arrow).

PHOTO 12. Starch gel electrophoresis of hemolysates prepared from peripheral blood of normal adult mice. Hemoglobin is separated into six fractions.

PHOTO 13. Betke staining of red blood cells of Rauscher leukemia.

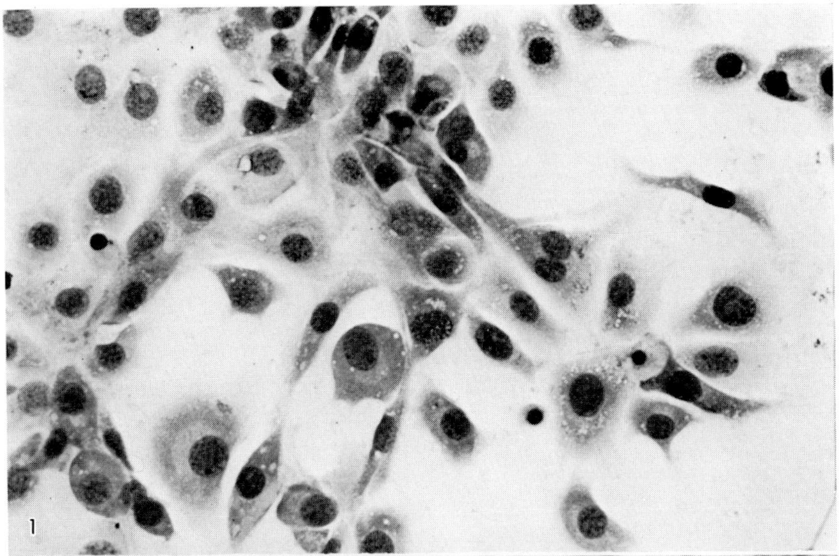
1

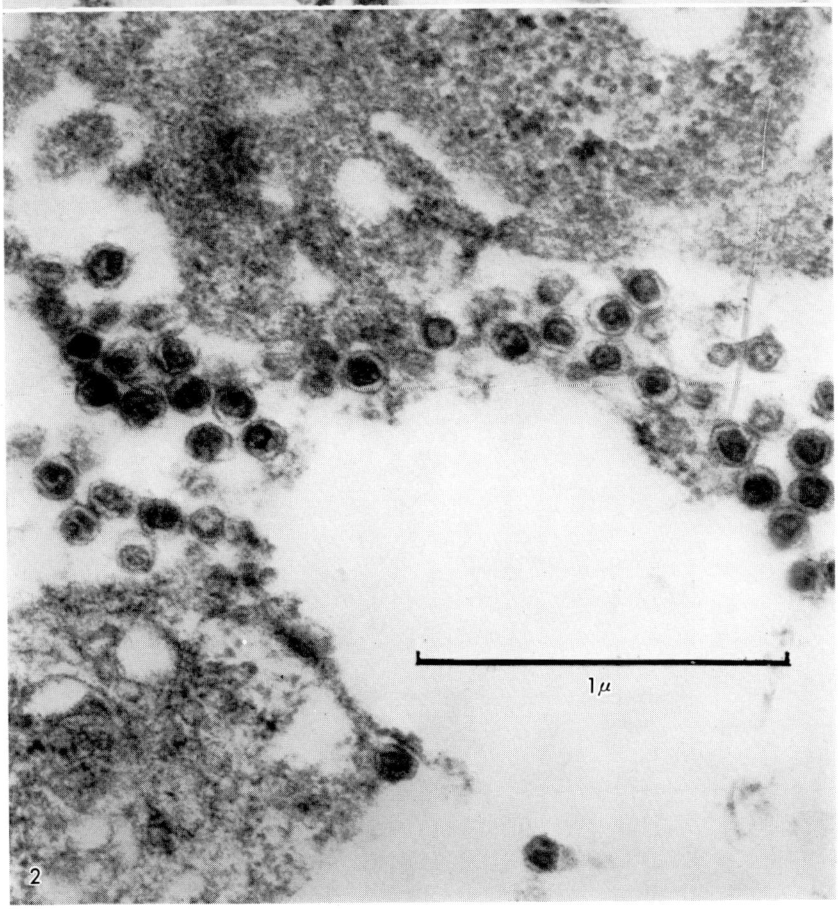
1μ
2

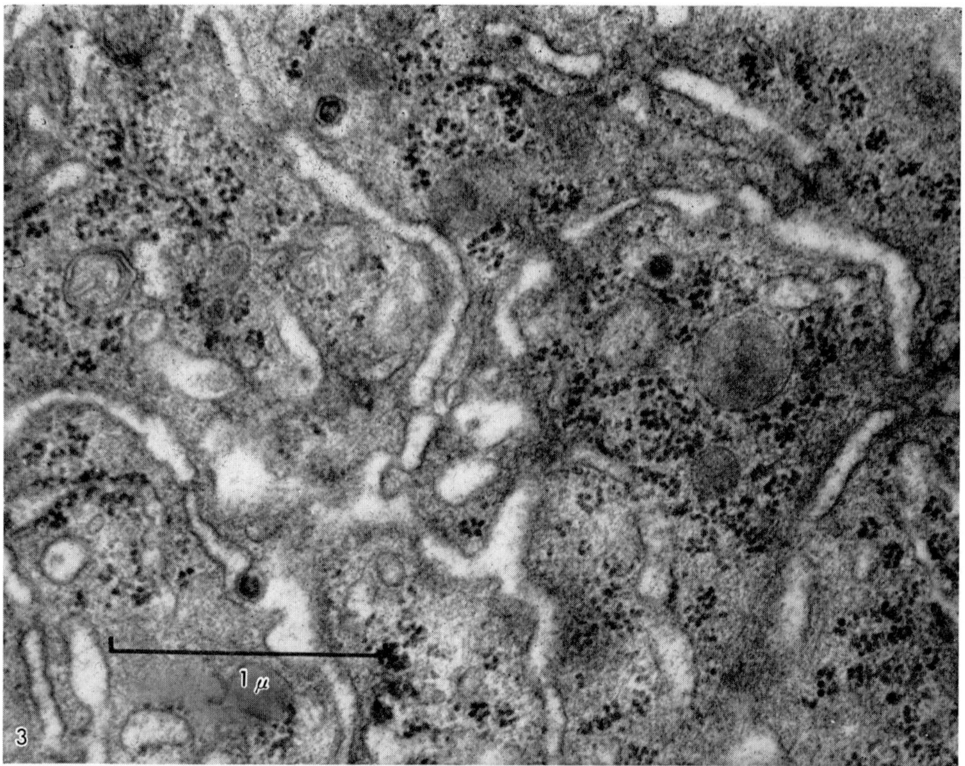
1 μ
3

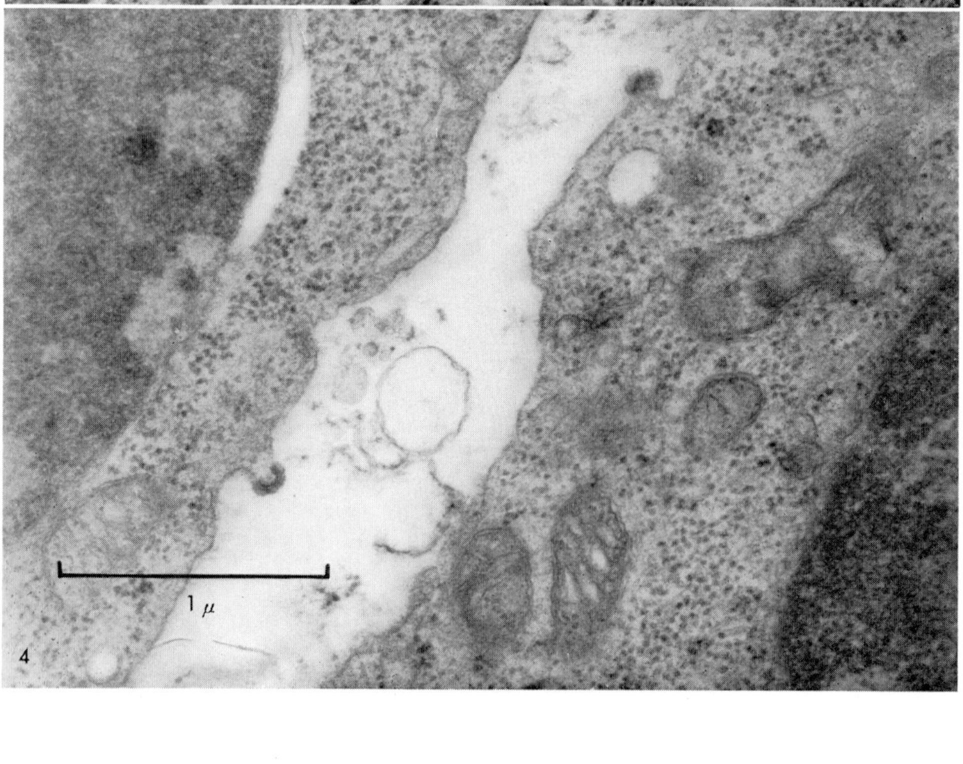
1 μ
4

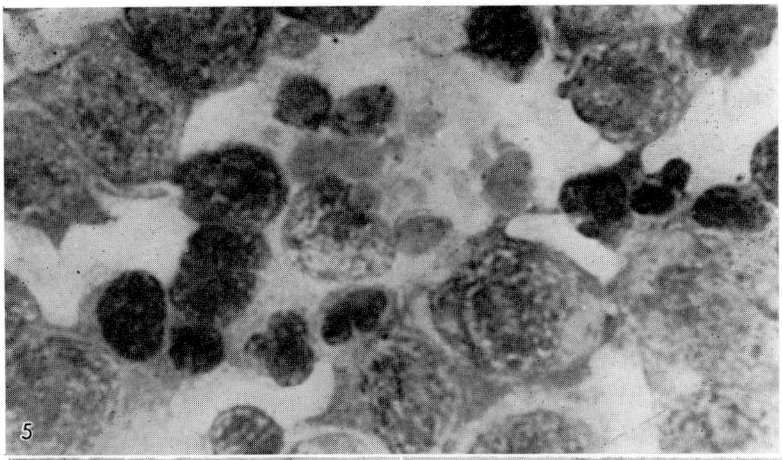
5

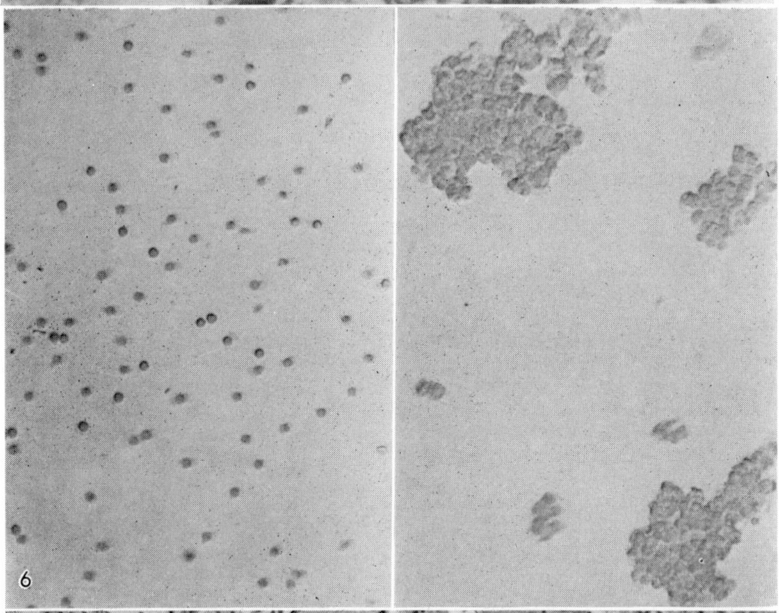
6

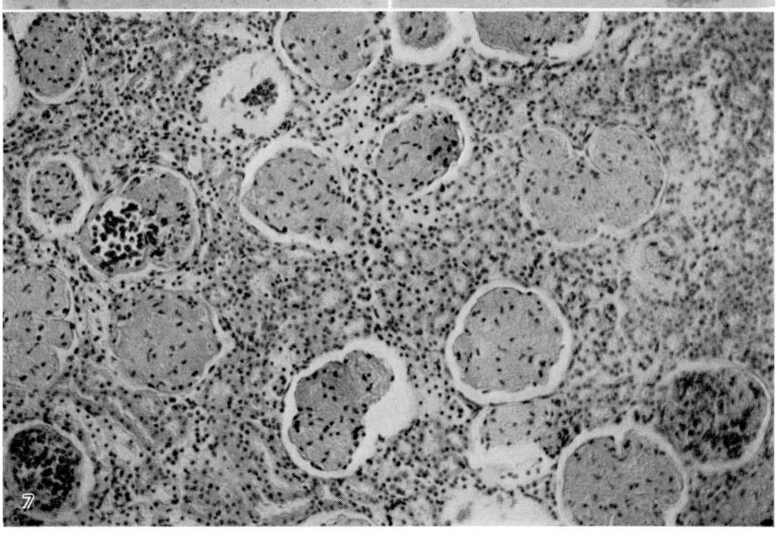
7

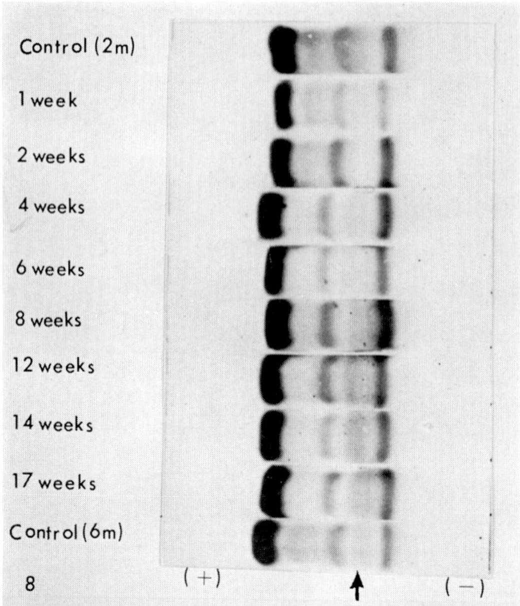

Control (2m)
1 week
2 weeks
4 weeks
6 weeks
8 weeks
12 weeks
14 weeks
17 weeks
Control (6m)
8
(+)
(−)

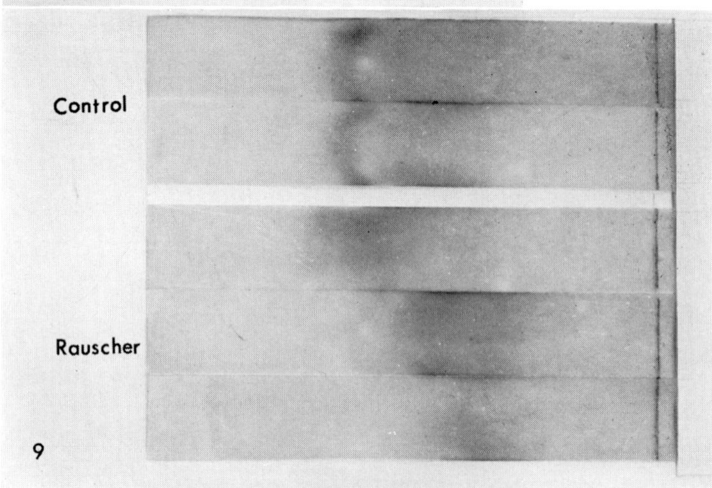

Control
Rauscher
9

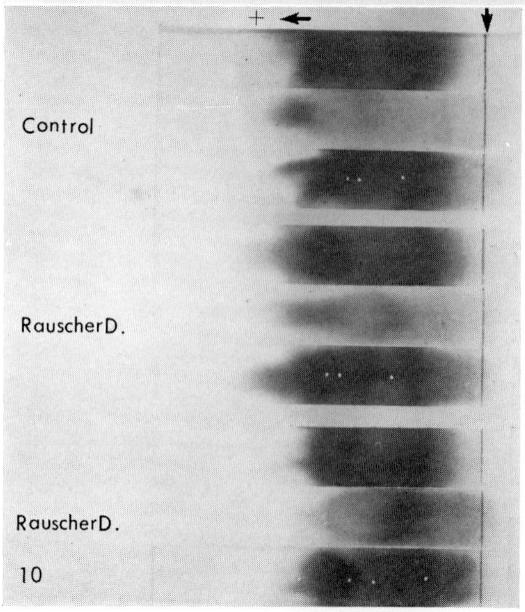

+
Control
RauscherD.
RauscherD.
10

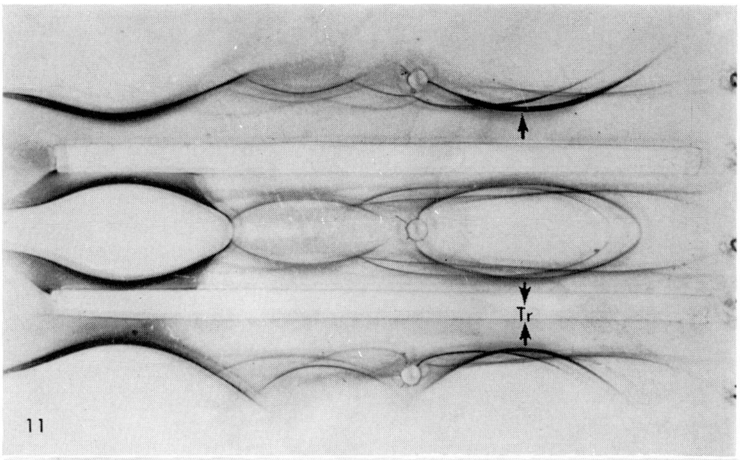
Tr
11

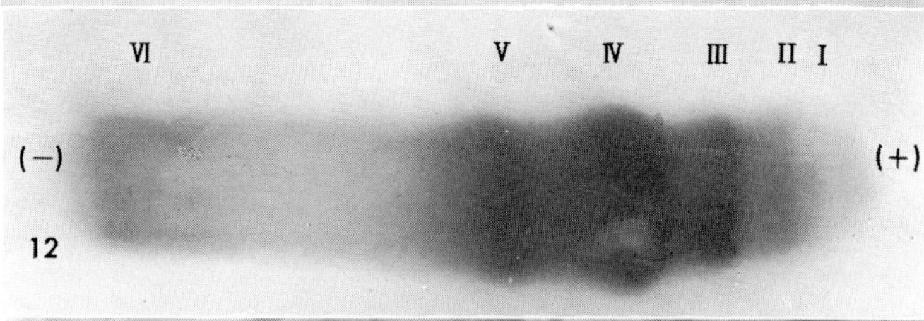
VI V IV III II I
(−) (+)
12

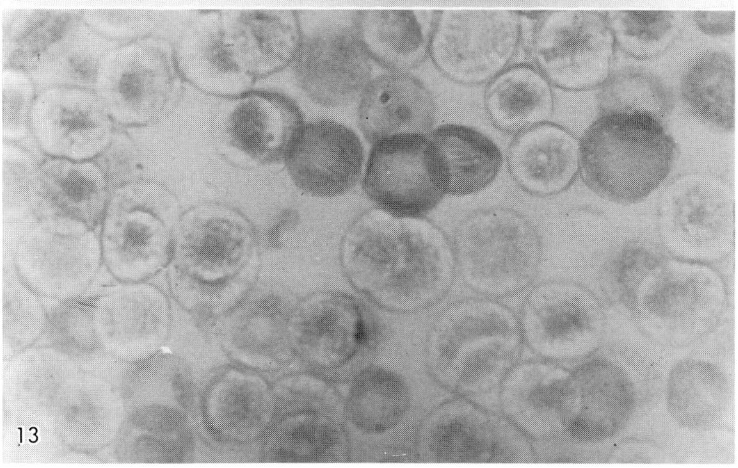
13

GANN Monograph on Cancer Research 12, 1972

PROPERTIES OF RAUSCHER VIRUS PROPAGATED IN C57BL/6 MOUSE CELLS *IN VIVO* AND *IN VITRO*

Isolation and Characterization of a Lymphatic Leukemia Virus

Akinori ISHIMOTO, Yohei ITO, and Michiyuki MAEDA

Laboratory of Viral Oncology, Aichi Cancer Center and Department of Tumor Virus, Institute for Virus Research, Kyoto University***

To determine whether Rauscher virus consists of more than one kind of murine leukemia virus, the leukemogenicity of the virus propagated in C57BL/6 lymphoma and the antigenicity of Rauscher virus-induced lymphoma were examined. A lymphoma that produces only lymphoma-inducible virus was isolated. However, both G (Gross) and FMR (Friend, Moloney, and Rauscher) antigens were found in the lymphoma. Infection and propagation of Rauscher virus in C57BL/6 spleen cells were examined *in vitro* where immunological reactions from the host could be excluded, in order hopefully to obtain cell clones producing only lymphoma-inducible virus or only erythroblastosis-inducible virus from the Rauscher virus-infected cells. However, Rauscher virus-infected cells produced viruses capable of inducing both erythroblastosis and lymphoma.

Rauscher virus induced erythroblastosis with rapidly progressing enlargement of spleens and livers in both newborn and weanling mice of the C3H, BALB/c, and Swiss strains. However, weanling mice of the C57BL/6 strain are almost completely resistant to Rauscher virus. When newborn C57BL/6 mice are inoculated with Rauscher virus, generalized lymphosarcomas and occasionally thymomas or myelogenous leukemia, develop without any sign of erythroblastosis, after relatively long incubation periods. Another striking contrast is that erythroblasts in the rapidly enlarged spleen of BALB/c, C3H, and Swiss mice are not transplantable, while the lymphoma cells of C57BL/6 mice are readily transplantable.

Many experiments have been performed in an unsuccessful attempt to elucidate this dual pathogenic potency of the Rauscher virus (*3*, *6*, *11*). Gross proposed that Rauscher virus consists of the Friend and Gross leukemia viruses. This proposal was based on the results of his experiments revealing that rat-adapted Rauscher virus did not induce erythroblastosis, even when inoculated into mice of the susceptible strains described above, and that the ability of this virus to induce lymphomas in C3H mice could be inhibited by anti-Gross virus rabbit serum (*3*).

* Kanokoden 81, Tashiro-cho, Chikusa-ku, Nagoya, 464 (石本秋稔, 伊藤洋平).

** Kawara-machi, Shogoin, Sakyo-ku, Kyoto 606 (前田道之).

Pluznik *et al.* (*11*) established 14 clones of Rauscher virus by 3 successive isolations from single splenic white colonies which had been induced by Rauscher virus. All these cloned viruses, however, could still produce both erythroid and myeloid leukemia. Such evidence suggests that the progeny obtained from a single colony-forming unit may contain 2 different leukemia viruses, or it may consist of single multipotent viruses capable of inducing erythroid and myeloid leukemia.

On the other hand, Old *et al.* (*10*) reported that lymphoma cells of C57BL/6 mice induced by Rauscher virus have a specific cytotoxic antigen designated as the Friend-Moloney-Rauscher (FMR) antigen which is not cross-reactive with Gross (G) leukemia. These new antigenic markers, G (Gross) and FMR antigens, made it feasible to attempt to analyze the components of the Rauscher virus complex. As to Gross *et al.*'s experiment, the question arises whether FMR antigen was demonstrable on the lymphomas cells induced with the Gross rat-adapted Rauscher virus.

To discover whether Rauscher virus is a mixture of some murine leukemia viruses, we examined the properties of Rauscher virus propagated in C57BL/6 mouse cells *in vivo* and *in vitro*. In particular we examined the antigenicity of the leukemic cells induced with the virus propagated in C57BL/6 lymphoma.

Leukemogenicity of Rauscher Virus Propagated in Originally Induced C57BL/6 Lymphomas

Standard Rauscher virus was inoculated into 113 newborn C57BL/6 mice (Table I). Generalized lymphomas developed in 46 C57BL/6 mice after a mean latent period of 198 days. Of 46 lymphomas, 28 were transplantable in C57BL/6 mice, 10 were not transplantable, and 8 were not tested. No lymphoma developed in BALB/c and SMA mice inoculated with the standard Rauscher virus. To determine the virus yield from C57BL/6 lymphomas originally induced by Rauscher virus, a crude homogenate (10%, w/v) of spleen and lymph nodes from 38 lymphomas was inoculated into SMA weanling mice. Except for a lymphoma designated RD-2, all originally induced lymphomas produced erythroblastosis-inducible virus, which was capable of inducing early hepatosplenomegaly in SMA mice.

To check the virus yield from the RD-2 lymphoma more precisely, cell-free supernatants prepared from originally induced and once transplanted RD-2 lymphoma were inoculated into newborn and weanling SMA, BALB/c, and C57BL/6 mice. As controls, cell-free supernatants from 3 lymphomas designated RD-8, RD-12, and RD-14 were also inoculated (*8*). Inoculations of cell-free extracts from RD-8, RD-12, and RD-14 lymphomas into newborn or weanling mice resulted in the same pathological changes as did the inoculations of the standard Rauscher virus. However, inoculations of cell-free extracts from RD-2 lymphomas did not produce such early splenomegaly but induced transplantable lymphomas in C57BL/6, and even in SMA and BALB/c mice. Inoculations of cell-free extracts from these C57BL/6, SMA, and BALB/c lymphomas induced by the extracts from RD-2 lymphomas again developed only lymphomas in all strains of mice.

TABLE I. Results of Inoculations of Standard Rauscher Virus

Mouse		Virus[a] dilution	No. of mice inoculated	Early splenomegaly with erythroblastosis[b]	Lymphoma
Strain	Age				
BALB/c	Newborn	10^0	50	50	0
	Weanling	10^0	10	10	0
C57BL/6	Newborn	10^0	113	0	46
	Weanling	10^0	20	0	0
SMA	Newborn	10^{-2}	8	8	0
	Newborn	10^{-3}	7	7	0
	Newborn	10^{-4}	7	7	0
	Newborn	10^{-5}	10	9	0
	Newborn	10^{-6}	8	3	0
	Newborn	10^{-7}	6	3	0
	Newborn	10^{-8}	32	0	0
	Newborn	10^{-9}	37	0	0
	Weanling	10^0	44	44	0

[a] A deep-frozen preparation was obtained through the courtesy of Dr. F. J. Rauscher. The Rauscher virus has been maintained by serial passages in BALB/c mice in our laboratory and it was designated as standard Rauscher virus in the present paper.

[b] Bioassay of leukemogenicity: unless otherwise noted, 0.05 ml of cell-free material was inoculated into newborn mice intraperitoneally. These mice were observed until death. To weanlings, 0.5 ml of crude homogenate of materials was inoculated intraperitoneally. At autopsy, enlarged spleen over 250 mg in weight were regarded as positive for early splenomegaly.

These lymphoma-inducible viruses obtained from RD-2 lymphomas were designated as RD-2 virus.

Antigenicity of Rauscher Virus-induced Lymphomas

The antigenicity of Rauscher virus-induced lymphomas was examined by the cytotoxic test and the immunofluorescent antibody technique. It was especially interesting to determine whether FMR antigen was still present in lymphomas that no longer produced erythroblastosis-inducible virus.

Both FMR and G antigens were detected in all Rauscher virus-induced lymphomas and RD-2 virus-induced lymphomas by both methods (Photo 1). The antigenicity of some leukemic cells tested is summarized in Table II.

Limiting Dilution of Rauscher Virus

The limiting dilution method was applied to Rauscher virus *in vivo* to separate the components. Serial 10-fold dilutions from 10^{-2} to 10^{-9} of standard Rauscher virus were inoculated into newborn SMA mice. Mice inoculated with virus diluted from 10^{-2} to 10^{-7} developed early splenomegaly with erythroblastosis and died within 2 months, without any lymphomas. Neither lymphomas nor erythroblastosis developed in any mice inoculated with highly diluted virus, *i.e.*, 10^{-8} and 10^{-9} dilutions (Table I).

TABLE II. Antigenicity of Leukemic Cells Detected by Cytotoxic[a] and Immunofluorescent Antibody Tests[b]

Leukemia	Antigenicity	
	G	FMR
Rauscher leukemia		
standard virus-induced leukemia	+	+
RD-2 virus-induced leukemia	+	+
Gross leukemia	+	−
AKR lymphoma	+	−
Moloney leukemia[c]	+	+
SL leukemia[c]	+	−

[a] The cytotoxic test was based on the technique of Gorer and O'Gorman (*2*). Equal volumes of cell suspension (3×10^6/ml), antiserum, and guinea pig serum (as a source of complement) were mixed and incubated for 90 min at 37°. The number of living cells was counted microscopically after the addition of Trypan Blue. Surviving cells in a test tube containing normal serum were counted as a control. A cytotoxic index was calculated for each sample as follows: the number of living cells in the control minus the number of living cells in the experiments, divided by the first figure. A cytotoxic index over 0.15 was considered positive (*4*).

[b] G and FMR antigens were shown by the indirect immunofluorescent antibody test according to the method of Möller (*9*) and Klein and Klein (*7*).

[c] See ref. (*5*).

Propagation of Rauscher Virus in C57BL/6 Spleen Cells in Vitro

Spleens from 28-day-old C57BL/6 mice were removed aseptically, and each spleen was separately minced with curved scissors. The minced fragments from each spleen were placed on the surface of a TD-40 flask. After the tissue fragments were attached firmly to the glass, culture medium was added. The caps of the TD-40 flasks were loosely wrapped with aluminum foil to avoid an air-tight situation. Incubation was carried out at 37° in a humidified atmosphere containing 5% CO_2. After the medium was changed on the third day, cultures were inoculated with 1 ml of the virus stock. Cultures without inoculation of the virus were maintained as controls.

Formation of small cell colonies around the tissue fragments attached to the glass was observed both in controls and in infected cultures. Cells forming the colonies were mainly spindle-shaped, with a few small, round cells. About 2 weeks after the virus infection, cells forming the small colonies in the virus-infected cultures began to proliferate extensively. Subcultivation of the virus-infected primary cultures was carried out 4 weeks after the virus infection. These subcultures were incubated at 37° in a regular incubator, and successive transfers were carried out every 2 weeks for 45 generations to date (December 1, 1970). In recent passages, cultures consisted of spindle-shaped cells, cells with some pseudopodia, and a few multinucleated giant cells (Photo 2). One of the cell cultures has been maintained for over 2 years. By contrast, the proliferation of the cells in the control cultures was faint and all subcultivations were unsuccessful. The infectivity of 10-fold serial dilutions of supernatant from the virus-infected cultures has been tested by intraperitoneal injection of 1 ml into weanling SMA mice. Mice inoculated with the supernatant developed early splenomegaly similar to that induced by standard Rauscher virus. The maximum dilution which induced splenomegaly in 50% of the inoculated mice was 10^{-2}. Inoculation of the supernatants into newborn C57BL/6 mice led to the development of lymphomas as in the case of inoculation with the standard virus. The oncogenic potential of the cell line has been tested occasionally by the injection of 200×10^4 cells/mouse inguinally into 7-days-old suckling C57BL/6 mice, and 50×10^4 cells/mouse subcutaneously into newborn C57BL/6 mice. However, no tumorous growth at the site of inoculation has yet been observed; G and FMR antigens were detected on all of the cells by the indirect immunofluorescent antibody techniques.

General Discussion

It was demonstrated that there were 2 kinds of Rauscher virus-induced C57BL/6 lymphomas. One is a lymphoma which produces both erythroblastosis- and lymphoma-inducible viruses. The other is a lymphoma which produces only lymphoma-inducible virus. Most originally induced lymphomas in C57BL/6 were of the former kind, and the RD-2 lymphoma demonstrated in our experiment was of the latter kind. Erythroblastosis-inducing virus was detected neither in the cell-free extracts from the originally induced RD-2 lymphoma nor in the extracts from the transplanted RD-2 lymphomas. Cell-free passages of this lymphoma-inducing virus, designated DR-2, were also successful without alteration of the leukemogenic properties. Possible origins of the RD-2 virus are; (a) an associated virus in the Rauscher virus complex; (b) a mutant of Rauscher virus which arises in C57BL/6 mice; or (c) a contaminant from other murine leukemia virus stocks. The antigenic properties of DR-2 lymphomas have many features in common with Moloney leukemia, which is known to be a lymphoma with FMR antigens. The possibility of contamination by Moloney virus in our laboratory can be excluded, because Moloney and Gross leukemias were not used until the major part of this experiment had been completed. It is also unlikely that RD-2 lymphoma was induced by viruses disseminated among the BALB/c or C57BL/6 mice, since no spontaneous lymphoma was observed among these strains in our mouse colony.

If Rauscher virus consists of Gross and Friend viruses, limiting-dilution methods might be applied to separate 1 component from another. But it was difficult in an experiment of this scale to apply the limiting-dilution methods to separate 2 components when the ratio of 1 component to the other was very low. The fact that mice inoculated with any 10-fold diluted virus do not develop lymphomas may suggest that the erythroblastosis-inducing virus in the standard Rauscher virus is more numerous than the lymphoma-inducing virus.

In our experiments, G and FMR antigens were found in all lymphomas including RD-2 lymphomas. These results are consistent with those of Gross (*3*) and Old *et al.* (*10*). Furthermore, the results of our experiment can be explained by the hypothesis that the lymphomatic transformation and G antigenicity were coded by the genome of Gross virus, while the erythroblastic transformation and FMR antigenicity of the cells were coded by the genome of Friend virus.

When more than 1 kind of virus is infectious to 1 cell at the same time, the frequent appearance of hybrid viruses can be expected, as is known in the case of observations on some other tumor viruses (*1*).

The standard Rauscher virus may consist of viruses that induce (a) only lymphoma, (b) only erythroblastosis, and (c) hybrid virus-inducible lymphoma and erythroblastosis. The relation of the genomes that code the neoplastic transformation and the antigenic transformations would make the analysis of Rauscher virus more complicated.

As to the components of RD-2 virus, there are 2 possibilities. One is that RD-2 virus consists of 1 kind of virus with genomes coding both neoplastic and antigenic transformations. The other is that RD-2 virus consists of many kinds of viruses, with the genome inducing only neoplastic transformation or only antigenic transformation.

Acknowledgments

The authors wish to acknowledge the able technical assistance of Mr. T. Yanagidani and Mr. M. Yasuda, of Kyoto University, and Miss S. Oota, Mrs. M. Mamiya, and Mrs. H. Yamanaka, of the Aichi Cancer Center. This work was supported in part by a Grant-in-Aid for Scientific Research from the Japanese Ministry of Education, and by Contract No. NIH-69-96 within the Special Virus Program of the National Cancer Institute, National Institutes of Health, U.S. Public Health Service.

REFERENCES

1. Boeye, A., Melnick, J. L., and Rapp, F. SV40-adenovirus " hybrids: " Presence of two genotypes and the requirement of their complementation for viral replication. *Virology*, **28**, 56–70 (1966).
2. Gorer, P. A., and O'Gorman, P. The cytotoxic activity of isoantibody in mice. *Transplant. Bull.*, **3**, 142–143 (1956).
3. Gross, L. The Rauscher virus: A mixture of the Friend virus and of the mouse leukemia virus (Gross)? *Acta Haematol.*, **35**, 200–213 (1966).
4. Hellström, K. E. Cytotoxic effect of isoantibodies on mouse tumor cells *in vitro*. *Transplant. Bull.*, **6**, 411–416 (1959).
5. Ishimoto, A. Antigenic relationship between SL-leukemia cells and other murine leukemia cells. *GANN*, **60**, 335–366 (1969).
6. Ishimoto, A., and Maeda, M. Studies on the susceptibility of C57BL/6 mice of Rauscher virus. I. Properties of Rauscher virus-induced C57BL/6 lymphomas. *J. Natl. Cancer Inst.*, **44**, 361–368 (1970).
7. Klein, E., and Klein, G. Antigenic properties of lymphomas induced by the Moloney agent. *J. Natl. Cancer Inst.*, **32**, 547–568 (1964).
8. Maeda, M., and Notake, K. *In vitro* culture of murine leukemia cell induced by Rauscher virus. *Ann. Rept. Inst. Virus Res. Kyoto Univ.*, **11**, 76–77 (1968).
9. Möller, G. J. Demonstration of mouse isoantigens at the cellular level by the fluorescent antibody technique. *J. Exp. Med.*, **114**, 415–435 (1961).
10. Old, B., Boyse, E. A., and Stocker, E. Typing of mouse leukemias by serological methods. *Nature*, **201**, 777–779 (1964).

11. Pluznik, D. H., Sachs, K., and Resnitzky, P. The mechanism of leukemogenesis by the Rauscher leukemia virus. *Natl. Cancer Inst. Monograph*, **22**, 3–14 (1966).

EXPLANATION OF PHOTOS

PHOTO 1. FMR antigen detected on RD-12 cells by the indirect immunofluorescent antibody test.

PHOTO 2. Rauscher virus-infected spleen cells of C57BL/6 mice. Phase contrast.

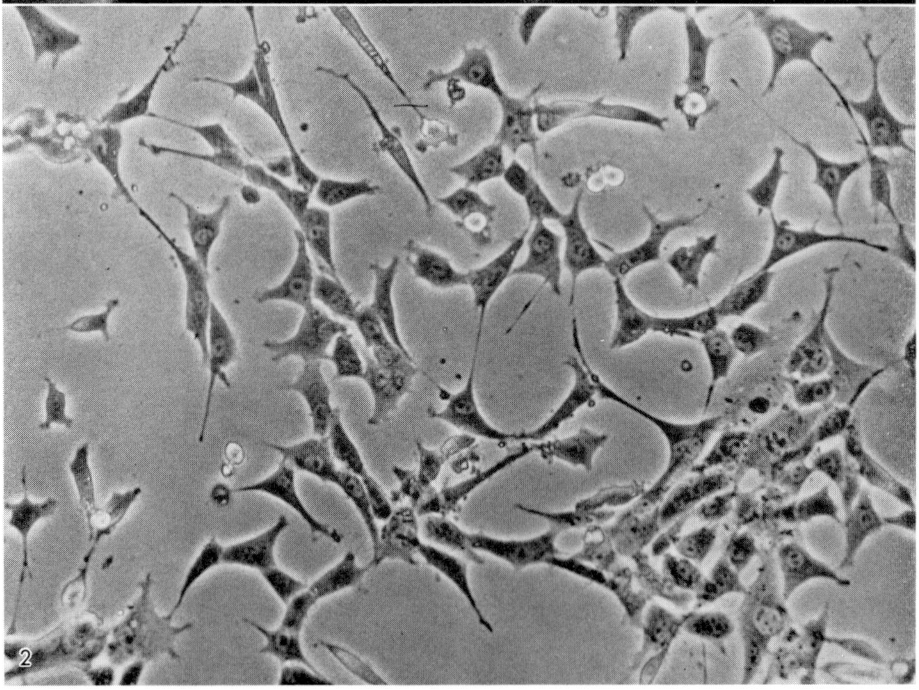

GANN Monograph on Cancer Research 12, 1972

CHARACTERISTICS OF FRIEND VIRUS-INDUCED TUMORS IN THE RAT COMPARED WITH THOSE IN THE MOUSE

Hiroshi KOBAYASHI, Noritoshi TAKEICHI,
Masuo HOSOKAWA, and Takao KODAMA
*Cancer Institute, Hokkaido University School of Medicine**

The authors compared Friend virus-induced leukemia in the rat with Friend virus-induced leukemia in the mouse and considered the nature of the differences in biological behavior. The following conclusions were reached: 1) When the Friend virus was injected into Wistar King Aptekman/Mk newborn rats, the target cell of the virus was the lymphocyte. The lymphocyte was transformed and lymphosarcomas developed in approximately 200 days after the virus injection. In the mouse the target cell was the erythroblast, and the biological differences in morphology, Friend virus production, electrophoretic mobilities, and chromosomal patterns between the Friend virus-induced tumors of the rat and those in the mouse may possibly be explained by the difference in the target cell. 2) Tumors of the rat induced by Friend virus do not grow well in isologous normal adult rats but they grow well in immunologically depressed rats or in rats made tolerant to the Friend virus. This may be because the Friend tumor cells in the rat possess a Friend virus-specific transplantation antigen on the surface of the tumor cell, which will be recognized as foreign to the host and will thus be rejected.

In previously reported studies, within 1 to 3 weeks after Friend virus was inoculated into mice, Friend leukemia developed and the mice died. Approximately 200 days after Friend virus was inoculated into rats within 24 hr after birth, Friend leukemia developed and the rats died (*1*, *3*, *27–29*). The leukemia in the rat, however, differed from that in the mouse both morphologically and biologically. In this report the authors will compare the leukemia of the rat with that of the mouse and will also analyze the nature of the differences between them.

Morphology of Friend Leukemia in the Mouse and Rat

It has been shown that dd/Om mice injected with Friend virus develop leukemia in 1 to 3 weeks. Wistar-King-Aptekman/Mk (WKA/Mk) adult rats, however, are not susceptible to Friend virus, and rats injected with Friend virus do not develop leukemia although lymphosarcoma will develop approximately 200

* Kita 14-jo, Nishi 7-chome, Sapporo 060 (小林　博, 武市紀年, 細川真澄男, 小玉孝郎).

TABLE I. Friend Virus-induced Tumors in Mice and Rats

Cases		Strain	Age when tumor developed (days)	Organs involved	Histological pattern
Friend virus-induced tumors in mice (MFT):					
Approx. 8,000 cases (incl. transplantable OFT–1)		dd/Om	7–21	S	Erythroleukemia, reticulum cell sarcoma
Friend virus-induced tumors in rats (RFT):					
FNR–1		WKA/Mk	194	T, L	Lymphosarcoma
FNR–2		Gifu	197	S, L	Reticulosarcoma
FNR–3		WKA/Mk	194	S	Reticulosarcoma
FNR–4		Gifu	190	S, T, L	Lymphosarcoma
FNR–5		W/Mk	163	T, L	Lymphosarcoma
FNR–6		W/Mk	194	S, T, L	Lymphosarcoma
FNR–7		WKA/Mk	229	S	Reticulosarcoma
FNR–8		WKA/Mk	270	S	Reticulosarcoma
FNR–9		WKA/Mk	242	S, L	Reticulosarcoma
FNR–10		W/Mk	233	S, T, L	Lymphosarcoma
FNR–11		W/Mk	200	S, T, L	Lymphosarcoma
FNR–12[a]		WKA/Mk	207	S, T, L	Lymphosarcoma
FNR–13		W/Mk	260	S, T, L	Lymphosarcoma
FNR–14	(WFT–1)[b]	WKA/Mk	244	S	Lymphosarcoma
FNR–15	—	WKA/Mk	257	S	Reticulosarcoma
FNR–16	(WFT–2)	WKA/Mk	269	S, T	Lymphosarcoma[c]
FNR–17	(WFT–3)	WKA/Mk	228[d]	S, T	Lymphosarcoma
FNR–18	(WFT–4)	WKA/Mk	240	S, T	Lymphosarcoma
FNR–19	(WFT–5)	WKA/Mk	177	S	Reticulosarcoma
FNR–20	(WFT–6)	WKA/Mk	190	S	Lymphosarcoma
FNR–21	(WFT–7)	WKA/Mk	220	S	Reticulosarcoma
FNR–22	(WFT–8)	WKA/Mk	165	S	Lymphosarcoma
FNR–23	(WFT–9)	WKA/Mk	199	S	Lymphosarcoma
FNR–24	(WFT–10)	WKA/Mk	165	S	Reticulosarcoma
FNR–25	(WFT–11)	WKA/Mk	183	S	(Not examined)
FNR–26	(WFT–12)	W/Mk	204	S, L	Lymphosarcoma
FNR–27	(WFT–13)	WKA/Mk	172	S, T, L	Lymphosarcoma(?)

S: spleen, T: thymus, L: lymph nodes.

[a] After FNR–12 primary tumors of all lines were transplanted into Friend-tolerant rats.

[b] Transplantable lines referring to WFT (WFT1–13) established. WFT means Friend tumors developed in Wistar KA/Mk rats.

[c] Corrected to lymphosarcoma from reticulosarcoma, the description given in *Cancer Res.*, **29**, 1385 (1969).

[d] Corrected to 228 from 288 days, the description given in the above reference.

days after Friend virus injection if the rats are inoculated within 24 hr after birth (*4*, *15*, *17*).

The only gross evidence of Friend leukemia in the mouse is enlargement of the spleen, and no other organs are involved (Photo 1). However, when rats are

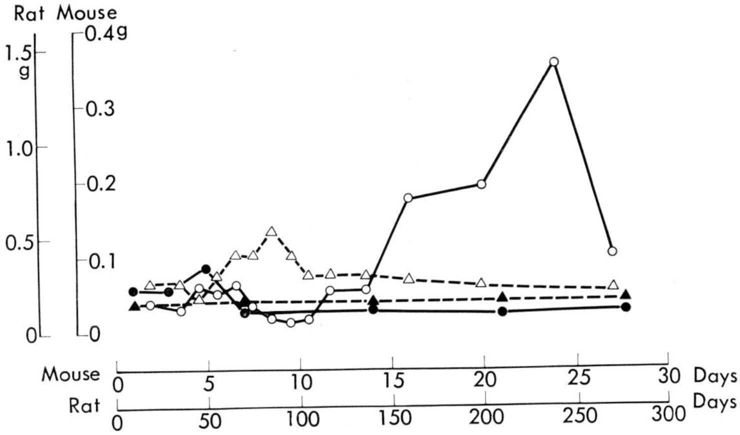

FIG. 1. Thymus weight of animals injected with Friend virus
○ WKA/Mk rats injected with Friend virus at birth ;
● dd/Om mice injected with Friend virus ;
△ normal WKA rats ; ▲ normal dd/Om mice.

inoculated with Friend virus at birth, enlargement of the thymus and lymph nodes may be observed in addition to enlargement of the spleen (Photo 2, Table I). Thus, out of 27 rats with Friend leukemia, 12 showed enlargement of the spleen only (S-type), 7 showed enlargement of the spleen, thymus, and lymph nodes (STL-type), 3 showed enlargement of the spleen and lymph nodes (SL-type), and 3 showed enlargement of the spleen and thymus (ST-type). Only 2 cases (FNR-1 and FNR-5 in Table I) showed enlargement of thymus and lymph nodes without involving spleen enlargement.

When thymus weights were taken daily after injection of Friend virus into mice, no variation was noted except for a slight increase in the thymus weight at about the fifth day (Fig. 1). By contrast, the thymus weight in rats injected with Friend virus at birth was slightly reduced between the 80th and 100th days. Thereafter the thymus in the Friend virus-injected rat increased gradually until it averaged around 1.4 g on the 150th day. Each point in Fig. 1 indicates the average weight of the thymus of 3 to 39 rats.

The spleen weight of mice injected with Friend virus increased gradually beginning around the tenth day after injection (Fig. 2). However, in rats injected with Friend virus at birth the spleen weight increased from the 80th to 100th day, then decreased around the 120th day. A second rapid increase occurred around the 150th day, so that the spleen weight in the rats showed 2 peaks. The significance of these 2 peaks in the spleen weight of the rat is not clear.

Our observations showed clearly that the same pattern of variation in organ weights was not found in mice with Friend leukemia. This may be because of the short survival period of mice injected with Friend virus, and also because some changes were not expressed in the mouse.

Microscopically, Friend leukemia in the mouse is considered to be erythroleukemia (*6*) or reticulum cell sarcoma (*30*), and that in the rat lymphosarcoma or,

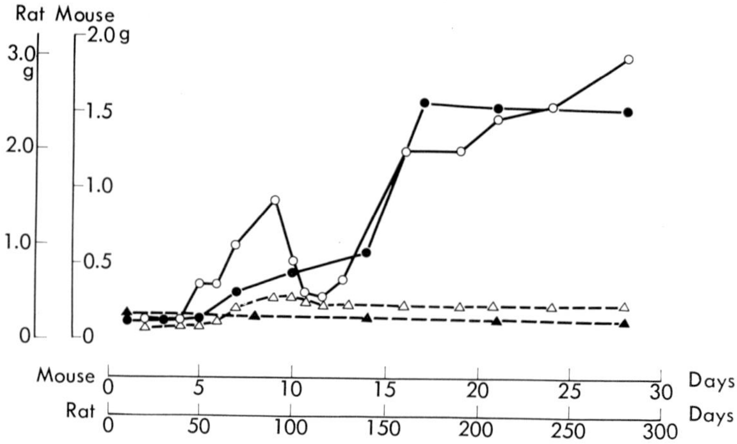

FIG. 2. Spleen weight of animals injected with Friend virus
○ WKA rats injected with Friend virus at birth ;
● dd/Om mice injected with Friend virus ;
△ normal rats ; ▲ normal mice.

rarely, reticulosarcoma (Photos 2 to 10). This indicates the difference in the target cells of the Friend virus in the mouse and rat. In rat leukemia there seems to be a significant relation between the histological pattern of Friend leukemia and the range of the involvement of organs. For example, Friend leukemia with spleen enlargement is often reticulum cell sarcoma, and Friend leukemia involving the thymus and lymph nodes in addition to spleen enlargement is lymphosarcoma (Table I). In WFT-1, for example, the starry sky picture was rarely observed (Photo 4). Most of the cases were characterized by enlargement of the spleen only, while in other cases, for example FNR-27 (WFT-13), there was generalized involvement of the liver, spleen, and lymph nodes. A chronic dilatation of the bronchi or bronchioles, probably resulting from the proliferation of leukemic cells, was also observed occasionally (Photo 8).

Attempts to Establish Transplantable Friend Virus-induced Tumors (Friend Tumors)

Repeated attempts have been made to obtain Friend virus-induced transplantable tumors in mice (Table II), but in only 1 of 332 mice have we succeeded in establishing a transplantable Friend tumor line from transfer of the enlarged splenic tissue. Many other attempts have failed, and the results in this one case have not been reproduced in our laboratory. One cause of this difficulty in obtaining transplantable Friend tumors in mice may be that the host injected with Friend virus dies of viremia before a transplantable tumor becomes established. Mice previously immunized with inactivated Friend virus have been used in order to prevent the occurrence of viremia that causes the early death of the host. Although we have tried 23 tumor lines using 86 mice, we have repeatedly failed so far. Splenectomized mice have also been used but all 8 lines failed and no transplantable mouse tumors have been obtained in these attempts.

TABLE II. Attempts at Establishing Transplantable Friend Tumors: Results of First Generation Transplantation from Primary Tumors into Isologous Host

Host	No. of lines established/ No. of lines tested	No. of hosts with lethal growth of tumors/ No. of hosts
Mice:		
Normal mice	1/89 (1.1%)	1/332 (0.3%)
Friend virus-immune dd/Om mice	0/23	0/86
Splenectomized dd/Om mice	0/8	0/23
Rats:		
Normal WKA/Mk rats	0/21	0/111
Friend virus-conditioned WKA/Mk rats	13/16 (81.3)	35/62 (56.5)

Attempts have also been made in rats. Using 111 isologous rats from 21 lines, we tried to obtain transplantable tumors from the spleen, thymus, and lymph nodes of the primary host suffering from Friend leukemia, but all efforts have failed. In 1 line only (FNR-4) we observed temporary growth of a tumor up to 0.5 cm, but this later regressed.

After FNR-12 appeared, all the primary tumors were transplanted into Friend virus-conditioned rats which had been injected with Friend virus at birth so that they may be tolerant to Friend-specific antigens. Using such Friend-tolerant rats, we succeeded in establishing transplantable Friend tumors in 13 of the 16 lines (81.3%). We did not succeed at all if they were transplanted into isologous normal adult rats.

We have concluded that the reason transplantable Friend virus-induced tumors in rats were easily obtained in Friend-tolerant rats but could not be obtained in the normal host may be some immunological mechanism, which will be described later. The reason transplantable Friend virus-induced tumors are difficult to establish in the mouse may be that the host dies of Friend leukemia before the development of a transplantable tumor. Another reason may be that the target cell of Friend leukemia in the mouse is the erythroblast, which might be difficult to establish as a transplant line, while the target cell of Friend leukemia in the rat is the lymphoblast, which may be easier to establish. Therefore, it is thought that the difference in target cells may play an important role in determining the successful production of transplantable Friend virus-induced tumors in the mouse and the rat.

Friend Virus Production

While a large amount of Friend virus is usually harvested from the splenic tissue ($<10^{6}$ ID_{50}/ml) or blood plasma ($<10^{4.0}$ ID_{50}/ml) of mice 1 to 2 weeks after injection of Friend virus, a poor harvest of Friend virus is observed in 1 to 2-month-old rats injected with Friend virus at birth: the average harvest of Friend virus was less than $10^{3.0}$ ID_{50}/ml from rat spleen and less than $10^{1.5}$ ID_{50}/ml from

TABLE III. Friend Virus Production from Primary Tumors Induced by Friend Virus

Experimental animal	Friend virus			
	Recovery (ID_{50}/ml)		FA antigen in spleen cells	Particles
	Spleen	Plasma		
dd/Om mice:	$<10^{6.0}$	$<10^{4.0}$	+++	+++
spleen-enlarged type (S)	$<10^{3.0}$	$<10^{1.5}$	+	+
WKA/Mk rats:				
spleen-, thymus-, and lymph node-enlarged type (STL)	$<10^{0.5}$	$<10^{0.5}$	–	–

blood plasma. A still poorer harvest of less than $10^{0.5}$ ID_{50}/ml of Friend virus was observed in the spleen of the rats when the thymus, lymph nodes, and spleen were also involved in the leukemia (Table III). Corresponding variations in results were obtained in immunofluorescence studies and electron-microscopic studies on the same groups of rats (Photos 11 and 12).

At present an A-type virus particle seen in the cytoplasm with the electron microscope is considered to be an immature form of the B- or C-type tumor virus in the mouse. We have reported that an accumulation of A-particles is observed frequently in transplanted Friend virus-induced tumor cells in mice, particularly when the tumor was transplanted into Friend virus-immune mice, or when the tumor was artificially exposed to Friend virus (*12*, *23*, *24*). However, A-particles have never been seen in transplanted Friend virus-induced tumors in rats. This might indicate that the rat is comparatively free of latent infection by the virus, compared with the mouse.

Electrophoretic Mobilities of Friend Tumor Cells

Determination of the electrophoretic mobilities of Friend virus-induced tumors in mice and rats was performed by Dr. K. Kojima, Aichi Cancer Center, Nagoya, in cooperation with us (Table IV) (*26*). While the electrophoretic mobilities of live mouse Friend tumor cells of SFAT mice indicated an increase in

TABLE IV. Electrophoretic Mobilities of Friend Virus-induced Tumors (Kojima *et al.*)

	Mobilities of cells, mean±S.D. (N/sec/V/cm)	
	Viable	Fixed
Friend virus-induced tumors in dd/Om mice:		
SFAT†	−1.257±0.043	−1.244±0.066
Friend virus-induced tumors in WKA/Mk rats:		
WFT-3	−0.897±0.053	−1.047±0.048
WFT-2A	−0.937±0.088	−1.123±0.074
WFT-2N	−0.960±0.069	−1.279±0.064
Normal lymphocytes in rats	−0.911±0.046	−0.904±0.076

† Kindly supplied by Dr. Y. Ikawa, Cancer Institute, Tokyo.

the negative charge, as the cells of transplantable tumors usually do, live rat Friend tumor cells of WFT-3, WFT-2A, and WFT-2N had nearly normal electrophoretic mobilities (−0.897 to −0.960) similar to normal rat lymphocytes (−0.911). The normal value of electrophoretic mobilities seen in rat Friend tumor cells may be a rather exceptional finding among several hundred lines of transplantable rat ascites tumor cells, in which a marked increase of the negative charge was usually observed. On the other hand, after fixing with 4% formalin, electrophoretic mobilities of the above lines of rat Friend tumors indicated an increase of the value of the negative charge. Though the value in the SFAT mouse Friend tumor and normal rat lymphocytes is still the same as that in live cells even after fixing the cells, the value of the rat Friend tumor cells from WFT-3, WFT-2A, and WFT-2N lines indicated an increase of the negative charge. This suggests that the positive electric charge which is inactivated by formalin solution may be markedly higher on the cell surface of rat Friend tumors than in other tumor cells tested or in normal rat lymphocytes. The details of the associated results will be published soon by Kojima *et al.*

Chromosomal Studies

Analysis of chromosomes of Friend virus-induced tumors was performed cooperatively by Dr. T. Sofuni, Atomic Bomb Casualty Commission, Hiroshima, and by Dr. M. Sasaki, Institute for Chromosome Research, Hokkaido University, Sapporo (*33*, *38*, *39*). Though their observations have not yet been completed, results obtained thus far show that chromosomal abnormalities are present more often in mouse Friend tumors (OFT-1, VPFT, and NVFT) (*13*) (Photo 13) than in rat Friend tumors (WFT-3, WFT-4, WFT-2A, and WFT-2N) (Photo 14). In other words, while the chromosome pattern of mouse Friend tumors, like the chromosome pattern in other tumors, differs markedly from that of normal cells, the pattern of rat Friend tumors is quite normal or shows minor abnormalities in only 3 of the 7 lines of rat Friend tumors so far examined. These findings on the electrophoretic mobilities and the chromosome pattern in rat Friend tumors, which are inconsistent with observations on most other tumors, cannot be explained adequately by a difference in the Friend tumors in the rat species, and it must be remembered that the Friend tumor cell originated from lymphocytes in the rat. It is known that the neoplastic lymphocytes in chronic lymphatic leukemia are often demonstrated to have a normal pattern of electric mobilities (live cells) or of chromosomes.

Transplantation of Friend Virus-induced Tumors into Normal Hosts

Both OFT-1 and OFT-2, transplantable tumors induced by Friend virus in dd/Om mice, proliferate well in both the ascites and solid form. They invariably kill the host if more than 10^6 cells are inoculated (Table V). Survival time and the growth curve do not vary with individual cases.

When the OFT-1 tumor was transplanted into dd/Om mice previously immunized by three inoculations with inactivated Friend virus, the growth of the

TABLE V. Transplantation of Friend Virus-induced Tumors into Normal Isologous Host

Tumor	No. of hosts with lethal growth of tumors/No. of hosts
Friend virus-induced tumors in dd/Om mice:	
OFT–1	85/85 (100%)
OFT–2	178/178 (100)
OFT–1[a] into immune mice	65/118 (55.1)
OFT–1[b] into immune mice	11/20 (55.0)
Friend virus-induced tumors in WKA/Mk rats:	
WFT–1	3/38 (7.9)
WFT–2A[c]	0/53
WFT–3	0/26
WFT–4	0/9
WFT–5	—
WFT–6	0/4
WFT–7	0/3
WFT–8	0/5
WFT–9	0/4
WFT–10	—
WFT–11	—
WFT–12	—
WFT–13	—
Total in WKA/Mk rats	3/142 (2.1)

[a] Transplanted into Friend virus-immune mice (immunized with 0.2% formalin-killed crude Friend virus).

[b] Transplanted into Friend tumor (OFT–1)-immune mice (immunized with 0.2% formalin-killed Friend tumor, OFT–1).

[c] Spontaneously regressed.

tumor was inhibited, since only about half of the mice (65 out of the 118) died of the tumor growth, while the remaining mice survived for more than 2 months. Results obtained in mice immunized with killed OFT-1 tumor cells were similar to those obtained in the mice immunized with killed Friend virus, and approximately half of the mice survived.

By contrast, when 13 different lines of Friend virus-induced tumors in rats were transplanted into isologous normal adult rats, tumors usually did not grow at all, and, if they did grow initially, they regressed later (WFT-2A). Three out of the 38 rats transplanted with WFT-1 died of tumor growth, but the cause of death could not be determined and there is some question whether it was really caused by the tumor. No later deaths of rats bearing the tumor have been observed in any lines of rats transplanted with rat Friend tumors. Only 2.1%, or 3 out of the 142 normal adult rats, died from the growth of rat Friend tumors. Subsequently, transplantation of tumors in order to maintain the rat Friend tumors has not been carried out with normal adult rats, since we have used only Friend-tolerant rats. These results will be described below. We can conclude that, although Friend virus-induced tumors in rats are histologically malignant, they will not grow at all or will regress spontaneously in isologous normal adult rats that have not been immunized with Friend virus. This is different from the results reported by other authors, and this curious "all-or-none" transplantation result appears to be unique, since it has not been observed in the transplantation of other tumors.

Transplantation of Friend Virus-induced Tumors from Rats into Immunologically Depressed or Friend Virus-tolerant Rats

Rat Friend tumors do not grow well in normal adult rats, but they grow well in immunologically depressed rats or in rats made tolerant to the Friend virus by injection of the virus at birth (Table VI). For example, of 9 WFT-1-line rats exposed to ^{60}Co 300 rad irradiation, none died, but all 4 WFT-1-line rats exposed to ^{60}Co 500 rad irradiation died. All 8 rats transplanted with WFT-2A and all 5 rats transplanted with WFT-3 when less than 24-hr-old died of tumor growth. When Friend virus-induced tumors from rats were transplanted into Friend-tolerant adult rats injected with live Friend virus at birth, the rat Friend tumors

TABLE VI. Growth of Friend Virus-induced Tumors in Immunologically Depressed and Friend-tolerant WKA/Mk Rats

Host (WKA rats)	Lethal growth of RFT (WFT-3)[a]	
^{60}Co 300R (WFT-1)	0/9	
^{60}Co 500R (WFT-1)	4/4	(100.0%)
Newborn		
1 day (WFT-1)	1/8	(12.5)
1 day (WFT-2A)	8/8	(100.0)
4 days (WFT-3)	5/5	(100.0)
Friend-tolerant[b]		
WFT-1	130/133[c]	(97.7)
WFT-2A	133/138	(96.3)
WFT-3	84/84	(100.0)
WFT-4	25/25	(100.0)
WFT-5	9/12	(75.0)
WFT-6	9/9	(100.0)
WFT-7	4/10	(40.0)
WFT-8	7/7	(100.0)
WFT-9	13/13	(100.0)
WFT-10	2/2	(100.0)
WFT-11	2/2	(100.0)
WFT-12	2/3	(66.7)
WFT-13	5/5	(100.0)
Total Friend tolerant	425/443	(95.9)

[a] Number of hosts with lethal growth of tumors/number of hosts.
[b] Injected with Friend virus at birth.
[c] Including the results in the rats at the first generation transplanted with primary tumors.

grow well and killed nearly all the hosts; for example, 130 out of 133 rats transplanted with WFT-1 died with generalized metastases 2 to 3 weeks after transplantation. The percentage of deaths in all lines of WFT-line tumors transplanted into Friend-tolerant rats was 95.9% (425 out of 443 rats). Twelve out of 13 lines of rat Friend tumors proliferate not only in solid form but also in ascites form and produce generalized metastases. Friend virus-tolerant rats 1–2 months old were used for maintaining the WFT tumors.

As previously reported, rat Friend tumors grow only in Friend-tolerant or immunologically depressed rats and do not grow in isologous normal adult rats. This may be because the Friend virus-specific transplantation antigen is located on the cell surface of Friend tumors and because this antigen located on the cell surface of Friend tumors is recognized as foreign by the normal host, whereas the same tumor antigen may not be recognized as foreign if the host is tolerant to the Friend antigen or if it is immunologically depressed. Other results in support of this concept are supplied by immunofluorescence and cytotoxic studies (*32*, *36*).

In any event, it can be said that, in order for leukemogenesis to be induced by Friend virus in the rat, a cellular neoplastic alteration must be brought about by the Friend virus infection and the host must be capable of accepting the new foreign antigen. In other words, the development of cancer cells alone does not assure that a neoplasm will develop, because Friend virus-induced tumors can grow only when the host is Friend-tolerant or immunologically depressed. The tumors, even if induced, will not grow in normal adult rats. Results such as these will occur only when the tumors are highly antigenic, as rat Friend tumors are in the rat.

DISCUSSION

Table VII presents a summary of all the experiments described above. Friend virus is highly infectious in most strains of mice, but it is not infectious in adult rats. However, when Friend virus is injected into newborn rats, Friend leukemia occurs approximately 200 days later. More variable forms of leukemia are observed after Friend virus inoculation in the rat than occur in the mouse. The target cell of the Friend virus in the rat is the lymphocyte, while in the mouse the erythroblast is the cell affected. This difference in target cells may partly explain the differences in the biological behavior of Friend virus-induced tumors in the two species.

A number of differences in biological characteristics have been noted in Friend virus-induced tumors in the mouse and rat. One concerns the ease with which transplantable Friend tumor lines can be established. This is very difficult in the mouse but is easy in the rat if Friend-tolerant rats are used. Other differences are that A-type virus particles are often observed in mouse Friend tumors but are not observed in rat Friend tumors. Electrophoretic mobilities have a normal pattern in rat Friend tumors and the chromosomes are also nearly normal in rat Friend tumors. Because the electrophoretic mobilities and the chromosome pattern of rat Friend tumor cells are normal, while growth of the Friend tumors does not occur in normal adult rats, the authors have proposed the phrase " noncancerous cancers " to designate rat Friend tumors.

TABLE VII. Summary of Friend Virus-induced Tumors in Mice and Rats

	Mice (dd/Om)	Rats (WKA/Mk)
Primary tumors:		
Period before development of the tumor	1–3 weeks	20–30 weeks[a]
Organs involved	spleen	spleen, thymus, lymph nodes
Histological pattern	erythroleukemia, reticulosarcoma	lymphosarcoma, reticulosarcoma
Transplantable tumors:		
Establishment of transplantable tumor	difficult	easy[b]
Friend virus production	++	+
A-type virus particles	+++	−
Increasing of electric mobilities	+++	−
Changes of chromosomes	++	− to +
Lethal growth in normal host	+++	−
Lethal growth in Friend-immune host	++	−[c]
Lethal growth in Friend-tolerant host	+++[c]	+++

[a] When Friend virus was injected into newborn rats.
[b] In Friend-tolerant host injected with Friend virus at birth.
[c] Probable data.

Next, the curious transplantation results of Friend virus-induced tumors in the rat, *i.e.*, their failure to grow or their early regression in the normal adult rat, may be due to the presence of the cellular antigen related to Friend virus, which on inoculation is initially not highly infectious to the entire adult rat but is persistently infectious to the cells of the tumor and thus caused a virus-specific antigen to develop on the membrane surface of the cell. It would seem that the difference between the species of the natural host of Friend virus and the species of the host to be injected with the virus plays the most important role in bringing about the curious transplantation results observed in Friend virus-induced tumors in the rat.

The spontaneous regression of the experimental tumors in the experiment on Friend virus-induced tumor suggested a subsequent experiment, in which regression of rat tumors, which had occurred spontaneously or had been induced by chemical carcinogens, was produced by an artificial infection of the tumors with Friend virus (*16*, *21*, *35*). In this experiment, the authors succeeded in producing regression of the rat tumors by infection with Friend virus (artificial xenogenization) (Fig. 3). If the same reasoning is followed, then the Friend virus-induced tumors in the rat are an example of " natural xenogenization " of tumor cells as compared with the " artificial xenogenization," because rat Friend tumors will not grow in normal adult rats, and no artificial procedures are needed to induce regression of the tumors.

On the other hand, the target cell of the Friend virus is a lymphocyte may lead to the development of the runting syndrome and subsequent death approximately 30 days after birth in rats when rather a small amount of Friend virus (approx. $10^{1.0}$ ID_{50}/ml) was injected (*40*, *41*). The mechanism of the runting syndrome may have resulted from the immunological incompatibility between lymphocytes

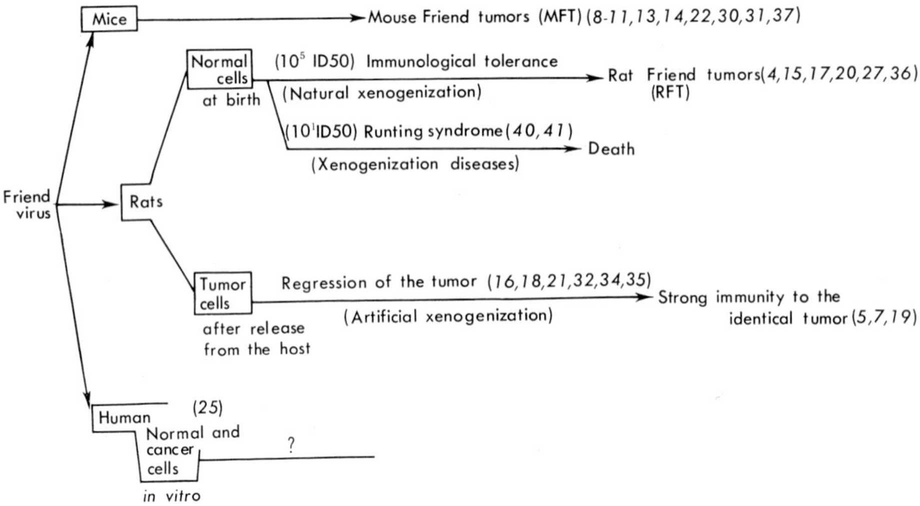

FIG. 3. Subsequent experiments after the mouse and rat Friend tumors

that had acquired the Friend virus-specific transplantation antigen and the uninfected cells. This is distinct from the case where the rat injected with a large amount of Friend virus acquires a Friend-tolerant state, in which the tumor grows normally. The runting syndrome and subsequent death produced by the Friend virus are designated as xenogenization disease. Details of these experiments will be published later.

REFERENCES

1. Dawson, P. J., Rose, W. M., and Fieldsteel, A. H. Lymphatic leukemia in rats and mice inoculated with Friend virus. *Brit. J. Cancer*, **20**, 114 (1966).
2. Dawson, P. J., and Fieldsteel, A. H. Pathogenesis of chronic Friend disease in hybrid BDF_1 mice. *Cancer Res.*, **29**, 1206 (1969).
3. Hosokawa, M., Kobayashi, H., Tanigaki, N., Kodama, T., and Kamibayashi, K. Neoplastic changes in rats induced by Friend virus. *Nippon Byōri Gakkai Kaishi* (*Trans. Soc. Pathol. Japon.*), **56**, 123 (1967).
4. Hosokawa, M., Takeichi, N., Sendo, F., Kodama, T., Shirai, T., Saito, H., and Kobayashi, H. Friend virus-induced transplantable tumors in rats (in Japanese). *Igaku no Ayumi*, **69**, 310 (1969).
5. Hosokawa, M., Sendo, F., Gotohda, E., and Kobayashi, H. Combination of immunotherapy and chemotherapy to experimental tumors in rats. *GANN*, **62**, 57 (1971).
6. Ikawa, Y., and Sugano, H. Spleen focus of Friend's disease. *GANN*, **58**, 61 (1967).
7. Kaji, H., Sendo, F., Shirai, T., Saito, H., Kodama, T., and Kobayashi, H. Immunological treatment of tumors by Friend virus-infected tumor cells in rats (in Japanese). *Saishin Igaku*, **24**, 1329 (1969).
8. Kobayashi, H., Kikuchi, K., Kodama, T., and Takeda, K. Inhibition of the growth of the Friend tumor cells in mice immunized with inactivated Friend virus. *J. Cancer Immunopathol.*, **1**, 55 (1965).

9. Kobayashi, H., Kodama, T., and Itoh, T. Significance of the co-existence of Friend virus in " Friend tumor." *Nature*, **212**, 939 (1966).
10. Kobayashi, H. Immunopathological studies on the Friend virus-induced ascitic tumor. *Acta Pathol. Japon.*, **16**, 79 (1966).
11. Kobayashi, H., Kodama, T., and Takeda, K. Electron microscopy of Friend tumor cell with special reference to the influence of Friend virus immunity on Friend tumor cell. *Nature*, **212**, 1260 (1966).
12. Kobayashi, H., Kodama, T., and Sendo, F. Electron microscopy of Friend virus-exposed Friend tumor cells; with special reference to the appearance of intracytoplasmic "A" particles. *GANN*, **58**, 395 (1967).
13. Kobayashi, H., Takeda, K., Kodama, T., and Itoh, T. Attempts to obtain a Friend virus-induced ascites tumor free of the virus. *Z. Krebsforsch.*, **69**, 10 (1967).
14. Kobayashi, H., and Takeda, K. Inhibition of the growth of Friend tumor cell in mice immunized with live Friend virus. *GANN*, **58**, 25 (1967).
15. Kobayashi, H., Hosokawa, M., and Takeichi, N. The role of virus in the growth of viral leukemia. *Acta Pathol. Japon.*, **18**, 372 (1968).
16. Kobayashi, H., Sendo, F., Shirai, T., Kaji, H., Kodama, T., and Saito, H. Modification in growth of transplantable rat tumors exposed to Friend virus. *J. Natl. Cancer Inst.*, **42**, 413 (1969).
17. Kobayashi, H., Hosokawa, M., Takeichi, N., Sendo, F., and Kodama, T. Transplantable Friend virus-induced tumors in rats. *Cancer Res.*, **29**, 1385 (1969).
18. Kobayashi, H., Kodama, T., Shirai, T., Kaji, H., Hosokawa, M., Sendo, F., Saito, H., and Takeichi, N. Artificial regression of rat tumors infected with Friend virus (xenogenization)—An effect produced by acquired antigen. *Hokkaido Med. J.*, **44**, 133 (1969).
19. Kobayashi, H., Sendo, F., Kaji, H., Shirai, T., Saito, H., Takeichi, N., Hosokawa, M., and Kodama, T. Inhibition of transplanted rat tumors by immunization with identical tumor cells infected with Friend virus. *J. Natl. Cancer Inst.*, **44**, 11 (1970).
20. Kobayashi, H., Shirai, T., Takeichi, T., Hosokawa, M., Saito, H., Sendo, F., and Kodama, T. Antigenic variant (WFT-2N) of a transplantable rat tumor induced by Friend virus. *Eur. Clin. Biol. Res.*, **15**, 426 (1970).
21. Kobayashi, H. Growth of rat tumor cells infected with Friend virus: An approach to the immunological treatment of cancer. *Immunity and tolerance in oncogenesis* (*IV Perugia Quadrennial International Conference on Cancer 1969*), **637**, (1970).
22. Kodama, T., and Kobayashi, H. Electron microscopic observations on transplantable Friend ascites tumor cells, with reference to the Friend virus. *GANN*, **57**, 527 (1966).
23. Kodama, T., Sendo, F., and Kobayashi, H. Electron microscopy of Friend tumor cell with special reference to the influence of Friend virus immunity on Friend tumor cell. *J. Cancer Immunopathol.*, **3**, 47 (1967).
24. Kodama, T., Sendo, F., and Kobayashi, H. Electron microscopy on Friend virus-exposed Friend tumor cells. *J. Cancer Immunopathol.*, **3**, 65 (1967).
25. Kodama, T., Kobayashi, H., Saito, H., Shirai, T., and Matsumiya, H. Electron microscopic studies on the cultured human cancer cells infected with Friend virus. *GANN*, **61**, 219 (1970).
26. Kojima, K., Takeichi, N., Kobayashi, H., and Maekawa, A. Electrokinetic charge

of transplantable Friend virus-induced tumors in rats. *Nagoya Med. J.*, **16**, 7 (1970).
27. Maruyama, K., and Oboshi, S. Carcinogenesis by Friend virus in rats (in Japanese). *Nippon Rinsho (Japan. J. Clin. Med.)*, **24**, 46 (1966).
28. Metcalf, D., Furth, J., and Buffett, R. F. Pathogenesis of mouse leukemia caused by Friend virus. *Cancer Res.*, **19**, 52 (1959).
29. Mirand, E. A., and Grace, J. T. Induction of leukemia in rats with Friend virus. *Virology*, **17**, 364 (1962).
30. Oboshi, S., Aoki, K., Sato, R., and Baba, T. Friend virus ascites sarcoma. *GANN*, **55**, 73 (1964).
31. Odaka, T., and Ikawa, T. Friend virus-induced transplantable tumors of C57-BL/6 origin containing usually minute amounts of infections virus. *Int. J. Cancer*, **3**, 211 (1968).
32. Saito, H. Immunofluorescence studies on the transplantable rat tumor cells infected with Friend virus. *GANN*, **61**, 253 (1971).
33. Sasaki, M., Mori, M., Kobayashi, H., and Takeichi, N. Cytologic studies of tumors. LII. Persistence of deploid stemlines in Friend virus-induced ascites tumors of rats. *Proc. Japan Acad.*, **46**, 792 (1970).
34. Sendo, F., Kaji, H., Shirai, T., Kodama, T., and Kobayashi, H. Modification in growth of transplantable rat tumors exposed to Friend virus (in Japanese). *Saishin Igaku*, **24**, 1118 (1969).
35. Sendo, F., Kaji, H., Saito, H., and Kobayashi, H. Antigenic modification of rat tumor cells artificially infected with Friend virus in the primary autochthonous host. *GANN*, **61**, 223 (1970).
36. Shirai, T., Kaji, H., Takeichi, N., Sendo, F., Saito, H., and Kobayashi, H. Cell surface antigens detectable by cytotoxic test on Friend virus-induced and Friend virus-infected tumors in the rat. *J. Natl. Cancer Inst.*, **46**, 449 (1971).
37. Siegler, R., and Rich, M. A. Pathogenesis of murine leukemia. *Natl. Cancer Inst. Monograph*, **22**, 525 (1966).
38. Sofuni, T., Yamada, K., Kobayashi, H., and Makino, S. A chromosome study of Friend virus-induced mouse ascites tumors. *Proc. Japan Acad.*, **43**, 161 (1967).
39. Sofuni, T., Makino, S., and Kobayashi, H. A study of chromosomes in Friend virus-induced mouse leukemias (in Japanese). *Proc. Japan Acad.*, **43**, 389 (1967).
40. Takeichi, N., Kuzumaki, N., Sendo, F., Hosokawa, M., and Kobayashi, H. Runting syndrome in rats infected with Friend virus. *Cancer Res.*, in press.
41. Takeichi, N., Kuzumaki, N., Kodama, T., Sendo, F., and Kobayashi, H. Immunological studies of runting syndrome infected with Friend virus. Submitted to *GANN*.

EXPLANATION OF PHOTOS

PHOTO 1. Macroscopic features of a mouse suffering from Friend leukemia. Note the enlargement of spleen.

PHOTO 2. Macroscopic features of a rat suffering from Friend leukemia. Note the enlargement of spleen, thymus, and lymph nodes (cervical and mesenteric).

PHOTO 3. Photomicrograph of the spleen in a Friend leukemic mouse. Note the diffuse proliferation of leukemia cells of probably erythroblastic origin. ×300

PHOTO 4. Photomicrograph of the thymus in a Friend leukemic rat (FNR 14=WFT-1). Note the starry sky picture. ×320

PHOTO 5. Spleen of a primary rat of the FNR 27 (WFT-13) tumor line. ×320

PHOTO 6. Thymus of a primary rat of the FNR 27 (WFT-13) tumor line. ×320

PHOTO 7. Lymph node of a primary rat of the FNR 27 (WFT-13) tumor line. ×320

PHOTO 8. A chronic dilatation of the bronchus or bronchioles due to the proliferation of Friend leukemia cells in the FNR 27 (WFT-13) tumor line. ×20

PHOTO 9. Electron micrograph of an OFT-1 line tumor with lobulated nuclei and large cytoplasm. Virus particles are observed intercellularly. ×3,500

PHOTO 10. Electron micrograph of a WFT-1 line tumor with poorly developed mitochondria and endoplasmic reticulum. ×3,500

PHOTO 11. Budding of a virus particle from the surface of a WFT-1 cell. ×80,000

PHOTO 12. Type C particles observed in the WFT-2A line. ×80,000

PHOTO 13. Karyotypes of cells from OFT-1 and NVP lines of mouse Friend tumors. A: OFT-1, 40 chromosomes including 4 marker chromosomes (M1, M2, M3, and M4). B: NVP, 40 chromosomes including 4 marker chromosomes (M1, M2, M3, and M4). C: OFT-1, 39 chromosomes including 5 marker chromosomes (3 M1, M2, and M4). D: NVP, 41 chromosomes including 6 marker chromosomes (M1, 2 M2, M3, M4, and M?).

PHOTO 14. Representative stemline karyotypes. A: WFT-3, showing a normal male karyotype. B: WFT-4. C: WFT-2A. D: WFT-2N. E: WFT-2N. Arrows indicate missing or additional elements, and markers.

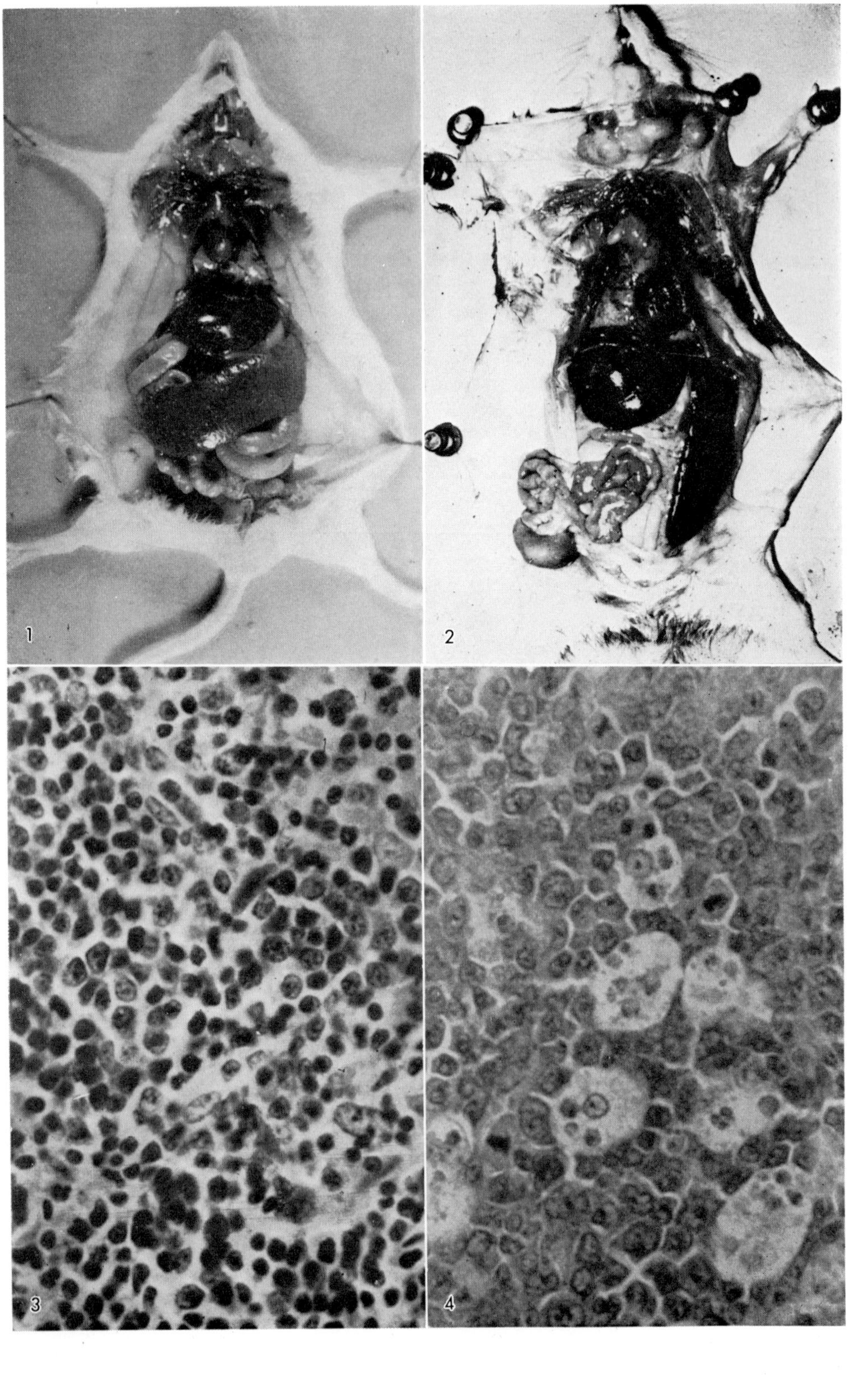

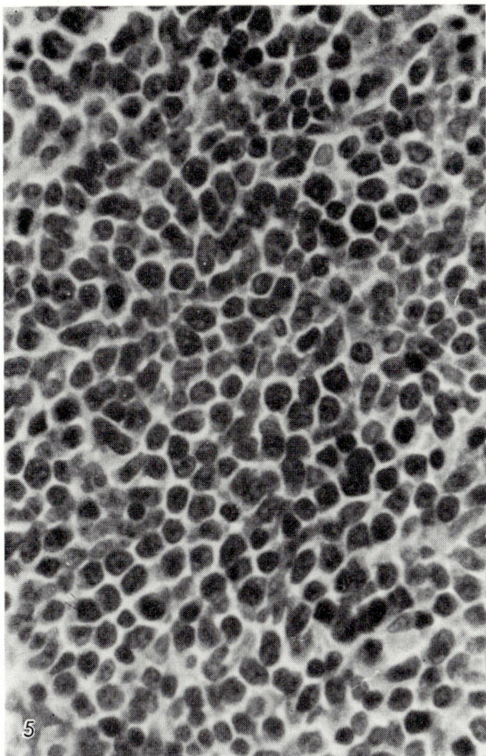
5

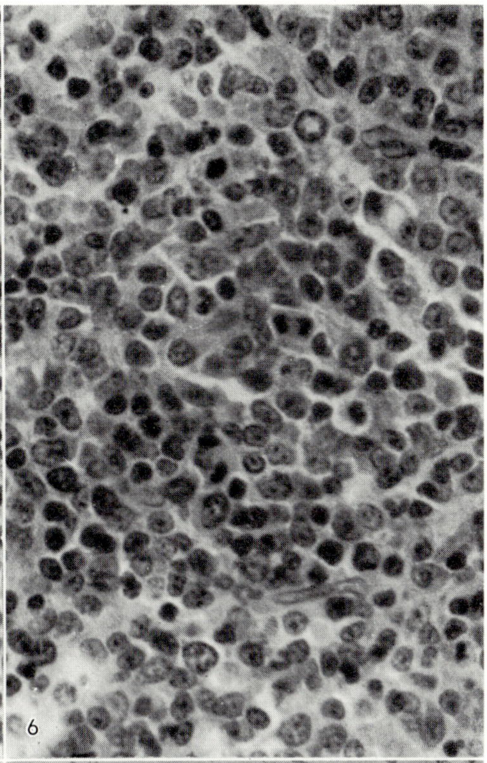
6

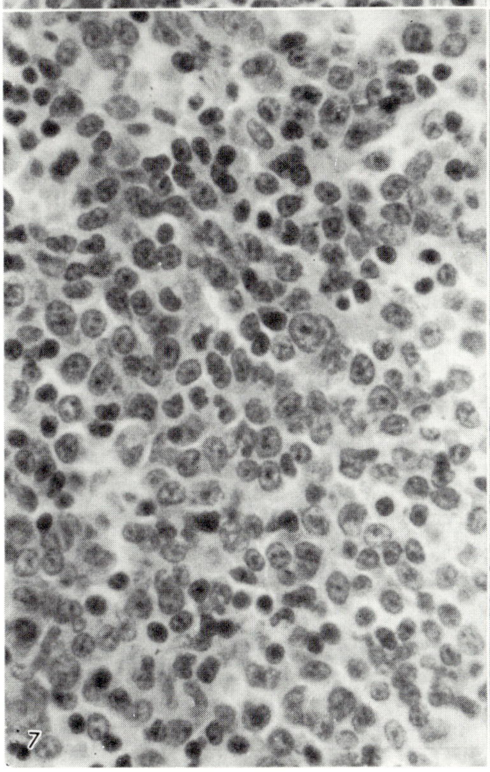
7

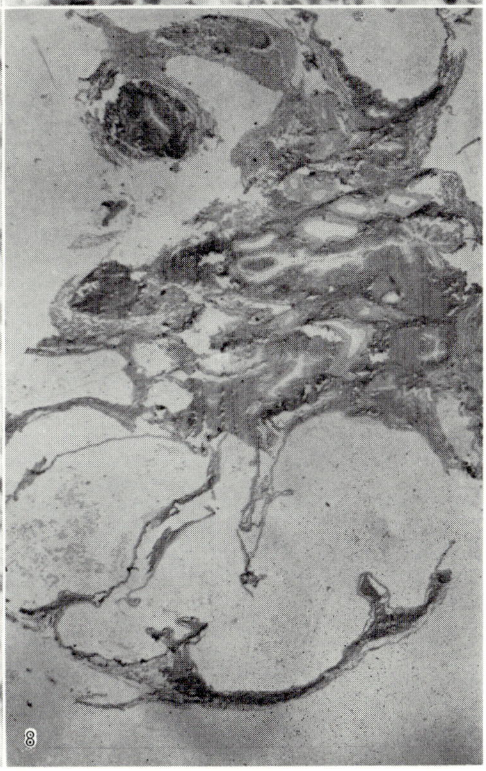
8

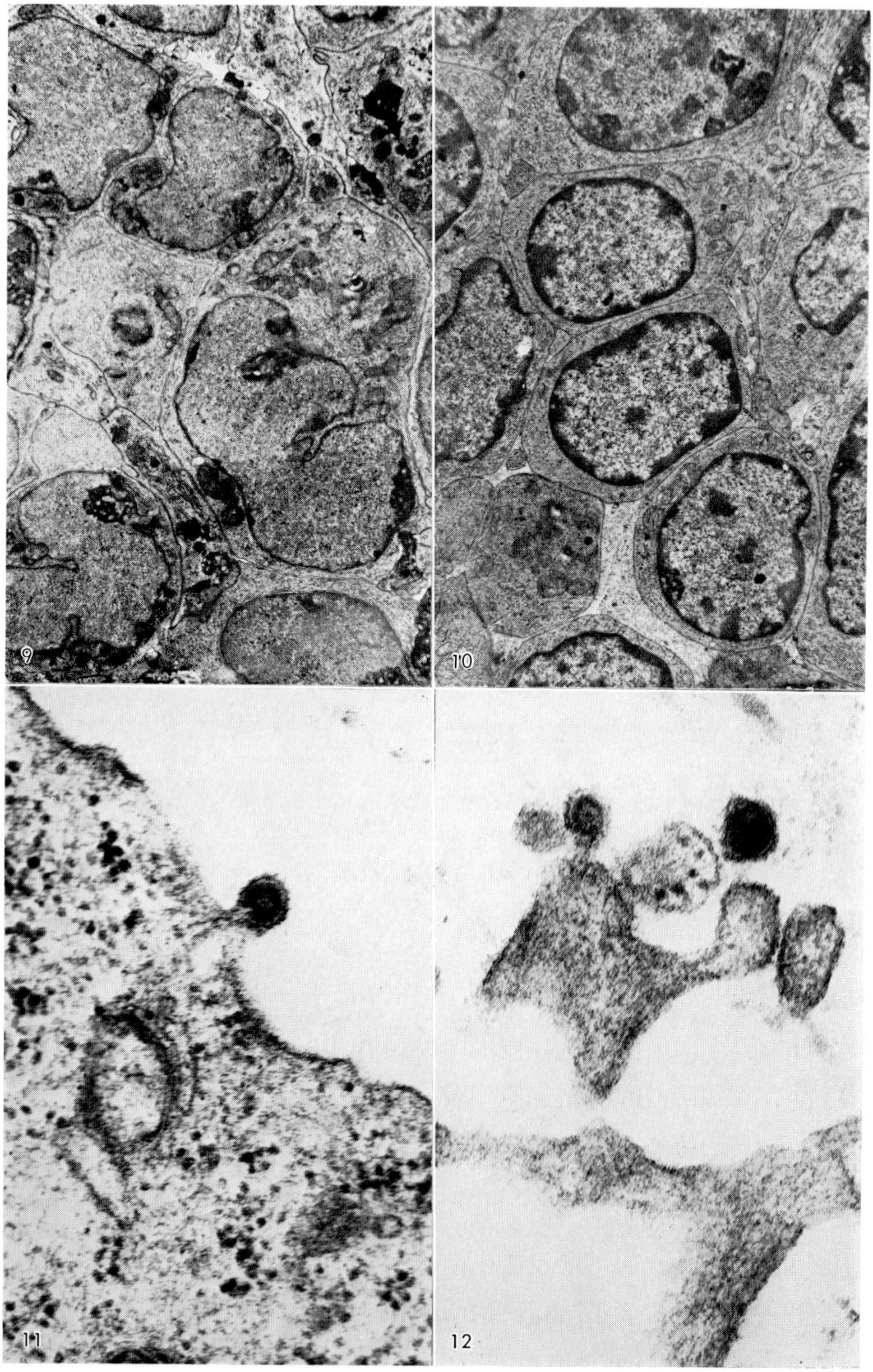
9
10
11
12

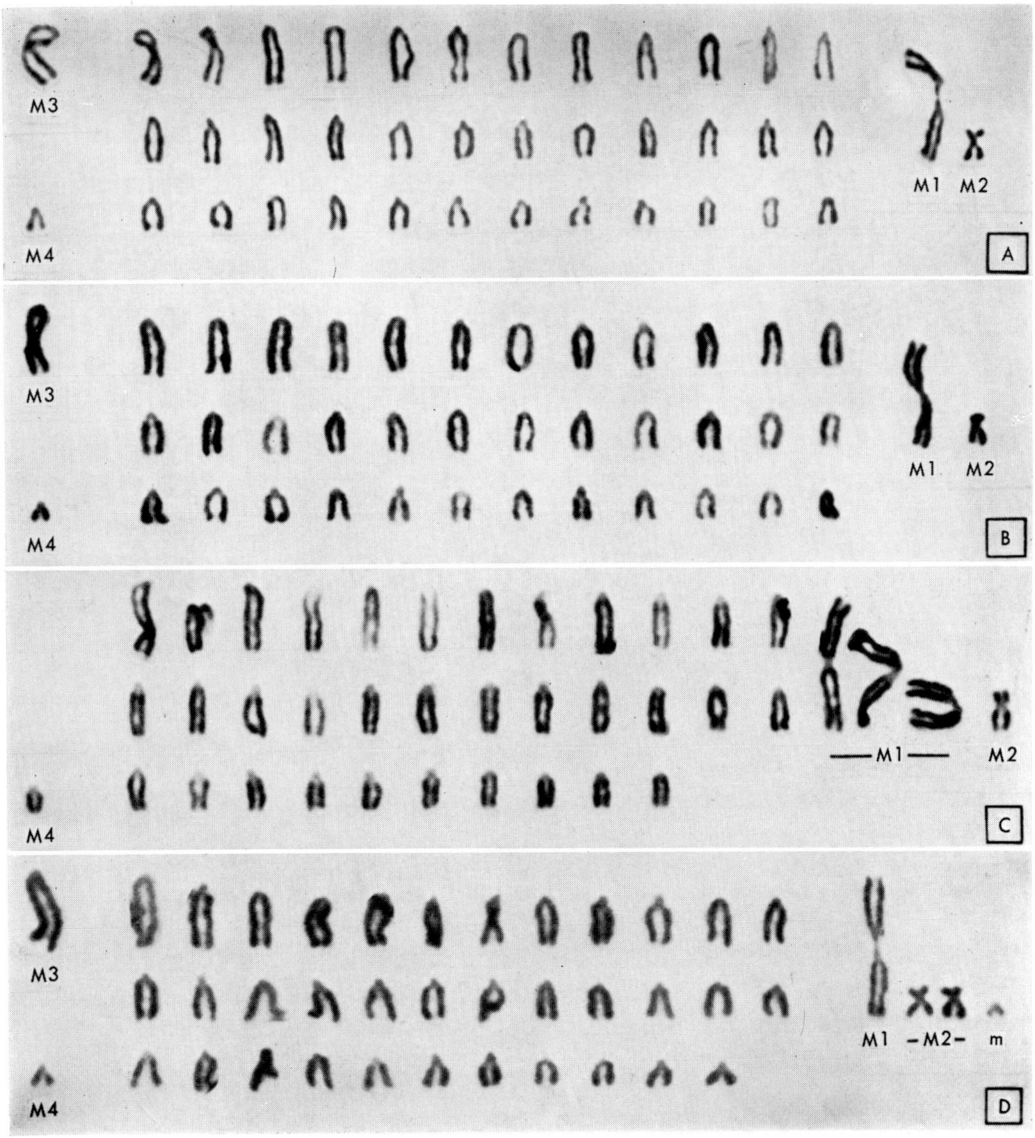

13

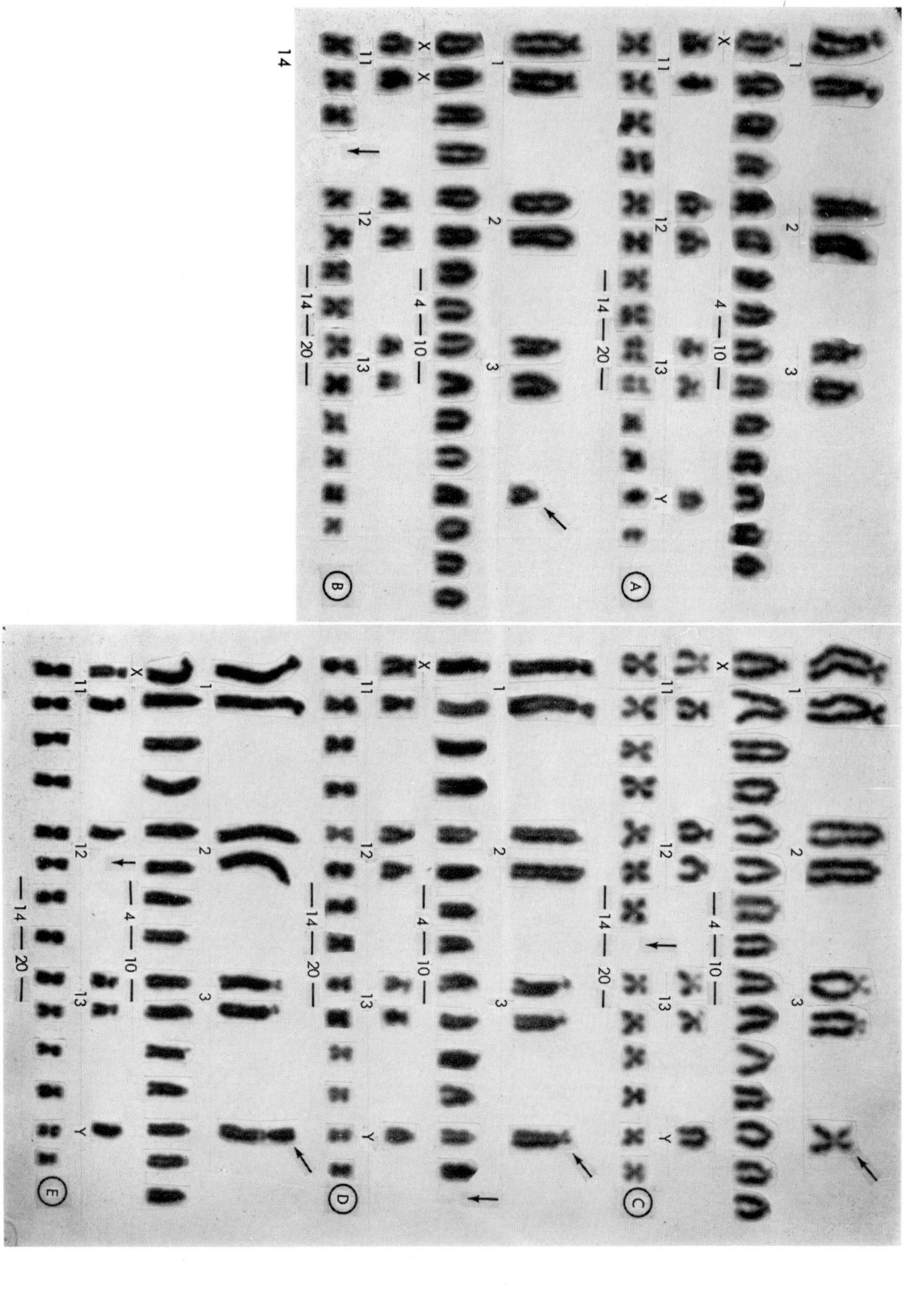

14

GANN Monograph on Cancer Research 12, 1972

INHERITANCE OF SUSCEPTIBILITY TO FRIEND LEUKEMIA VIRUS IN MICE

Takeshi ODAKA
Institute of Medical Science, University of Tokyo*

A single autosomal locus, *Fv*, controls susceptibility to Friend leukemia virus in mice, and its effect is expressed in cells derived from bone marrow. Two new strains congenic with standard inbred strains except for the locus *Fv* have been established, and some of their characteristics are described.

Spontaneous leukemia is observed frequently in some inbred strains of mice but very rarely in others. The fact indicates the involvement of genetic constitution in leukemia development. Previous genetic cross experiments could not provide clear-cut information on the number of genes concerned (*12*).

The mouse leukemia virus (FLV) isolated by Friend (*7*) in 1957 has advantages in studies on genetic susceptibility. It can induce marked splenomegaly in adult mice of susceptible strains after a short latent period, but C57BL mice are refractory to the infection. This paper summarizes the genetic studies carried out in our laboratory.

A virus-infected Swiss mouse was obtained in 1960 through the courtesy of Dr. W. Nakahara. The virus was passed in ddD and then in DDD mice in our laboratory. The DDD mice were established in our institute as an inbred strain by Dr. K. Suzuki from ddD mice which had originally come from Germany. They are albino mice (color gene: ccAABBDDSS) and their histocompatibility type is unknown. Both mammary tumor and leukemia spontaneously develop in old mice (*13*). They are highly susceptible to FLV, developing splenomegaly within 10 days after inoculation with 0.2 ml of the 10% extract from the infected spleens.

Mice of the C57BL/6 strain are highly resistant to FLV. The virus is rapidly eliminated when it is inoculated into old mice. In young adult mice it may grow, but no macroscopical alterations are observed in these mice. When inoculated within 1 week after birth, the mice are persistently infected with the virus and develop splenomegaly after an unusually long latent period (*14*). The relative susceptibility of other strains is shown in Table I.

A Major Locus, Fv

To clarify the marked differences in innate susceptibility to FLV among mouse strains, genetic cross experiments were carried out. In the first one, RF

* Shirokanedai 4-6-1, Minato-ku, Tokyo 108 (小高　健).

TABLE I. Susceptibility of Various Mouse Strains to FLV

Virus dilution[b]	Susceptibility[a]			
	DDD	DBA/2	BALB/c	C57BL/6
10^{-1}			14/15	0/10
10^{-2}			0/15	
10^{-3}	8/8	4/4		
10^{-4}	8/8	8/8		
10^{-5}	0/4	1/4		
10^{-6}	0/4	0/4		

Four-to five-week-old mice were inoculated with FLV which had been adapted to DDD mice. They were observed for 1 month for the development of splenomegaly ($\geqq$0.6 g).
[a] Number of mice with splenomegaly / number of mice inoculated.
[b] 0.2 ml of 10% extract of the spleens of infected DDD mice.

and C57BL/6 mice were crossed (*21*), and in the second, DDD mice were used instead of RF (*23*). When 20 to 30 days old, hybrid mice were inoculated with 0.2 ml of 10% extract obtained from the enlarged spleens of infected DDD mice. The mice were killed when their spleens became remarkably palpable. The remaining ones were killed on the 21st day of the infection and their spleens were weighed. Mice with spleens weighing less than 0.6 g were considered resistant, and those with enlarged spleens susceptible.

Two series of experiments gave the same results. All of the F_1, about one-half of the BC ($F_1 \times$C57BL/6), and about three-quarters of the F_2 mice were susceptible. Neither hair color nor sex had any relation to susceptibility. This finding indicates that a single major autosomal locus controls the early splenomegalic response to FLV in mice. The locus was named *Fv*, the alleles controlling susceptibility and resistance being Fv^s and Fv^r, respectively (*15*).

Such genetic control of susceptibility was also observed in the incidence of foci which appeared on the spleen surface 9 days after the FLV infection (*1*, *22*).

Congenic Strains

In studying the control mechanism of the gene, information based on comparative studies of resistant and susceptible mice might be misleading, because the effects of other genes which play no essential role in pathogenesis could be considered significant. A pair of congenic strains which have a common genetic background except for the gene of interest is useful for this purpose. The establishment of the congenic strain itself should be the most conclusive evidence for the single-gene hypothesis.

Since 1964, an attempt has been made to place the gene of susceptibility (Fv^s) from DDD mice into the genetic background of C57BL/6, and to place the gene of resistance (Fv^r) from C57BL/6 into that of DDD. Two different systems were adopted, a backcross system for the former purpose and a cross-intercross system for the latter. These systems depended on the assumption that unrelated genes could be diluted out on successive crosses, introducing the selected genes

Fv^s and *Fv*^{r} into the genetic background of C57BL/6 and DDD mice, respectively. To establish the congenic strains, it was necessary to select appropriate mice without infecting them with the virus. This was possible by determining their genotypes by means of progeny tests. Individual mice to be tested were crossed with C57BL/6 mice (genotype *Fv*^{r}/*Fv*^{r}) and their progeny were tested for susceptibility to FLV. If the tested mouse has the *Fv*^{s}/*Fv*^{s} genotype, all its progeny should be of the *Fv*^{s}/*Fv*^{r} genotype, susceptible to FLV. If the mouse is heterozygous, both susceptible mice (*Fv*^{s}/*Fv*^{r} genotype) and resistant ones (*Fv*^{r}/*Fv*^{r}) should appear among the progeny in a 1: 1 ratio. If the mouse is of the *Fv*^{r}/*Fv*^{r} genotype, all its progeny should be resistant. This progeny test was shown to be reliable. During the course of the successive crosses, segregation in both phenotype and genotype almost always occurred as expected on the basis of the single-gene hypothesis. The congenic strains, C57BL/6-*Fv*^{s} (*15*) and DDD-*Fv*^{r} (*16*), have thus been established.

The DDD-*Fv*^{r} mice are resistant to FLV and do not develop typical splenomegaly within 3 weeks after infection, but, the virus grows considerably in their spleen (*16*). The C57BL/6-*Fv*^{s} mice are susceptible to FLV. When compared quantitatively, introduction of the *Fv*^{r} gene into DDD mice increased their resistance by more than 10^5-fold, and the introduction of the *Fv*^{s} gene into C57BL/6 mice increased their susceptibility by at least 10^2-fold. Although the *Fv* locus was selected in the above-mentioned crosses, some minor histocompatibility gene seemed to have been introduced together with the *Fv* allele, but the identity of the *Fv* locus with the histocompatibility locus or the linkage relationship between them is still unknown.

The *Fv* locus or some locus closely linked to it appears to control the early splenomegalic response to Rauscher leukemia virus also (Table II).

The possible interference of Kaplan leukemia virus which is known to be congenitally transmitted in C57BL as the cause of resistance to FLV could be eliminated by comparing the incidence of radiation-induced leukemia in C57BL/6 and C57BL/6-*Fv*^{s} mice. Mice were irradiated four times with 200 or 175 R of ^{60}Co at weekly intervals and were observed for over 300 days for the development of leukemia. As shown in Table III, leukemia developed in C57BL/6-*Fv*^{s} mice.

TABLE II. Susceptibility to Rauscher Leukemia Virus

Virus dilution[b]	Susceptibility[a]			
	DDD	DDD-*Fv*^{r}	C57BL/6	C57BL/6-*Fv*^{s}
10^{-1}		0/10	0/5	4/6
10^{-2}	7/7	0/4		1/6
10^{-3}	3/4			2/7
10^{-4}	1/4			0/7
10^{-5}	0/4			

Mice aged 21 to 30 days were inoculated with Rauscher virus which had been passed 3 times in DDD mice. They were observed for 1 month for the development of splenomegaly ($\geqq$0.6 g).

[a] Number of mice with splenomegaly / number of mice inoculated.

[b] 0.2 ml of 10% extract of the spleens of infected DDD mice.

TABLE III. Induction of Leukemia by Whole-body ^{60}Co Irradiation

Strain	Radiation dose (R)	Incidence of leukemia†
C57BL/6	200×4	20/30
	175×4	10/20
	0	0/36
C57BL/6-*Fv*^{s}	200×4	18/39
	175×4	9/25
	0	0/41

Mice were irradiated 4 times at weekly intervals and observed for 300 days. At the first irradiation, they were 30 to 40 days old.

† Number of cases of leukemia / number of mice surviving 100 days after the first irradiation.

Bone Marrow-derived Cells as a Site of Gene Expression

There is accumulating evidence that the proliferating cells in early splenomegaly in Friend virus infection are primitive erythroid cells (*2*, *26*). If the effect of the locus *Fv* is expressed on hemopoietic cells, the innate resistance or susceptibility could be enhanced or decreased by the transfer of bone marrow cells from donor mice with appropriate genotypes. To test this, 2 pairs of congenic mouse strains, DDD—DDD-*Fv*^{r} and C57BL/6—C57BL/6-*Fv*^{s}, were used. Mice of each strain were exposed to 700–900 R of whole-body irradiation with ^{60}Co, inoculated with 10^6–10^7 bone marrow cells taken from either a syngenic or a congenic strain, and tested later for the susceptibility to FLV. The transfer of syngenic bone marrow cells did not qualitatively alter the response of the recipient to FLV. However, when *Fv*^{s}/*Fv*^{s} mice had received transplants of bone marrow cells taken from *Fv*^{r}/*Fv*^{r} mice, the spleens remained small after the virus inoculation. In contrast, *Fv*^{r}/*Fv*^{r} mice receiving *Fv*^{s}/*Fv*^{s} cells responded to the virus with marked spleen enlargement (*20*).

These results indicate that cells derived from bone marrow determine the type of response to FLV. The hosts contributed little or not at all to the response observed. Since irradiation of less than 200 R is ineffective in inducing such alteration in response, the altered response seems to be due to repopulation of destroyed tissues by the transplanted bone marrow cells.

Bone marrow is now known to contain precursors for various cell lines. Therefore, the bone marrow grafts mentioned above could alter the response to FLV in 2 alternative ways: by providing either (i) the cells participating in the defense mechanism, or (ii) the target cells, susceptible or resistant to FLV according to the *Fv* genotype. This study does not provide any direct evidence for either reconstitution of the defense mechanism or replacement of target cells. To obtain some clue on this point, *Fv*^{s}/*Fv*^{s} bone marrow cells were mixed with the same number of cells of *Fv*^{r}/*Fv*^{r} mice and inoculated into the heavily irradiated recipients. When C57BL/6 or C57BL/6-*Fv*^{s} mice were the recipients, the spleen enlargement after FLV infection was somewhat slower in the case of a transfer of mixed cells than in that of *Fv*^{s}/*Fv*^{s} bone marrow cells only, but no such delay was

TABLE IV. Development of Splenomegaly after FLV Infection in Bone Marrow-restored Mice

Genotype of bone marrow donor	Recipient	
	DDD or DDD-*Fv*^{r}	C57BL/6 or C57BL/6-*Fv*^{s}
Fv^s/*Fv*^{s}	1.22±0.54 (12)†	0.99±0.20 (9)
Mixture	0.95±0.24 (10)	0.44±0.21 (11)
Fv^r/*Fv*^{r}	0.17±0.06 (9)	0.10±0.03 (7)

One day after ^{60}Co irradiation (800 R), the recipient mice were injected intravenously with 3–5× 10^6 bone marrow cells obtained from either *Fv*^{s}/*Fv*^{s} or *Fv*^{r}/*Fv*^{r} mice, or with a mixture of them. The donors for DDD or DDD-*Fv*^{r} mice were DDD (*Fv*^{s}/*Fv*^{s} genotype) or DDD-*Fv*^{r} (*Fv*^{r}/*Fv*^{r}) mice, while those for C57BL/6 or C57BL/6-*Fv*^{s} mice were C57BL/6-*Fv*^{s} (*Fv*^{s}/*Fv*^{s}) or C57BL/6 (*Fv*^{r}/*Fv*^{r}) mice. The recipients were challenged with FLV 7–12 days after the bone marrow graft and killed 10–11 days (in the case of DDD and DDD-*Fv*^{r}) or 18 days (C57BL/6 and C57BL/6-*Fv*^{s}) after the infection in order to weigh the spleen.

† Mean weight of spleen ±1 S.D.; figures in parentheses indicate the number of mice.

observed in DDD and DDD-*Fv*^{r} recipients. In any case, most recipient mice developed splenomegaly upon FLV infection (Table IV). This experiment suggests that *Fv*^{r}/*Fv*^{r} bone marrow cells are inert and that *Fv*^{s}/*Fv*^{s} cells are the target cells for the development of splenomegaly. However, this conclusion awaits further confirmation.

DISCUSSION

The presence of the single locus, *Fv*, was shown in the above experiments. However, the resistance of C57BL/6 mice to FLV cannot be completely explained by the *Fv*^{r} allele. With respect to spleen enlargement, both C57BL/6 and DDD-*Fv*^{r} are resistant to FLV and have the same genotype, *Fv*^{r}/*Fv*^{r}. However, the virus grows actively in DDD-*Fv*^{r} but very poorly or irregularly in C57BL/6 mice. Furthermore, the DDD strain is more susceptible to FLV than is C57BL/6-*Fv*^{s}, although both strains have the same genotype, *Fv*^{s}/*Fv*^{s}. These facts could be explained by assuming 2 independent groups of cells (*16*): 1) bone marrow-derived cells which are able to proliferate upon FLV infection in mice with *Fv*^{s}/*Fv*^{s} or *Fv*^{s}/*Fv*^{r} genotypes, and 2) cells of unidentified type(s) which are not involved in the development of splenomegaly. Irrespective of an allele on the *Fv* locus, the genetic constitution of DDD is favorable for FLV multiplication in cells of group 2 (as described above), whereas background of the C57BL/6 is not. According to this assortment of cells, FLV might grow in DDD in cells of both groups 1 and 2, in DDD-*Fv*^{r} in cells of group 2 only, in C57BL/6-*Fv*^{s} in cells of group 1 only, and in C57BL/6 very poorly in both groups of cells. This assumption could account for the higher level of FLV in DDD-*Fv*^{r} than in C57BL/6 and also for the higher susceptibility of DDD than C57BL/6-*Fv*^{s}. It should be stressed that, as shown in the case of DDD-*Fv*^{r} FLV multiplication alone does not lead to the early splenomegaly which is typical of Friend leukemia.

Another possible explanation for the difference in susceptibility between DDD and C57BL/6-*Fv*^{s} or between DDD-*Fv*^{r} and C57BL/6 is to postulate that a mechanism is operating in C57BL/6 and also in C57BL/6-*Fv*[s] to eliminate the virus or to inhibit virus multiplication. Disappearance of infectious FLV from transplantable Friend tumor of C57BL/6 origin was repeatedly observed (*19*), whereas Friend tumors of DDD and A origin constantly yield the infectious virus (*18*). The difficulty of adapting the virus to C57BL/6 mice may be relevant to this phenomenon. During the past 4 years, FLV has been passed in newborn or suckling C57BL/6 mice, and it is now in the 30th passage. Even with this preparation, it is difficult to induce splenomegaly in adult C57BL/6 mice in a short latent period (*17*). The virus that was adapted to C57BL/6 mice by Steeves *et al.* (*25*) also grows poorly in C57BL/6. In contrast, it is not difficult to adapt the virus to resistant A or BALB/c mice (*9*, *17*). Considered together, mouse strains can be divided into 3 groups with respect to FLV susceptibility: 1) highly susceptible, DBA/2, ICR/Ha, C3Hf/Bi, and DDD, 2) resistant, BALB/c and A, and 3) refractory, C57BL/6 (*9*).

Friend virus is now being passed in various mouse strains in different laboratories. Using 2 FLV strains, Lilly found 2 loci, *Fv-1* and *Fv-2* (*11*). Which of them is identical to *Fv* has not yet been determined. Furthermore, he observed that histocompatibility type affected the response to FLV under some experimental conditions (*10*). With C57BL-adapted virus, the effect of the *W* (*24*) and *Sl* (*4*) loci (both affecting hereditary anemia in mice) on FLV susceptibility was noticed. Another anemia gene, *f*, seems to affect the susceptibility also (*2*). It is interesting that anemia genes operating by different mechanisms or at different stages of erythroid maturation influence the susceptibility to FLV.

Although the effect of the *Fv* locus is apparent, its exact control mechanism is unknown. Innate resistance of hosts to several animal viruses was shown to be controlled by a single major gene. The gene responsible for resistance to arbovirus B (*8*) or hepatitis virus (*3*) in mice is expressed on macrophages, whereas penetration or uncoating of Rous sarcoma virus is blocked in genetically resistant chicken cells (*5*). Recently, Crittenden *et al.* (*6*) found that the gene controlling the susceptibility to Rous sarcoma virus of group B is closely linked with or identical to the gene controlling blood group in chicken. Since the FLV-mouse system is the most clear-cut example of Mendelian control in tumor virus infection in mammals, an *in vitro* method for study of the *Fv* locus is eagerly awaited.

REFERENCES

1. Axelrad, A. Genetic control of susceptibility to Friend leukemia virus in mice: Studies with the spleen focus assay method. *Natl. Cancer Inst. Monograph*, **22**, 619–621 (1966).
2. Axelrad, A. Genetic and cellular basis of susceptibility or resistance to Friend leukemia virus infection in mice. *Can. Cancer Conf.*, **8**, 313–343 (1968).
3. Bang, F. B., and Warwick, A. Mouse macrophages as host cells for mouse hepatitis virus and the genetic basis of their susceptibility. *Proc. Natl. Acad. Sci. U.S.*, **46**, 1065–1075 (1960).
4. Bennett, M., Steeves, R. A., Cudkowicz, G., Mirand, E. A., and Russell, L. B.

Mutant Sl alleles of mice affect susceptibility to Friend spleen focus-forming virus. *Science*, **162**, 564–565 (1968).
5. Crittenden, L. B. Observations on the nature of a genetic cellular resistance to avian tumor viruses. *J. Natl. Cancer Inst.*, **41**, 145–153 (1968).
6. Crittenden, L. B., Briles, W. E., and Stone, H. A. Susceptibility to an avian leukosis-sarcoma virus: Close association with an erythrocyte isoantigen. *Science*, **169**, 1324–1325 (1970).
7. Friend, C. Cell-free transmission in adult Swiss mice of a disease having the character of a leukemia. *J. Exp. Med.*, **105**, 307–318 (1957).
8. Goodman, G. T., and Koprowski, H. Macrophages as a cellular expression of inherited natural resistance. *Proc. Natl. Acad. Sci. U.S.*, **48**, 160–165 (1962).
9. Lilly, F. Susceptibility to two strains of Friend leukemia virus in mice. *Science*, **155**, 461–462 (1967).
10. Lilly, F. The effect of histocompatibility-2 type on response to the Friend leukemia virus in mice. *J. Exp. Med.*, **127**, 465–473 (1968).
11. Lilly, F. Fv-2: Identification and location of a second gene governing the spleen focus response to Friend leukemia virus in mice. *J. Natl. Cancer Inst.*, **45**, 163–169 (1970).
12. MacDowell, E. C., Potter, J. S., and Taylor, M. J. Mouse leukemia. XII. The role of genes in spontaneous cases. *Cancer Res.*, **5**, 65–83 (1945).
13. Matsuzawa, A., Yamamoto, T., and Suzuki, K. Studies on DDD mouse with special reference to mammary gland tumors. *Japan. J. Exp. Med.*, **40**, 159–181 (1970).
14. Odaka, T. Inheritance of susceptibility to Friend mouse leukemia virus. IV. Persistence of Friend leukemia virus in C57BL/6 mice. *Japan. J. Exp. Med.*, **37**, 71–72 (1967).
15. Odaka, T. Inheritance of susceptibility to Friend mouse leukemia virus. V. Introduction of a gene responsible for susceptibility in the genetic complement of resistant mice. *J. Virol.*, **3**, 543–548 (1969).
16. Odaka, T. Inheritance of susceptibility to Friend mouse leukemia virus. VII. Establishment of a resistant strain. *Int. J. Cancer*, **6**, 18–23 (1970).
17. Odaka, T. Unpublished data.
18. Odaka, T., and Ikawa, Y. Friend virus-induced transplantable tumors of C57BL/6 origin containing unusually minute amounts of infectious virus. *Int. J. Cancer*, **3**, 211–222 (1968).
19. Odaka, T., Ikawa, Y., and Takizawa, K. Disappearance of infectious virus from Friend virus-induced C57BL/6 tumors. *Int. J. Cancer*, **4**, 403–415 (1969).
20. Odaka, T., and Matsukura, M. Inheritance of susceptibility to Friend mouse leukemia virus. VI. Reciprocal alteration of innate resistance or susceptibility by bone marrow transplantation between congenic strains. *J. Virol.*, **4**, 837–843 (1969).
21. Odaka, T., and Yamamoto, T. Inheritance of susceptibility to Friend mouse leukemia virus. *Japan. J. Exp. Med.*, **32**, 405–413 (1962).
22. Odaka, T., and Yamamoto, T. Inheritance of susceptibility to Friend mouse leukemia virus. II. Spleen foci method applied to test the susceptibility of cross-bred progeny between a sensitive and a resistant strain. *Japan. J. Exp. Med.*, **35**, 311–314 (1965).
23. Odaka, T., and Yamamoto, T. Inheritance of susceptibility to Friend mouse leukemia virus. III. Susceptibility of F1 and genotypes of F2 and backcross progeny. *Japan. J. Exp. Med.*, **36**, 23–31 (1966).

24. Steeves, R. A., Bennett, M., Mirand E. A., and Cudkowicz, G. Genetic control by the W locus of susceptibility to (Friend) spleen focus-forming virus. *Nature*, **218**, 372–374 (1968).
25. Steeves, R. A., Mirand, E. A., Bulba, A., and Trudel, P. J. Spleen foci and polycythemia in C57BL mice infected with host-adapted Friend leukemia virus. *Int. J. Cancer*, **5**, 346–356 (1970).
26. Zajdela, F. Contribution à l'étude de la cellule de Friend. *Bull. Assoc. Fr. Etude Cancer*, **49**, 351–373 (1962).

ONCOGENESIS OF MURINE LEUKEMIA-SARCOMA VIRUS COMPLEX *IN VIVO* AND *IN VITRO**

Yoshihiko TSUBURA and Keiji TOYOSHIMA
*Department of Pathology, Nara Medical College***

The shift of oncogenicity of murine leukemia-sarcoma virus in *in vivo* and *in vitro* studies is reported. Inoculation of M-MLV into three strains of mice revealed that BALB/c and BC [(C57×DD)×DD] mice were more susceptible to M-MLV than DD strain mice, suggesting a possible interfering effect of MTA on MLV. A moderately pure manifestation of generalized lymphoid leukemia was recognized in DD mice at an incidence of 33%, but 7% of M-MLV-inoculated DD mice developed sarcomatous lesions in the spleen or lymph node. On the other hand, M-MSV-induced sarcoma in BALB/c mice at the site of inoculation with an average latent period of 19 days after inoculation. When inoculated mice survived longer, they occasionally developed leukemia, with an incidence of 3%. In *in vitro* studies, release of more numerous C-type particles than with *in vivo* tumor was recognized electron-microscopically in culture cells derived from M-MSV-induced tumor. When culture cells derived from whole embryonic A and BALB/c mice were infected with M-MSV *in vitro*, morphological transformation was evident 3 months after the infection. It was determined electron-microscopically that they also released C-type particles, as seen in MSV-induced tumor cells in culture. An attempt to infect cultured mammary and pulmonary tumor cells with M-MSV *in vitro* was unsuccessful. The oncogenicity of particles released in culture was assayed by inoculating culture fluid into newborn BALB/c or A mice, and sarcomagenic activity was demonstrated in the fluids obtained from cultured embryonic cells infected with M-MSV and from cultured cells of MSV-induced tumor. After 1 year's cultivation, these fluids lost their sarcomagenic activity, and their oncogenicity was converted to leukemogenesis. Superinfection of these cells with M-MSV was not successful. Possible causes of the shift of oncogenesis in both *in vivo* and *in vitro* studies of murine leukemia-sarcoma virus complex are discussed.

Several types of tumor in mice are known to be caused by tumor viruses, and mammary tumor agent (MTA) was the first such virus to be discovered in the murine group. We were originally interested in spontaneous tumor in mice and attempted to establish the high mammary tumor DD strain (*10*) from non-inbred

* This work was supported by Grants-in-Aid for Scientific Research from the Ministry of Education of Japan, Nos. 94134, 94178, 9244, 9039, 9289, and 9267.
** Shijo-cho 840, Kashihara-city, Nara 634 (螺良義彦, 豊島桂次).

dd mice. Though MTA was evident in this strain, further viral studies encountered difficulties because of the lack of an adequate culture system to maintain MTA *in vitro* (*36*), and the time-consuming assay method for MTA. Meanwhile, a series of leukemia viruses (MLV) have been isolated from mice during the last 20 years. Both MTA and MLV are RNA-type tumor viruses; therefore, a common biological background may be expected in viral oncogenesis of both mammary tumor and leukemia in mice. The recent discovery of murine sarcoma virus (MSV) from leukemia virus has also provided evidence comparable to that found in chicken tumor viruses. Studies on leukemia-sarcoma virus complex in mice would help to clarify the complicated mechanism of RNA viral oncogenesis not only in mice but also in other species, including human beings.

In Vitro *Study of Murine Leukemia Virus*

Though MLV has a moderately short latent period for inducing leukemia in mice, it takes more than several weeks, sometimes over a year. In addition to the long experimental period required for MLV *in vivo* studies, another technical problem has been the lack of an adequate culture system for MLV. Pioneering work in this field was reported by Ichikawa (*13*) who described the suspension culture of SL leukemia cells where continuous release of virus was demonstrated by electron microscopy. Antibody was prepared by the virus particles collected from the culture medium, and the fluorescent antibody technique revealed the presence of antigens on the surface of culture cells, but leukemogenic activity was not present in the culture fluid (*14*). Maintenance of the Moloney murine leukemia virus (M-MLV) in serial passage *in vitro* has been reported by Manaker (*20*) though its infectivity was lost after 5 successive subcultures of M-MLV-induced leukemic cells. A similar attempt of ours has also been in vain. Long-term propagation of M-MLV in an established cell line (MT-77) was reported later by Manaker (*21*). Cells derived from the spleens of suckling BALB/c AnN strain mice continuously released leukemogenic virus for 4 years after infection with M-MLV *in vitro*. No overt cytopathic changes were noted in virus-releasing MT-77 cells. Inoculation of the cells into homologous hosts resulted in the development of reticulum cell sarcoma, and no conclusion can be drawn concerning the role of MLV in the neoplastic transformation.

These earlier studies indicated that the establishment of an *in vitro* system for MLV was somewhat more difficult than might be expected, and a reliable quantitative method was not available because of the absence of cytopathic changes. However, the recent discovery of the plaque assay technique using XC cells (*30*) has brought progress in the quantitative study of MLV.

Murine Sarcoma Virus

In 1964, Harvey (*7*) noted the development of sarcoma in mice in the course of a routine passage of M-MLV. Plasma, obtained form M-MLV-induced leukemic rat, was stored at −70° for 3 months and was inoculated into newborn BALB/c mice after diluting it 1 in 30 with Hanks' solution. The tumors induced were of 2 main types, solid and firm, or cystic and filled with blood.

Two years later, Moloney (*25*) reported the isolation of a sarcoma agent derived from sarcomas in BALB/c mice following inoculation with high doses of M-MLV. Though Harvey's strain (H-MSV) and Moloney's isolate (M-MSV) were both derived from M-MLV, they differed in their host range: M-MSV was not effective in untreated rats, hamsters, or guinea pigs, whereas H-MSV was able to induce sarcomas, angiomas, and leukemias similar to the Rauscher and Friend diseases in mice, rats, and hamsters. Both agents can be maintained in tissue culture systems for extended periods (*28*) and can produce foci of altered cells in cultures (*2*). Titration of MSV in culture was established by focus assay (*6*). Further study revealed that focus-forming M-MSV is defective, and it requires helper virus for focus production, and that helper virus is identified as nonfocus-forming leukemia virus (*11*).

Behavior of Murine Leukemia and Sarcoma Virus in Vivo

We obtained lyophilized Moloney leukemia virus (M-MLV, LT(V)-17) in 1959 through the courtesy of Dr. Moloney, and, after reconstitution with distilled water, virus was inoculated into DD mice (*22*). Afterward, virus was extracted by Moloney's method and routine passage was carried out in DD and other strains of mice, inoculating newborn mice with 0.1 ml of the concentrate, equivalent to 25 mg of leukemia tissue.

Mice were kept in aluminum cages measuring 32×23×11 cm and were given MNF pellets (Oriental Yeast Co.) and tap water *ad libitum*. The animal room was air-conditioned to maintain a room temperature of 22°±1° and a relative humidity over 40%.

Though, as was reported by Moloney (*24*), M-MLV is not strain specific, the susceptibility was different in 3 strains of mice, as shown in Table I. Compared with milk agent-carrying DD strain mice, agent-free BALB/c and BC [(C57BL×DD)×DD] mice were more susceptible to M-MLV, suggesting a possible interfering effect of MTA on MLV (*34*). Similar evidence was noted by Squartini *et al.* (*32*) and by Matsuzawa *et al.* (*23*), who have a paper concerning this problem in the present volume.

TABLE I. Serial Passage of MLV in DD, BC, and BALB/c Mice

Virus passage	Strain of mice	No. of mice inocul.	Leukemia cases	Incidence of leukemia	Av. latent period[a] (days)	Tumor-free mice	Av. survival days after inoculation (days)
1 to 15th	DD	261	87	33%	131	174	143
3 to 4th	BC[b]	25	17	68	74	8	86
16th	DD	13	4	31	152	11	213
	BALB	8	7	88	138	1	67
17th	BALB	19	15	79	113	4	198

[a] Latent period means time-to-death with leukemia after virus inoculation.
[b] (C57BL×DD)×DD

TABLE II. Type of Tumor Induced in DD Mice by M-MLV

Type of tumor	Incidence	Av. latent period (days)
Lymphoid leukemia	93%	126
Fibrosarcoma	7	160

TABLE III. Serial Passage of MSV in BALB/c Mice

Virus passage	No. of mice	Cases of sarcoma	Av. latent period† (days)	Cases of leukemia	Av. latent period† (days)
Origin	14	14	18	—	—
1	7	6	43	—	—
2	15	15	17	—	—
3	20	20	13	—	—
4	29	29	14	—	—
5	12	12	15	—	—
6	11	9	43	2	112
7	21	21	24	—	—
8	28	28	13		
9	31	31	14	—	—
10	39	39	16	—	—
11	20	20	11	—	—
12	16	16	23	—	—
13	22	17	36	5	383
14	10	1	101	4	120

† Latent period means time-to-death with tumor after virus inoculation.

Usually, a moderately pure manifestation of lymphoid leukemia was seen in mice inoculated with M-MLV (*26*, *33*), but sarcomatous lesions were occasionally found (Table II) in the spleen or lymph nodes (Photo 1). An attempt to isolate sarcoma virus from these lesions failed.

In contrast to M-MLV, occasional development of leukemia was recognized in M-MSV-inoculated mice. Sarcoma virus was obtained from Dr. Moloney as the lyophilized material SV-221, and serial passage was conducted with BALB/c mice. The routine method for virus passage was almost identical to that described above for MLV, except for the site of inoculation and strain of mice. M-MSV-induced tumor (Photo 2) at the site of inoculation after an average 18.8 day's latent period (time to death after the inoculation) which sometimes extended over a month, especially in the later generations of virus passage. When inoculated mice survived longer, they occasionally developed leukemia (Photos 8 and 9), as shown in Table III.

The type of tumor induced by MLV or MSV *in vivo* depends mainly on the type of tumor virus, but some influence by the host is also anticipated. Therefore, the question arises whether sarcoma and leukemia are different entities or are variations of a single pathological entity. Pathological manifestations of MSV- and MLV-induced tumor in regard to their latent period are illustrated in Fig. 1;

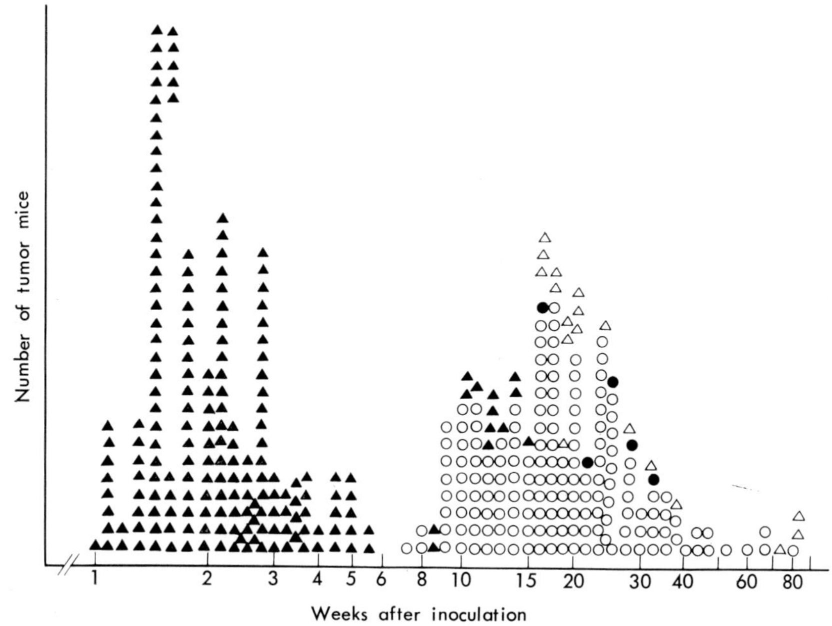

FIG. 1. Latent periods and types of tumors in mice produced by MSV or MLV

	Sarcoma	Leukemia
MSV	▲	△
MLV	●	○

sarcoma usually develops within a month, while leukemia has a longer latent period. Further, MSV induces sarcoma at the site of inoculation while leukemia develops systemically regardless of the site of inoculation. Histologically, sarcoma (Photo 3) derives from striated muscle cells and fibroblasts, and leukemic cells derive from lymphoid cells or stem cells. These findings suggest that virus-induced sarcoma and leukemia in mice are different tumor entities, and the results of *in vivo* experiments suggest that the viruses used in this study are a mixture of MLV and MSV.

Maintenance of MSV in Vitro

Though it was not easy to produce an MLV carrier state culture, a similar attempt on MSV was successful, and, in addition, cultured whole embryonic cells were converted to malignant for a moderately short period after infection with MSV *in vitro.*

Primary culture: Aseptically obtained tissue was minced with scissors and was digested in 0.25% trypsin for 1 hr by stirring with a magnetic stirrer. Separated cells thus obtained were washed twice with phosphate-buffer saline (PBS) (−) solution and planted in TD-40 flasks with Eagle's minimum essential medium (MEM) supplemented with 20% calf serum containing 100 units/ml of penicillin. Flasks were incubated at 37°. The medium was changed twice a week.

Subculture: When culture cells had grown to cover almost the entire surface of the glass, cells were collected with a rubber cleaner, and the cells separated by pipetting were planted in new flasks with fresh medium. No trypsinization was applied to the subculture.

1. *MSV-induced sarcoma cells* in vitro

Tissue culture: When virus-induced sarcoma cells were introduced into the culture, fibroblastic cells began to grow within 24 hr; then polyhedral and multinucleated cells became evident in the early stage of culture (Photo 4). After 1 month's cultivation, the variety of cell types in culture shifted toward spindle-shaped fibroblastic cells, which grew with random orientation, piling up in some places (Photo 5). Fine granules were evident in the cytoplasm, and cinematography revealed that they were the result of pinocytosis. Sometimes eosinophilic bodies were seen in the cytoplasm of the cells. Culture cells grew so active that a serum content of less than 10% in the medium was enough to maintain cell growth equal to that at a higher content.

Transplantability: Approximately 10^6 cells collected from a culture flask were suspended in 0.1 ml of saline solution and inoculated into adult BALB/c mice subcutaneously.

As shown in Table IV, cells in early stages of culture were not transplantable, but further cultivation resulted in a sarcoma (Photo 10) representing a histology (Photo 11) similiar to that used as the source of culture. After long-term culture, transplantation of cells resulted in the development of leukemia. As described below, cells release virus continuously, so the tumor grown in the host is not only derived from inoculated cells, but may also be induced by released virus, which will be discussed later.

Electron microscopy: Culture cells were collected with a rubber cleaner and washed twice with PBS (−). After centrifugation at 1,000 rpm for 10 min, the pellet was fixed in osmic acid and glutaraldehyde, and, after dehydration and embedding in methacrylate resin, sections were cut with a Leitz ultramicrotome. Sections stained by uranyl acetate were observed under a JEOL type-6 electron microscope.

Photograph 12 shows an electron micrograph of an MSV-induced tumor in

TABLE IV. Back-transplantation of Cultured MSV-Induced Tumor Cells

Culture cells			Recipient		
Designation	Passage	Days in culture	No.	Tumor	Latent period† (days)
MSV-BAL_2–30	6	156	1	—	79
MSV-BAL_2–44	8	184	1	—	94
MSV-BAL_2–65	18	243	1	Sarcoma	95
MSV-BAL_2–138	27	367	1	Sarcoma	75
MSV-BAL_2-MSV–11	39	451	1	Leukemia	198
MSV-BAL_2-MSV–63	51	571	1	Leukemia	60

† Latent period means time-to-death after transplantation.

which C-type particles are observed on the surface of cells. When the tumor was cultured, C-type particles were more numerous (Photo 13) than in the *in vivo* tumor, as shown in Photo 12.

2. *Culture cells infected with MSV* in vitro

Cultivation of whole embryonic tissues: The 18-day-old embryo of a strain A mouse was cultured following the method described above, and an attempt was made to infect it with MSV in vitro.

Infection with MSV in vitro: After 2 weeks of cultivation, cells (Photo 6) were infected with MSV extract equivalent to 1 g of sarcoma per culture flask, after contact with the virus for 48 hr, the medium was replaced with a fresh one, and the next medium change was performed as described above. Culture cells

TABLE V. *In Vitro* MSV Infection of Culture Strains of Whole Embryo, Mammary Carcinoma, and Pulmonary Adenoma

Culture cells						Recipients inoculated culture fluid		
Origin of cell		Designation	After contact with MSV			No. of mice in-oculated	No. of mice developed tumor	Latent period† (days)
Cell type	Strain of mice		Days in culture	Passage	Medium change			
Whole embryo	A	WNE-14	3	—	0	1	1	13
		WNE-21	17	1	5	2	2	13
		WNE-42	49	4	12	1	1	35
		WNE-58	86	7	21	2	2	61
		WNE-68	86	10	25	2	2	83
		WNE-94	147	18	41	1	1	59
Mammary carcinoma	DD	MC-2 10682	130	6	45	3	—	—
Pulmonary adenoma	A	PA-78	135	5	40	2	—	—

† Latent period means time-to-death after inoculation of medium.

TABLE VI. Virus-like Particles found in Cultured Cells and Back-Transplants

Culture cells	Particle	Recipient		Particle in back-transplanted tumor
		Strain	Mouse No.	
MSV+BAL_2-5	+	BALB/c	12754	+
MSV+BAL_2-17	—			
PA7+MSV-46	—	A	12167	—
PA7+MSV-55	—			
MC2+MSV-10663	—	DD	12290	—
MC2+MSV-10668	—	DD	12291	—
		DD	12299	—
WNE+MSV-42	+	BALB/c	12296	+

TABLE VII. Back-Transplantation of Cultured Whole Embryonic Cells (A/Jax) Infected with MSV

Culture cells			Recipient		
Designation	Passage	Days in culture	Strain	Tumor	Latent period (days)
WNE-MSV-14	3	13	BALB	Sarcoma	13
WNE-MSV-27	4	16	BALB	Sarcoma	13
WNE-MSV-68	10	81	A	Regression	—
WNE-MSV-90	12	147	A	Sarcoma	30
WNE-MSV-109	8	164	A	Sarcoma	132
WNE-MSV-123	10	181	BALB	Sarcoma	7
WNE-MSV-142	14	204	A	Regression	114
WNE-MSV-164	15	214	A	Sarcoma	11
WNE-MSV-175	15	218	A	Sarcoma	17
WNE-MSV-156	36	478	A	—	—
WNE-MSV-154	38	478	A	—	—

before infection are shown in Photo 6. When the cells were in contact with MSV, small refractile spindle-shaped cells became evident, but no foci of altered cells were recognized. Three months after infection, cells had grown in a multilayered pattern, and random orientation and piling-up were predominant, indicating the malignant transformation (Photo 7). A similar attempt was carried out on the established cell lines derived from mammary tumor of DD mouse and transplantable pulmonary adenoma of strain A mouse (Table V), but no morphological transformation was recognized in these cell lines.

Transplantability: Transplantation of MSV-infected culture cells was done to examine whether transformation is malignant or not. As shown in Table VII, culture cells were inoculated into either strain A or BALB/c mice. Though BALB/c mice are not homologous with culture cells, they developed sarcoma, probably not from the cells but from the virus released by the cells. When the cells were transplanted into homologous strain A mice, most of the recipients developed tumors, while some showed regression. All the recipients were adult, not newborn mice, and this may be responsible for the regression of transplants.

Electron microscopy: After infection with MSV *in vitro*, cells released numerous virus-like particles (Photo 14), as seen in MSV-induced tumor cells in culture. Particles were seen on the surface of the cells, and most of them possessed electron-dense nucleoid bodies, whereas some immature particles were also recognized. Electron-microscopically, particles were not detected in mammary carcinoma and pulmonary adenoma cells after contact with MSV (Table VI).

Oncogenicity of Particles Released in Culture

Since a reliable titration system for MLV and MSV *in vitro* has not yet been established in this laboratory, the oncogenicity of particles was assayed by inoculating them into newborn BALB/c mice. Particles were collected from the culture

TABLE VIII. Oncogenic Activity of Culture Fluid from the Culture of MSV-induced Tumor

Culture cells				Inoculation of supernatant of medium		
Designation	Passage	Days in culture	Medium change	Strain of mice	No. of mice inoc./No. of developing tumor	Latent period† (days)
MSV-BAL-1	Primary	3	0	A	1/1	9
	Primary	21	7	BALB/c	2/2	30.5
MSV-BAL-12	4	97	32	BALB/c	2/2	37.0
MSV-BAL-13	4	77	25	BALB/c	2/2	32.5
MSV-BAL-15	3	28	8	A	3/3	60.6
MSV-BAL-17	2	29	9	BALB/c	2/2	28.5
MSV-BAL-27	5	96	31	BALB/c	2/2	63.5

† Latent period means time-to-death with leukemia after inoculation.

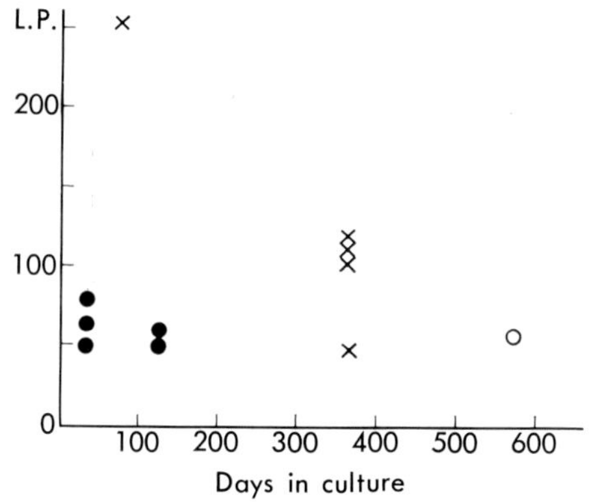

FIG. 2. Shift of oncogenicity of culture fluid from long-term cultivation of MSV-induced tumor to newborn mice

● sarcoma ; ○ leukemia ; × none.

fluid by graded centrifugations and extract equivalent to 1 TD-40 flask was inoculated into the thigh of each BALB/c mouse. The recipients were sacrificed when a noticeable tumor had developed; otherwise they were allowed to live as long as possible.

When MSV-induced tumor cells were cultured for a long time, they released sarcomagenic virus for several months (Table VIII), but later on bioassay revealed the decrease of oncogenicity and then demonstrated leukemogenic activity (Fig. 2). Histologically, all the leukemias were of the lymphoid cell type.

Similar findings were observed in the cells cultivated for a long time after infection with MSV. During 20 months' culture period, bioassay of the culture fluid showed sarcomagenic activity, and prolongation of latent period or lowering of sarcoma incidence was not recognized. Bioassay after 20 months' culture revealed leukemogenesis as shown in Fig. 3, where some of the recipients developed leukemia accompanied by sarcoma at the site of inoculation.

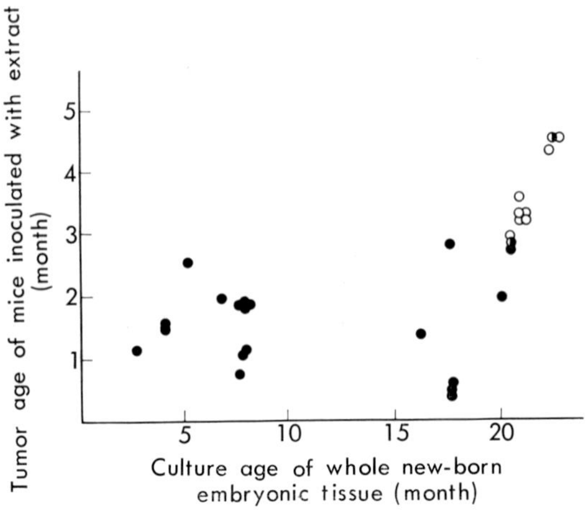

FIG. 3. Oncogenicity of cell-free extract from the medium of cultured whole embryonic tissue infected with MSV to newborn mice
● sarcoma; ◑ sarcoma and leukemia; ○ leukemia.

TABLE IX. Rescue of Virus from MSV-BAL_2 Cells Superinfected with MLV or MSV

Culture passage before infection	Days in culture before infection	Infected with	Culture passage after infection	Days in culture after infection	No. of recipients inoculated culture medium	No. of mice developing sarcoma	No. of mice developing leukemia	Av. latent period of leukemia† (days)
31	406	MLV	1	3	3	0	0	
			5	24	3	0	2	115
			14	86	5	0	5	120
			20	160	1	0	1	60
34	430	MSV	1	2	3	0	3	166
			10	62	4	0	4	125
			44	91	1	0	1	94
44	519	MSV	76	186	5	0	4	125
			108	396	4	0	1	148

† Latent period means time-to-death after the inoculation of culture medium.

In these two *in vitro* systems, one was derived from *in vivo* induced-tumor cells, the other from *in vitro* infected cells, and both resulted in a similar oncogenic pattern; they released MSV first, for approximately a year, then oncogenicity converted to leukemogenicity.

When the medium from culture cells had lost its oncogenic activity, cells were infected again with MSV or MLV *in vitro* and the results of fluid bioassay are shown in Table IX. After the cells came into contact with MLV, the culture fluid exhibited leukemogenic activity. This result does not indicate superinfection with MLV, because leukemogenic activity was also noted in the cells that contacted MSV.

DISCUSSION

Establishment of an *in vitro* titration system for MSV revealed that MSV is a defective virus, requiring MLV as a helper for replication (*6*). *In vitro* studies also indicate that MSV is always associated with MLV, and a rescue experiment on defective M-MSV genomes from noninfectious hamster tumor revealed that Gross, Friend, or Rauscher virus behaves as a helper (*11*). Similar defective nature was also reported in Kirsten's sarcoma virus K-MSV (*19*) but not in H-MSV (*8*), though it shares the same origin as M-MSV.

Murine leukemia virus exerts a relatively poor cytopathic effect on culture cells, but malignant transformation *in vitro* by MLV has been reported by several investigators dealing with Friend virus (*27*), Gross virus (*15*) and Rauscher virus (*4, 29, 37*). Instead, MSV can transform the cells *in vitro* in a moderately short period, and malignancy was confirmed by transplantation into the host. Production of particles in culture was also confirmed by electron microscopy and bioassay where oncogenicity was shifted from sarcoma to leukemia. There are several possible explanations of this phenomenon. As MSV is associated with MLV, one possible explanation is that the balance of these 2 viruses in culture was shifted by some unknown experimental condition. Another possibility is the spontaneous release of leukemia virus by culture cells. Electron microscopy revealed the presence of C-type particles even in germ-free mice (*16*), and widespread contamination of C-type RNA virus in mice is pointed out by Huebner (*12*). Hall (*5*) reported that 7 out of 8 cell lines of mice are contaminated with leukemia virus, and spontaneous release of leukemia virus has been reported by Aaronson (*1*). Because the present studies were designed only as qualitative assays, further quantitative experiments are necessary to explain the mechanism of this phenomenon.

A similar phenomenon was also observed in *in vivo* studies. Compared with Friend or Rauscher virus or Kirsten's erythroblastosis virus, M-MLV usually induces moderately uniform lymphoid leukemia *in vivo*. Therefore, development of tumors other than leukemia was checked in mice inoculated with M-MLV, and 7% incidence of fibrosarcoma was discovered (*35*). Though the histology of these tumors is not identical to M-MSV-induced tumor, the presence of M-MSV in M-MLV is anticipated. Meanwhile, *in vivo* serial passage of M-MSV revealed the development of leukemia, especially in the later stages of passage. Moloney's original report (*25*) states that M-MSV apparently does not include lymphocytic leukemia virus, but the present investigation suggests that M-MSV is accompanied by MLV. A similar fact has been reported by several investigators. When H-MSV was inoculated into BALB/c and C3H/Bi mice or Sprague Dawley rats, some of them ultimately developed generalized lymphocytic leukemia instead of sarcoma (*9*). Harvey and East described 2 types of tumor, early response and late response, indicating that sarcoma develops earlier than leukemia. In their report, factors influencing the response are also discussed; inactivation of H-MSV by ether treatment or inoculation of a reduced titer of H-MSV tended toward leukemogenesis. Sano (*31*) reported that dilution of M-MSV, intravenous inoculation, or inoculation of MSV with MTA also resulted in leukemogenesis. The influence of the host is also anticipated; older animals tend to develop leukemia instead of sarcoma (*18*). Dose response depending on the type of virus-induced tumor is reported by Kirsten and Mayer (*17*), who isolated mouse erythroblastosis virus (K-MEV) from C3H/Gs mice. When W/Fu rats were given graded doses of MEV, higher dosis resulted in erythroblastosis, sarcoma, and osteolytic lesion, while dilution of the virus to 10^{-4} resulted mainly in leukemogenesis. As shown in *in vitro* studies, MSV requires helper virus for replication, and a similar phenomenon was found in *in vivo* study: sarcomagenesis in mice was enhanced by leukemia virus, as reported by Harvey and East (*9*) and Chirigos *et al.* (*3*).

The similarity of the phenomena observed in *in vivo* and *in vitro* studies may offer some answers to the question of viral leukemogenesis and sarcomagenesis.

REFERENCES

1. Aaronson, S. A., Hartley, J. W., and Todaro, G. J. Mouse leukemia virus: "Spontaneous" release by mouse embryo cells after long-term *in vitro* cultivation. *Proc. Natl. Acad. Sci. U.S.*, **64**, 87–94 (1969).
2. Bassin, R. H., Simons, P. J., Chesterman, F. C., and Harvey, J. J. Murine sarcoma virus (Harvey): Characteristics of focus formation in mouse embryo cell cultures, and virus production by hamster tumor cells. *Int. J. Cancer*, **3**, 265–272 (1968).
3. Chirigos, M. A., Perk, K., Turner, W., Burka, B., and Gomez, M. Increased oncogenicity of the murine sarcoma virus (Moloney) by co-infection with murine leukemia virus. *Cancer Res.*, **28**, 1055–1068 (1968).
4. Dug-Nguyen, H., Rosenblum, E. N., Wivel, N. A., and Smith, M. V. A. Malignant transformation by Rauscher strain murine leukemia virus. *Nature*, **214**, 815–817 (1967).
5. Hall, W. T., Andresen, W. F., Sanford, K. K., and Evans, V. J. Virus particles and murine leukemia virus complement-fixing antigen in neoplastic and nonneoplastic cell lines. *Science*, **156**, 85–88 (1967).
6. Hartley, J. W., and Rowe, W. P. Production of altered cell foci in tissue culture by defective Moloney sarcoma virus particles. *Proc. Natl. Acad. Sci. U.S.*, **55**, 780–786 (1966).
7. Harvey, J. J. An unidentified virus which causes the rapid production of tumours in mice. *Nature*, **204**, 1104–1105 (1964).
8. Harvey, J. J. Replication of murine sarcoma virus-Harvey (MSV-H) in tissue cultures of virus induced sarcomas. *J. Gen. Virol.*, **3**, 327–336 (1968).
9. Harvey, J. J., and East, J. Biological activity and separation of a leukaemogenic virus from murine sarcoma virus-Harvey (MSV-H) *Int. J. Cancer*, **4**, 655–665 (1969).
10. Heston, W. E., Vlahakis, G., and Tsubura, Y. Strain DD, a new high mammary tumor strain, and comparison of DD with strain C3H. *J. Natl. Cancer Inst.*, **32**, 237–251 (1964).
11. Huebner, R. J., Hartley, J. W., Rowe, W. P., Lane, W. R., and Capps, W. I. Rescue of the defective genome of Moloney sarcoma virus from a noninfectious hamster tumor and the production of pseudotype sarcoma viruses with various murine leukemia viruses. *Proc. Natl. Acad. Sci. U.S.*, **56**, 1164–1169 (1966).

12. Huebner, R. J., and Todaro, G. J. Oncogenes of RNA tumor viruses as determinants of cancer. *Proc. Natl. Acad. Sci. U.S.*, **64**, 1087–1094 (1969).
13. Ichikawa, Y. Electron microscopic observations on leukemia and lymphosarcomatosis in SL and Ak strain mice, with special reference to the distribution of viral particles as possible causative agents. *Annu. Rep. Inst. Virus Res.*, **1**, 197–220 (1958).
14. Ichikawa, Y., and Notake, K. Studies on the intracellular location of SL leukemia virus antigen by fluorescent antibody. *Annu. Rep. Inst. Virus Res.*, **5**, 103–117 (1962).
15. Ioachim, H. L. Neoplastic transformation of rat thymic cells induced *in vitro* by Gross leukemia virus. *Science*, **155**, 585–587 (1967).
16. Kajima, M., and Pollard, M. Detection of virus-like particles in germ-free mice. *J. Bacteriol.*, **90**, 1448–1454 (1965).
17. Kirsten, W. H., and Mayer, L. A. Morphologic responses to a murine erythroblastosis virus. *J. Natl. Cancer Inst.*, **39**, 311–335 (1967).
18. Kirsten, W. H., and Mayer, L. A. Malignant lymphomas of extrathymic origin induced in rats by murine erythroblastosis virus. *J. Natl. Cancer Inst.*, **43**, 735–746 (1969).
19. Kirsten, W. H., and Sommers, K. D. Murine sarcoma virus: Titration patterns and interference by a murine leukemia virus. *Int. J. Cancer*, **4**, 697–704 (1969).
20. Manaker, R. A., Strother, P. C., Miller, A. A., and Piczak, C. V. Behavior *in vitro* of a mouse lymphoid leukemia virus. *J. Natl. Cancer Inst.*, **25**, 1411–1419 (1960).
21. Manaker, R. A., Jensen, E. M., and Korol, W. Long-term propagation of a murine leukemia virus in an established cell line. *J. Natl. Cancer Inst.*, **33**, 363–368 (1964).
22. Matsumoto, K. Pathology of lymphatic tumor in ddO mice produced by Moloney's leukemia virus (in Japanese). *J. Nara Med. Assoc.*, **12**, 565–593 (1961).
23. Matsuzawa, A., Yamamoto, T., and Suzuki, K. Studies on DDD mouse with special reference to mammary gland tumors (in Japanese). *Japan. J. Exp. Med.*, **40**, 159–181 (1970).
24. Moloney, J. B. Biological studies on a lymphoid-leukemia virus extracted from sarcoma 37. I. Origin and introductory investigations. *J. Natl. Cancer Inst.*, **24**, 933–951 (1960).
25. Moloney, J. B. A virus-induced rhabdomyosarcoma of mice. *Natl. Cancer Inst. Monograph*, **22**, 139–142 (1966).
26. Nakazawa, M. Morphological characteristics of Moloney leukemia virus-induced tumor cell (in Japanese). *J. Nara Med. Assoc.*, **13**, 155–172 (1962).
27. Osato, T., Mirand, E. A., Grace, J. T., and Price, F. *In vivo* malignant transformation of cells by Friend virus. *Nature*, **209**, 779–782 (1966).
28. Perk, K., and Moloney, J. B. Pathogenesis of a virus-induced rhabdomyosarcoma in mice. *J. Natl. Cancer Inst.*, **37**, 581–590 (1966).
29. Rhim, J. R., Huebner, R. J., and Ting, R. C. Transformation of hamster embryo cells *in vitro* by Rauscher leukemia virus. *J. Natl. Cancer Inst.*, **42**, 1053–1060 (1969).
30. Row, W. P., Pugh, W. E., and Hartley, J. W. Plaque assay techniques for murine leukemia viruses. *Virology*, **42**, 1136–1139 (1970).
31. Sano, S. Oncogenicity of Moloney sarcoma virus *in vivo* and *in vitro* (in Japanese). *J. Nara Med. Assoc.*, **19**, 626–644 (1968).
32. Squartini, F., Olivi, M., Bolis, G. B., Ribacchi, R., and Giraldo, G. Reciprocal

interference between mouse mammary tumour virus and leukemia virus. *Nature*, **214**, 730–732 (1967).

33. Tsubura, Y. Pathology of tissue response to Moloney leukemia virus. *Acta Pathol. Japon.*, **11** (Suppl.), 449–463 (1961).
34. Tsubura, Y., Kimura, I., Ohta, T., and Nakazawa, M. Interference between the occurrences of Moloney virus-induced leukemia and spontaneous mammary tumor in mice (in Japanese). *Proc. Japan. Cancer Assoc.*, **21**, 268–269 (1962).
35. Tsubura, Y., Toyoshima, K., and Sano, S. Viral leukemogenesis in mice (in Japanese). *Acta Haematol. Japon.*, **28**, 834–847 (1965).
36. Tsubura, Y., Toyoshima, K., Sano, S., and Watanabe, T. Fate of B particles of mouse mammary tumor *in vivo* and *in vitro*. *In* " Cancer Cells in Culture," ed. by H. Katsuta, University of Tokyo Press, Tokyo, pp. 216–230 (1968).
37. Tyndall, R. L., Teeter, E., Otten, J. A., Bowles, N. D., Vidrine, J. G., Upton, A. C., and Walburg, H. E., Jr. Further observations on *in vitro* cytopathic effects associated with murine leukemia virus infection. *Int. J. Cancer*, **1**, 565–572 (1966).

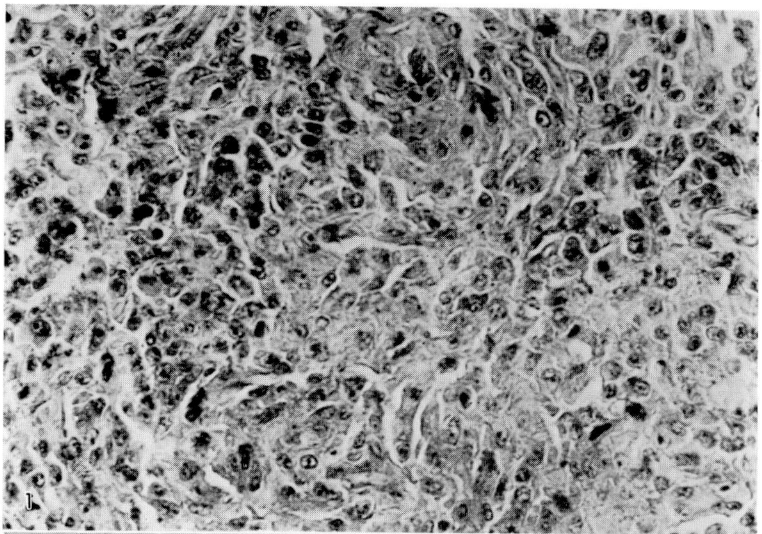

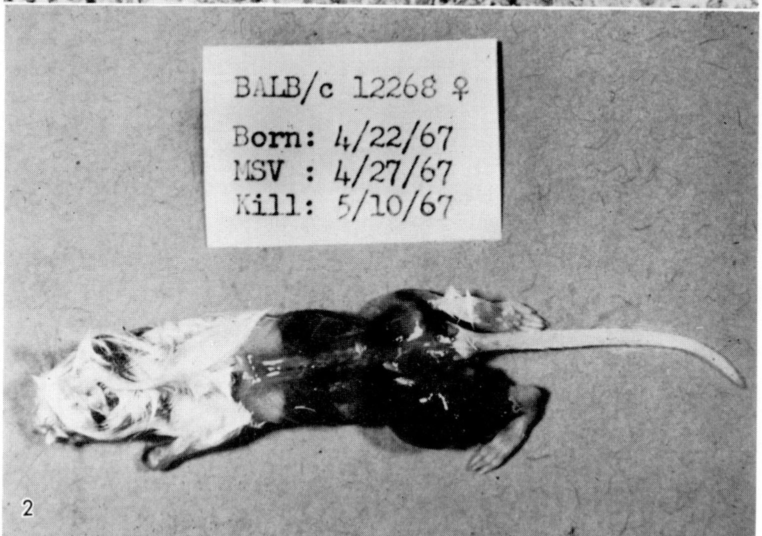
BALB/c 12268 ♀
Born: 4/22/67
MSV : 4/27/67
Kill: 5/10/67
2

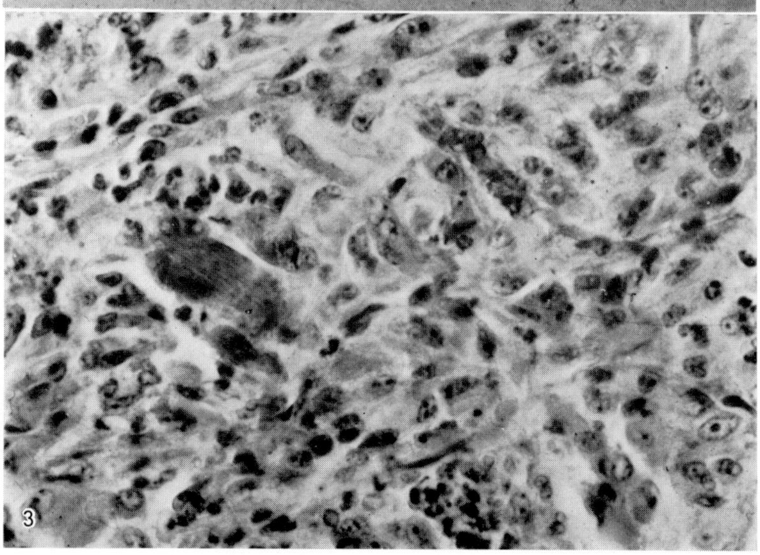

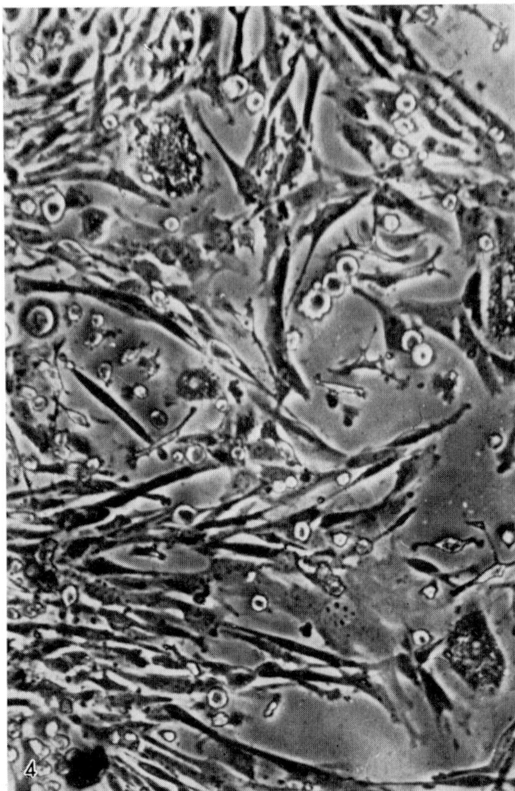
4

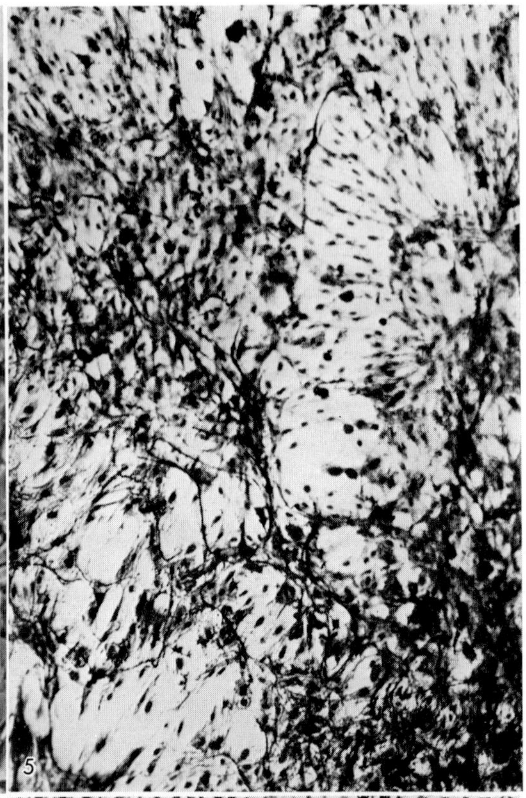
5

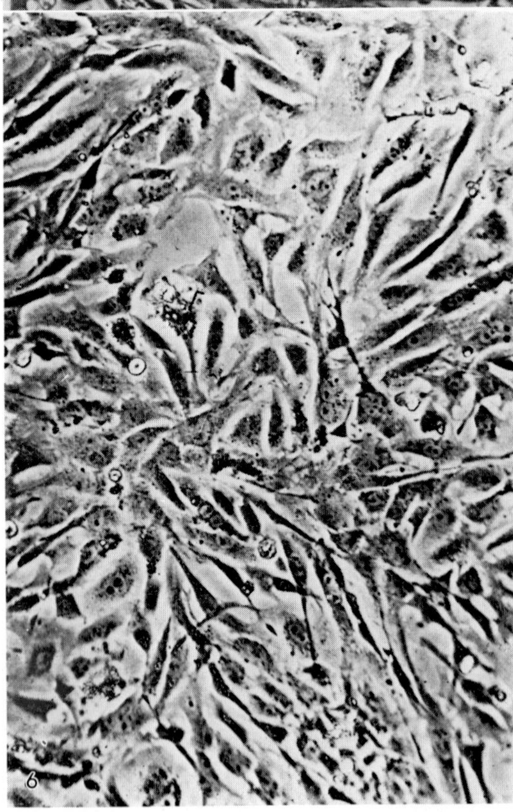
6

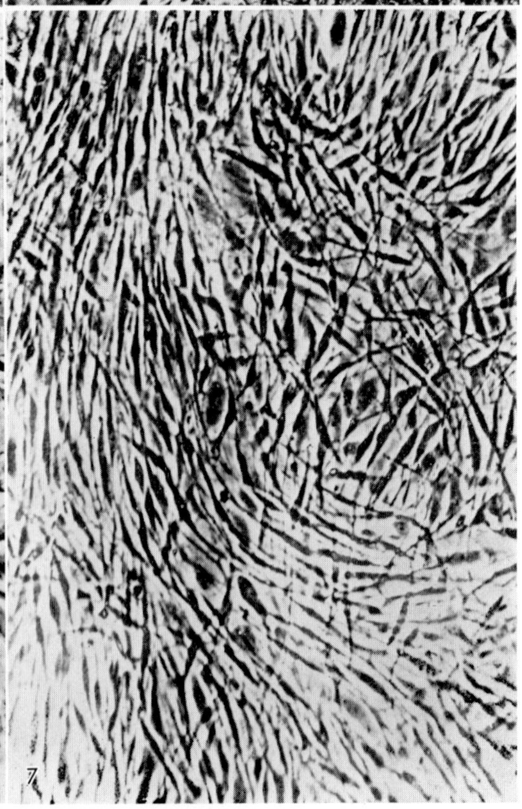
7

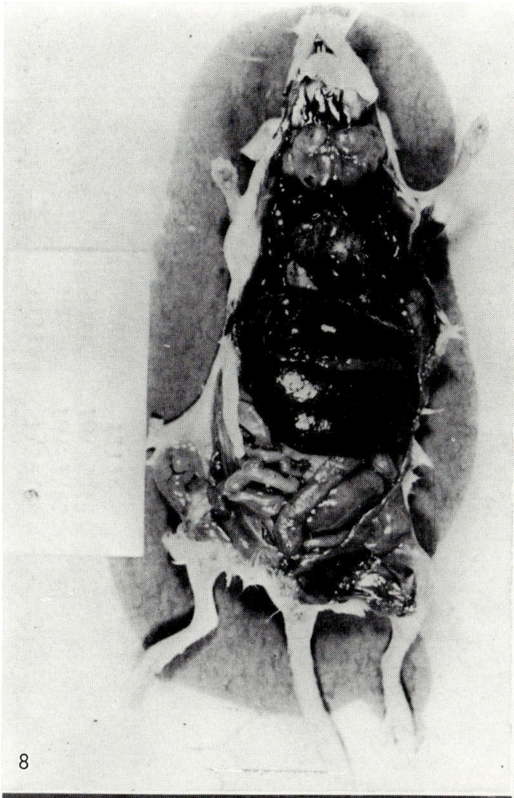
8

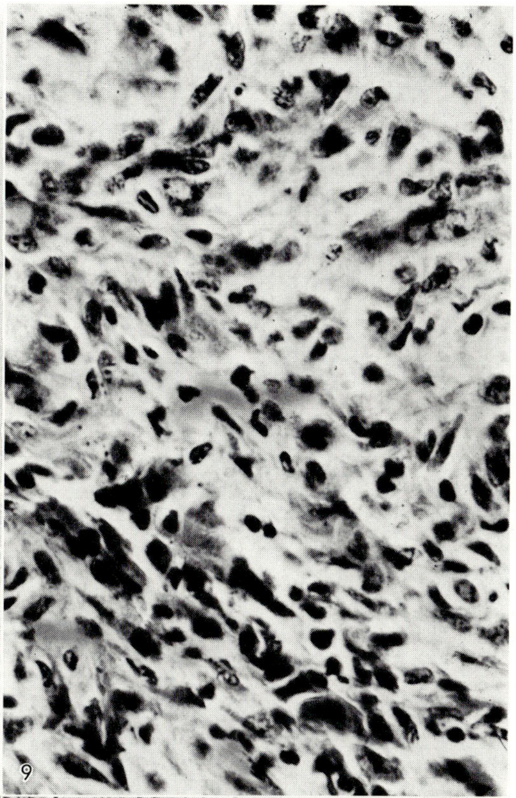
9

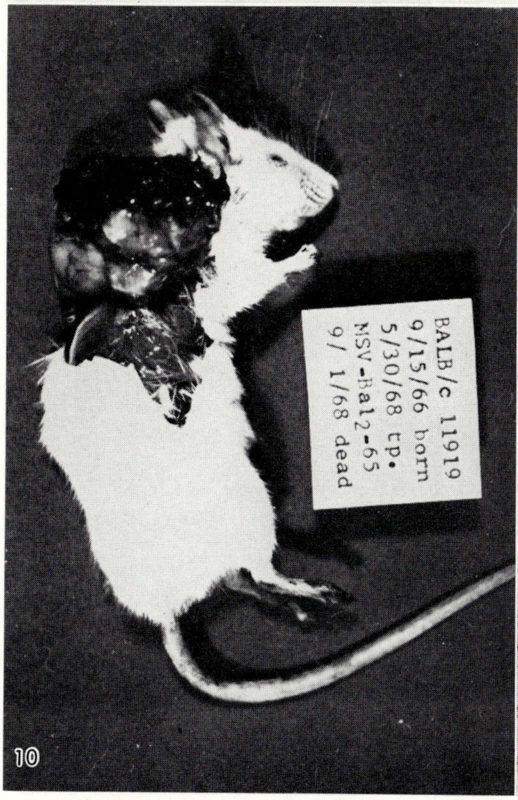
BALB/c 11919
9/15/66 born
5/30/68 tp.
MSV-Bal2-65
9/ 1/68 dead
10

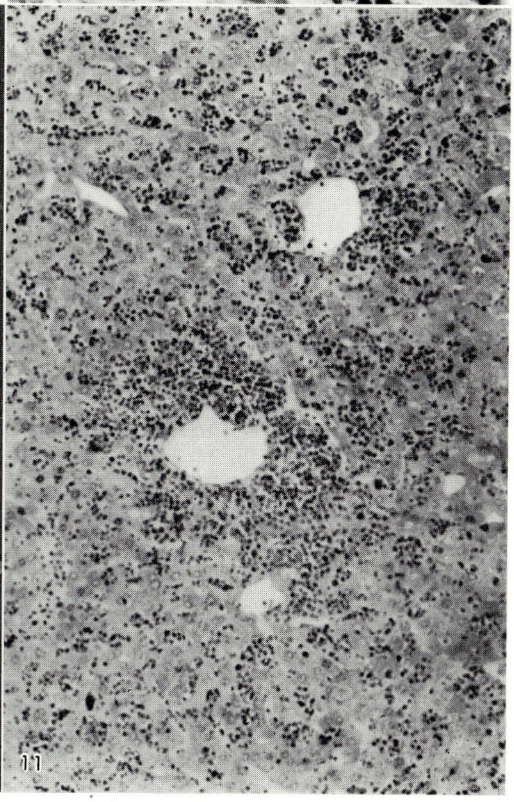
11

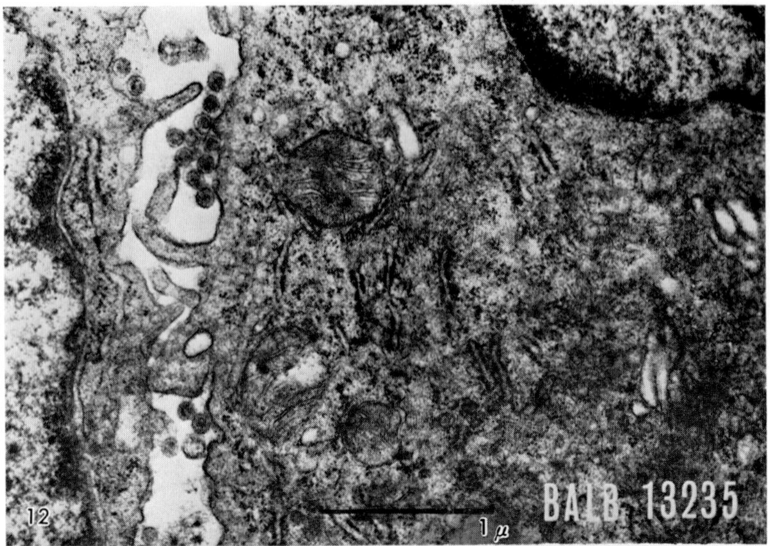
12
1 μ
BALB 13235

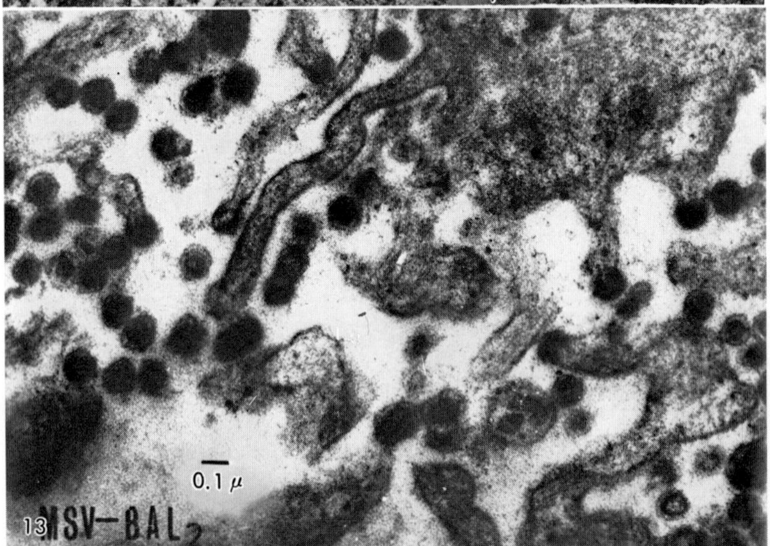
0.1 μ
13
MSV-BAL

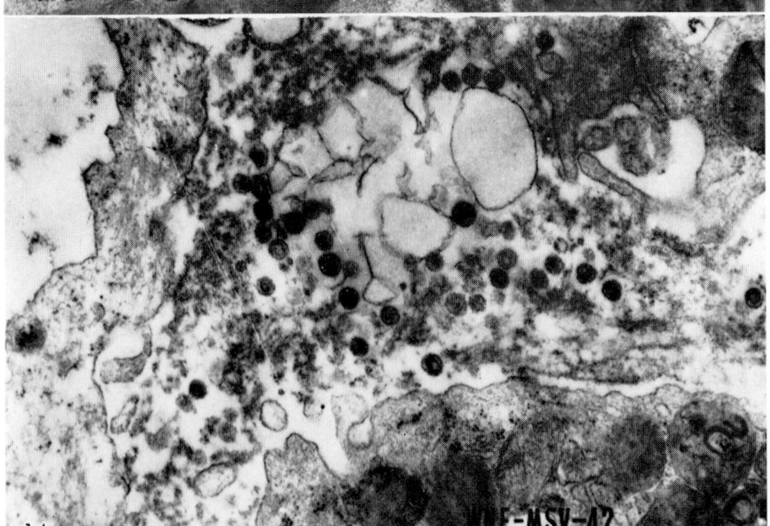
14
0.1 μ
1 μ
NE-MSV-42

AN ANALYSIS OF CAUSES FOR SPONTANEOUSLY DECREASED MAMMARY TUMOR INCIDENCE IN DDD MOUSE

Akio MATSUZAWA and Tadashi YAMAMOTO

*Department of Oncology, Institute of Medical Science,** *University of Tokyo*

Mammary tumor incidence decreased markedly for a short time in DDD mice. By contrast, the incidence of reticular tissue neoplasms increased. However, DDD mothers transmit MTV, strongly oncogenic in BALB/c mice, to their offspring through milk. In view of the fact that it can induce hyperplastic alveolar nodules, mammary plaques, and pregnancy-dependent mammary tumors, the MTV of this strain is regarded as belonging to the category of plaque-inducing viruses (MTV-P), designated by Bentvelzen and Daams. It is very interesting from the genetic point of view that MTV of this type is found only in genetically related strains of mice, RIII, DD, GR, BR6, and DDD, all of which originated in Europe. MTV activity was detected in mammary glands and hemopoietic tissues.

The reticular tissue neoplasm incidence appeared to increase when MTV was removed. Irradiation with ^{60}Co reduced the age of reticular tissue neoplasms by an average of 6.5 months but did not influence their incidence.

In the BALB/c line established by foster-nursing with DDD mothers, mammary tumors became very rare in the third generation and thereafter, and splenomegaly occurred unexpectedly in several animals at the fourth and fifth generation. This observation suggests that DDD mice bear an MLV-like agent which they transmit *via* milk.

In consideration of the above results, an attempt is made to explain the spontaneously decreased mammary tumor incidence on the basis of Squartini's hypothesis.

It is well known that mouse mammary tumor incidence and age vary between mother strain and substrain, and among strains (*51*). Numerous authors have tried to explain this phenomenon on genetical, endocrinological, and virological bases. Blair observed that A/Crg breeders developed mammary tumors at an average age of 4 months younger than those of its substrain, A/Crg/3 (*7*). She attributed this change to a mutation in mammary tumor virus (MTV). Lee indicated that there exists a genetic difference between T and TN substrains derived from BR_6 strain in response to MTV, namely, the latter was more resistant to MTV

* Shirokanedai 4-6-1, Minato-ku, Tokyo 108 (松沢昭雄, 山本　正).

(*25*). The sudden halt in mammary tumor development was explained by Smith as spontaneous loss of active MTV in C3H/StWi mice (*45*). Andervont and Dunn also observed the same phenomenon in RIII mice (*1*). In addition, they produced evidence that MTV introduced from a C3H mother can also disappear from, or persist as an inapparent infection, in strain RIII mice (*2*). On the other hand, to explain the tendency for disappearance of MTV in RIII and BALB/cfRIII mice, Squartini suggested the possibility that MTV and mouse leukemia virus (MLV), which are probably transmitted through milk together, may interfere with each other in mice (*48*); this hypothesis was based on the finding that RIII mice developed a number of lymphoid tumors when free from MTV (*42*). When they were foster-nursed by RIII mothers, a high incidence of lymphatic leukemia was unexpectedly observed in BALB/c mice with a usually low incidence of leukemia (*46, 49, 50*). And the presence of a cell-free leukemogenic agent was proved in BALB/cfRIII mice (*46*). In addition, Squartini proved experimentally the existence of reciprocal interference between MTV and MLV (*48*).

Recently, we observed a decreased mammary tumor incidence along with an increased incidence of the reticular tissue neoplasms of Dunn's definition (*10*) in DDD-strain mice established by Dr. K. Suzuki in 1962 at this institute from the dd colony originating in Germany (*27*). According to our observations, the DDD strain bears a striking resemblance to RIII in mammary tumor properties, and both strains originated in Central Europe. Experiments are, therefore, being performed to explain this phenomenon in relation to Squartini's hypothesis. The results obtained, though far from conclusive in this respect, are presented here to stimulate discussion.

Incidence of Mammary Tumors and Reticular Tissue Neoplasms

The incidence of mammary tumors and reticular tissue neoplasms was observed in forcibly bred DDD, virgin DDD, and forcibly bred DDDfC3H/He mice. DDDfC3H/He mice were obtained by getting newborn DDD mice suckled by C3H/He mothers from within the first 48 hr of life until weaning at the age of 4 weeks. Almost all C3H/He breeders develop mammary tumors by the age of 9 months at this institute. In forcibly bred tests, 2 females were kept with a male in a metal cage and their babies were removed within the first 48 hr of life. Seven to 10 virgins were placed in each metal cage for observation. All animals were given Funabashi Laboratory Chow (Funabashi Nojo Co.) and tap water *ad libitum* and were examined for mammary tumors and enlargement of the spleen and peripheral lymph nodes once weekly. When animals became poor in condition they were killed for autopsy.

The results observed are presented in Table I. It should first be noted that there was a significant difference in mammary tumor incidence ($\chi^2=16.8$; $P<0.001$) between forcibly bred mice born in 1965 and those born in 1967: 71.4% of the former developed mammary tumors at an average age of 11.9 months, while 14.4% of the latter developed mammary tumors at an average age of 13.7 months. Though foster-nursing by C3H/He mothers produced an approximately 2-fold increase in mammary tumor incidence, this increase was not

TABLE I. Incidence of Mammary Tumors and Reticular Tissue Neoplasms in DDD Mouse

Year of birth	Condition of animals	No. of animals observed	Animals with mammary tumors		Animals with reticular tissue neoplasms		Animals dead from other causes	
			%	Mean age ±S.D.[a] (months)	%	Mean age ±S.D. (months)	%	Mean age ±S.D. (months)
1965	Forcibly bred	14	71.4	11.9	14.3	16.0	14.3	17.1
1967	Forcibly bred	42	14.3	13.7±2.2	28.6	16.8±2.3	57.1	14.8±3.9
	Virgin	67	7.5	14.4±3.8	34.4	16.4±3.8	58.1	17.3±3.8
	Foster-nursed[b] on C3H/He mother and forcibly bred	49	24.5	11.2±2.9	18.4	16.0±2.6	57.1	16.1±4.7

[a] S.D.=standard deviation

[b] Foster-nursing began within 48 hr after birth and was continued thereafter until weaning at the age of 4 weeks.

significant ($\chi^2=1.352$; $P>0.20$). In this respect this strain differs from RIII, which showed a high mammary tumor incidence when exposed to C3H MTV (*5*). In explanation of this observation, 2 hypotheses can be introduced: a) MTV introduced from C3H/He is inactivated by some factors in DDD mice, or b) DDD mice become genetically resistant to MTV. However, in view of the fact that mammary tumor incidence was higher in the group in which the incidence of reticular tissue neoplasms was lower (Table I) and also considering Squartini's above-mentioned hypothesis, the first hypothesis is more feasible.

MTV Properties Carried by DDD Mouse

1. Occurrence of hyperplastic alveolar nodules

Hyperplastic alveolar nodules as precursors of mammary tumors have been extensively studied by numerous investigators (*19*, *21*, *30*) since Apolant first reported them in 1906 (*3*). They have been proved to be caused by MTV (*40*), nodular-inducing virus (*41*), hormonal stimulation (*29*), and chemical carcinogens (*12*), and to give rise to tumors under appropriate hormonal conditions (*32*, *33*).

The number of hyperplastic nodules was counted under a dissecting microscope in whole-mount preparations of the third mammary glands of DDD virgins of various ages and of all mammary glands of multiparous mice with 5 litters and of DDD and DDDfBALB/c virgins treated with noduligenic pellets according to the schedule of Nandi's nodular test (*36*). The results are presented in Table II. An average number of 2.2 and 25.5 hyperplastic nodules per mouse were found respectively, in about 20% of 58 virgins aged 9 months and upward, where only the third mammary glands were examined, and in all 6 multiparous mice where all mammary glands were observed about a month after the end of the last lactation. Though no hyperplastic nodules occurred spontaneously in any of the 81 virgins under 6 months of age, an average of 7.2 were induced by noduligenic treatment

TABLE II. Occurrence of Hyperplastic Alveolar Nodules (HAN) in Various Kinds of DDD Mice

Condition of animals	No. of animals examined	No. (%) of animals with HAN	Average No. of HAN per animal with HAN
4- or 6-month-old virgins	81[a]	0 (0)	—
9-, 12-, or 15-month-old virgins	58[a]	12 (20.7)	2.2
Multiparous females[c]	6[b]	6 (100)	25.5±S.D. 17.5
Virgins treated with noduligenic pellets[d]	25[b]	25 (100)	7.2±S.D. 5.3
MTV-free virgins[e] treated with noduligenic pellets[d]	15[b]	0 (0)	—

[a] Only the third mammary glands were examined.
[b] All mammary glands were examined.
[c] These animals bore 5 litters and were examined about a month after the last lactation.
[d] A noduligenic pellet consisting of 0.16 mg 17 β-estradiol, 39.92 mg deoxycorticosterone, and 9.92 mg cholesterol was implanted subcutaneously at the age of 4 to 5 weeks. It was removed and a fresh pellet was implanted contralaterally after 6 weeks. The second pellet was removed 6 weeks thereafter. Animals were killed for examination 30 to 35 days after the removal of the second pellet.
[e] Babies taken by Caesarean section were foster-nursed on a BALB/c mother, and mice coming from a pair of them were used.

in all 25 virgins aged approximately 4 months. DDDfBALB/c virgins did not developed any hyperplastic nodules even when treated with noduligenic pellets. In addition, BALB/cfDDD mice were all nodular-test-positive (*27*) and B-particles believed to be MTV (*5*) were detected in mammary tumors of DDD mice with an electron microscope (*27*).

The above results suggest that MTV and B-particles are transmitted predominantly by means of milk but probably not via eggs or males in this strain, in contrast to GR-strain mice (*53*). It should be noted that mammary tumor incidence was very low in forcibly bred mice (Table I) in contrast to the 100% incidence of hyperplastic nodules in multiparous mice born in the same year. This point is very important in considering an explanation of the decrease in mammary tumor incidence in this strain, for Squartini indicated that hyperplastic noduligenesis was also supressed by MLV in BALB/cfC3H mice (*1*).

2. *Occurrence of mammary plaques*

Mammary plaques are typical histological structures responsive to pregnancy which were first described in C57BL×RIII and reciprocal hybrids, and their offspring, by Foulds (*15–17*). This change was also reported in DD (*20*), RIII (*47*), and GR mice (*31*). It is very interesting, genetically speaking, all these strains originated in Europe. As DDD mice also came from Europe, we investigated whether this histological structure develops in pregnant mice of this strain. All mammary glands from 20 female mice killed late in the fifth or sixth pregnancy were embedded in paraffin and sectioned serially at 10 μ parallel to the skin surface. The sections were selected at regular intervals and stained with hematoxylin and eosin for microscopic examination. The results obtained are presented in

TABLE III. Occurrence of Mammary Plaques in DDD Females Examined Late in the Fifth or Sixth Pregnancy

No. of animals examined	No. of animals with mammary plaques	Average No. of mammary plaques per animal with plaques
20	2	1.5

Table III. The plaque structure was unexpectedly rare: only 2 out of 20 pregnant mice had plaques, and the number was only 1 or 2.

3. Comparison of oncogenicity of MTV from DDD mice and C3H/He mice in BALB/c mice

It is peculiar to DDD mice that they have a low mammary tumor incidence, though they transmit MTV from mother to offspring through milk. Whether or not this is due to a defect in MTV itself was examined. BALB/c newborns free from and highly sensitive to MTV were removed from their mother within the first 48 hr of life and then foster-nursed on DDD or C3H/He mothers. After weaning at the age of 1 month, the mice were housed, 2 females and 1 male per metal cage, and were examined for tumors once weekly throughout the experimental period. Their babies were discarded. As Table IV shows, mammary tumors developed in 71.5% of the BALB/cfDDD mice at an average age of 9.8 months and in 90.0% of the BALB/cfC3H/He mice at an average age of 8.5 months. Though the MTV from DDD mice appeared to be slightly less oncogenic than that from C3H/He, this strain resembling GR in this respect (*4*), it showed a markedly stronger tumorigenicity in BALB/c mice than in its own host. The low mammary tumor incidence in mice of this strain was, therefore, not because of a mutation of MTV, as suggested by Blair (*7*), but due to other causes.

TABLE IV. Comparison of Oncogenicity of MTV from DDD Mice and C3H/He Mice in BALB/c Mice, Using the Force-breeding Test

Foster mother[a]	No. of animals observed	Animals with mammary tumors		Animals with reticular tissue neoplasms	
		No.	Mean age ± S.D.[b] (months)	No.	Mean age (months)
DDD	21	15	9.8±2.8	2[b]	11.7
C3H/He	10	9	8.5±2.6	0	—

[a] Foster-nursing was done within the first 48 hr of life and thereafter.
[b] One of them also had mammary tumor.

4. Pregnancy-dependence of mammary tumors

Pregnancy-dependent mammary tumors have been reported in RIII×C57BL and reciprocal hybrids (*14*), RIII (*47*), GR (*52*), and BR6 mice (*26*), the last of these mouse strains resulting from a cross between a C57BL female and an RIII male (*13*), and are believed to arise not from hyperplastic alveolar nodules but from mammary plaques (*31*). This characteristic appears to have a genetic basis, for the

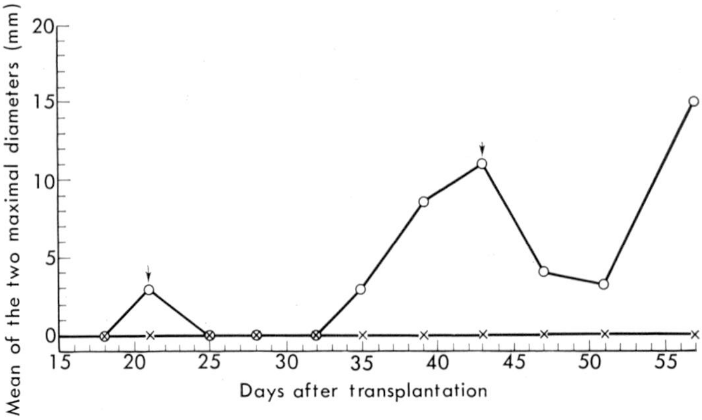

FIG. 1. Pregnancy-dependence of the growth pattern of a mammary tumor of a DDD mouse

Arrow shows the time at which the mouse gave birth. ○ breeder; × virgin.

above-mentioned mouse strains all came from Europe. Considering this point, a plan was made to examine the growth and progression of mammary tumors in DDD mice for pregnancy-dependence. For this purpose, we searched for mammary tumors in all breeders retired at the end of the fifth or sixth lactation, usually between 8 and 12 months of age. Blocks measuring approximately $2 \times 2 \times 2$ mm were cut from the mammary tumors obtained and implanted into the inguinal fat pads of 10 DDD virgins 8 to 9 weeks old. Half of them were kept with 2 males throughout the observation period, their litters being removed, and the other half as virgins. The 2 maximal diameters of each tumor were measured with calipers twice weekly. However, as reported before (*27*), mammary tumor incidence was extremely low in mice below 1 year of age, so only 4 tumors have been tested to date. One of them showed a completely pregnancy-dependent growth pattern (Fig. 1). This characteristic remained at the third transplantation generation (*28*). Though only a very small number of mammary tumors have been examined, this strain appears to be similar to RIII with respect to the pregnancy-dependence of mammary tumors (*47*).

Considering the above-mentioned results collectively, MTV transmitted by DDD mice is regarded as belonging to the category of plaque-inducing viruses (MTV-P) proposed by Bentvelzen and Daams (*4*).

Influence of ^{60}Co Irradiation and Removal of MTV on Reticular Tissue Neoplasm Incidence

Many investigators have observed an increase in the incidence of thymic lymphoma after ionizing irradiation (*18*, *23*, *24*). Though thymic lymphoma is very rare in DDD mice, the influence of ^{60}Co irradiation was examined. Five-week-old DDD virgins were exposed to systemic ^{60}Co irradiation at a dose of 600 R. At the same time, reticular tissue neoplasm incidence was observed in DDDfBALB/c virgins. Animals dying within 5 months after birth were excluded from the observation.

TABLE V. Influence of ^{60}Co Irradiation and Removal of MTV on Reticular Tissue Neoplasm Incidence in DDD Mouse

Properties of animals	No. of animals observed	Animals with reticular tissue neoplasms		Animals with mammary tumors		Animals dead from other causes	
		%	Mean age ±S.D. (months)	%	Mean age ±S.D. (months)	%	Mean age ±S.D. (months)
MTV+	78	39.8	15.9±3.8	3.9	16.0±2.5	56.3	16.5±4.3
MTV+ ^{60}Co+	53	35.9	9.4±2.9	7.5	10.3±2.1	54.8	9.9±3.0
MTV−	33	51.5	15.8±2.4	0	—	48.5	12.4±3.8

^{60}Co-Irradiation was generally performed at a dose of 600 R at the age of 35 days.
All animals used remained virgin. Animals that died before the age of 5 months were excluded.

Reticular tissue neoplasms occurred at an average age of 15.9 months in 39.8% of DDD virgins (MTV+), at an average age of 9.4 months in 35.9% of ^{60}Co-irradiated DDD virgins (MTV+), and at an average age of 15.8 months in 51.5% of DDDfBALB/c virgins (MTV−) (Table V). It was found that ^{60}Co irradiation reduced the mean tumor age significantly (t value=6.240; $P<0.001$) but did not influence tumor incidence. The incidence of reticular tissue neoplasm in DDDfBALB/c virgins was slightly higher than that in DDD, though not significant ($\chi^2=1.104$; $P>0.20$). However, compared with that in forcibly bred DDDfC3H/He mice, in which MTV is regarded as proliferating actively (Table I), it was significantly higher ($\chi^2=9.889$; $P<0.01$). It remains to be confirmed whether or not this finding is related to the interference between MTV and MLV observed by Squartini (*48*).

MTV Activity in Various Organs and Tissues from Lactating Females

Nandi has proposed a hypothetical life cycle for MTV (*35*) on the basis of his group's observations (*37*, *39*, *44*); see (Fig. 2). MTV activity is detected in spleens from completely mammectomized female mice (*11*). The existence of MTV antigens in spleen cells and other hemopoietic tissues was proved by immunofluorescence techniques (*8*). These observations also suggest that the MTV genome proliferates in hemopoietic tissues.

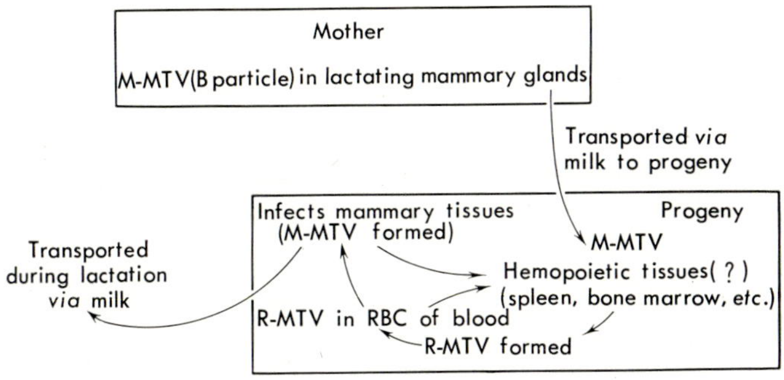

FIG. 2. Hypothetical life cycle of MTV according to Nandi (*42*)

TABLE VI. Detection of MTV Activity in Various Organs and Tissues from Lactating DDD Females by Nodular Test

Expt. No.	Organs or tissues examined	Kinds of test animals used	No. of animals with positive test / No. of animals used
49	Saline solution	BALB/c	0/15
50	Mammary gland[a]	BALB/c	6/15
51	Mesenteric gland[a]	BALB/c	0/9
52	Spleen[a]	BALB/c	0/9
55	Liver[a]	BALB/c	0/9
57	Red blood cells[b]	BALB/c	0/8
58	Red blood cells[b]	(BALB/c × DDDf) F_1	5/12
59	Bone marrow cells[c]	BALB/c	2/4
60	Saline solution	(BALB/c × DDDf) F_1	0/17
61	Mammary tumors from C3H/He[a]	BALB/c	10/10

[a] MTV extract was prepared by the method of Blair (*50*) and kept at −70° until tested. Each test mouse was given an intraperitoneal injection of 200 mg equivalents of the extract in a volume of 0.2 ml.

[b] Blood collected from the heart with a heparinized syringe was centrifuged at 3000 rpm. The pellet was suspended in 10 volumes of saline solution and 0.2 ml of it was injected intraperitoneally into a test mouse.

[c] The bone marrow cells obtained from the femurs of 2 mice were injected intraperitoneally into a test mouse.

The distribution of MTV activity in lactating DDD females was examined by Nandi's nodular test (*36*). In view of the fact that MTV borne by red blood cells (R-MTV) is strain-specific in its infection (*38*), which is explained by the histocompatibility-2 locus (*34*), test mice were selected, as presented in Table VI. The MTV activity unrelated to the histocompatibility-2 locus was detected in mammary glands and in bone marrow tissue. Special attention, however, should be paid to the fact that in the latter case living cells themselves were injected intraperitoneally into 4-week-old BALB/c females, whereas in other organs the fraction corresponding to the MTV fraction of Blair (*6*) was used, because the virus genome can be transferred directly from cell to cell without the participation of complete viruses. The existence and the strain specificity of R-MTV were also proved. Finally, it was concluded that the MTV genome proliferates in mammary glands and hemopoietic tissues in this strain.

On the other hand, Domochowski *et al.* (*9*) observed C-particles in milk from various strains of mice under an electron microscope. Accordingly, the interference between MTV and MLV observed by Squartini (*48*) can also occur in mammary glands and/or hemopoietic tissues in this strain.

Mammary Tumors and Splenomegaly in BALB/cfDDD Breeders

A high mammary tumor incidence was observed in forcibly bred BALB/cfDDD females (Table IV). However, the question arose whether or not this

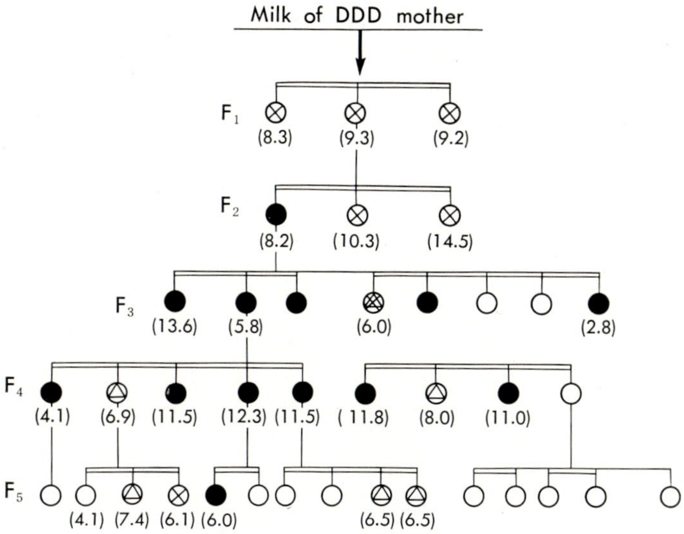

FIG. 3. Mammary tumors and splenomegaly in BALB/cfDDD line from F_1 to F_5

⊗ mammary gland tumors ; ◬ splenomegaly ; ● dead or killed from other causes ; ═══ littermates.
( ) : age in months.

tendency would be maintained through subsequent generations. Since this observation was started, mammary tumor incidence has been seen to decrease at the third generation and thereafter, and splenomegaly of more than 500 mg has been recorded in several animals at the fourth and the fifth generation (Fig. 3). The reticular tissue neoplasm incidence is very low in the mother BALB/c strain (*27*). These preliminary results suggest that an MLV-like agent, probably borne by DDD mice, was transmitted to BALB/c newborns through milk and adapted to and propagated in its new hosts through several generations to produce splenomegaly. If it exists, this agent may also be transmitted *via* the placenta and/or on a genetic basis like chromosomes, because DDDfBALB/c line showed a high reticular tissue neoplasm incidence (Table V). This interpretation is not unexpected, because Domochowski *et al.* showed C-particles with an electron microscope in the milk from various low- or high-leukemia strains of mice (*9*), Ida *et al.* proved the milk transmission of Moloney leukemia virus in A/LN and BALB/c mice (*22*), and, furthermore, Squartini and Rossi (*50*) reported an increasing incidence of lymphatic leukemia in subsequent generations of males of the BALB/cfRIII strain. By contrast, Rich concluded from a survey of the literature that the spontaneous, high-leukemic lines of mice (*e.g.*, AKR, C58) do not transmit the disease through milk (*43*).

Preliminary observations have proved the existence of tumor-specific transplantation antigens common to LD 34 lymphoma established from a spontaneous lymphoma of a DDD female and to LB 1 lymphoma coming from a spontaneous lymphoma of a BALB/cfDDD female. The presence of gs antigen was detected in all 6 DDD mouse reticular tissue neoplasms examined. These findings also suggest the existence of an MLV-like agent in the DDD strain. If such an agent actually exists, interference between MLV and this agent may also occur in this strain. However, a great deal of work remains to be done before we can reach a final conclusion on this point.

REFERENCES

1. Andervont, H. B., and Dunn, T. B. Studies of mammary tumor agent of strain RIII mice. *J. Natl. Cancer Inst.*, **28**, 159–185 (1962).
2. Andervont, H. B. and Dunn, T. B. Further studies of the mammary tumor agent of strain RIII mice. *J. Natl. Cancer Inst.*, **35**, 39–54 (1965).
3. Apolant, H. Die epithelialen Geschwülste der Maus. *Arb. Kgl. Inst. Exp. Therapie Frankfurt*, **1**, 7–64 (1906).
4. Bentvelzen, P., and Daams, J. H. Hereditary infections with mammary tumor viruses in mice. *J. Natl. Cancer Inst.*, **43**, 1025–1035 (1969).
5. Bernhard, W. The detection and study of tumor viruses with electron microscope. *Cancer Res.*, **20**, 712–727 (1960).
6. Blair, P. B. Serologic comparison of mammary tumor viruses from 3 strains of mice. *Proc. Soc. Exp. Biol. Med.*, **103**, 188–190 (1960).
7. Blair, P. B. A mutation in mouse mammary tumor virus. *Cancer Res.*, **20**, 635–642 (1960).
8. Daams, J. H., Calafat, J., Lasfargues, E. Y., Kramarsky, B., and Bentvelzen, P. Mammary tumor virus associated antigens on the membrane of infected mouse spleen cells. *Virology*, **41**, 184–186 (1970).
9. Domochowski, L., Langford, P. L., Williams, W. C., Liebel, R. A., and Liebel, A. G. Electron microscopic and bioassay studies of milk from mice of high and low mammary cancer and high and low leukemia strain. *J. Natl. Cancer Inst.*, **40**, 1339–1358 (1968).
10. Dunn, T. B. Normal and pathologic anatomy of the reticular tissue in laboratory mice. *J. Natl. Cancer Inst.*, **14**, 1281–1433 (1954)
11. Dux, A., and Mühlbock, O. Propagation of the mammary tumor agent (Bittner virus) in the absence of mammary glands in mice. *J. Natl. Cancer Inst.*, **40**, 1309–1312 (1968).
12. Faulkin, L. J. Hyperplastic lesions of mouse mammary glands after treatment with 3-methylcholanthrene. *J. Natl. Cancer Inst.*, **36**, 289–297 (1966).
13. Foulds, L. Mammary tumors in hybrid mice: Presence and transmission of the mammary tumor agent. *Brit. J. Cancer*, **3**, 230–239 (1949).
14. Foulds, F. Mammary tumors in hybrid mice: Growth and progression of spontaneous tumors. *Brit. J. Cancer*, **3**, 345–375 (1949).
15. Foulds, F. The histologic analysis of mammary tumors of mice. II. The histology of responsiveness and progression: The origins of tumors. *J. Natl. Cancer Inst.*, **17**, 713–753 (1956).
16. Foulds, F. The histologic analysis of mammary tumors of mice. III. Organoid tumors. *J. Natl. Cancer Inst.*, **17**, 755–781 (1956).
17. Foulds, F. The histologic analysis of mammary tumors of mice. IV. Secretion. *J. Natl. Cancer Inst.*, **17**, 783–799 (1956).
18. Furth, J., and Furth, O. B. Neoplastic diseases produced in mice by general

irradiation with X-rays. I. Incidence and types of neoplasms. *Am. J. Cancer*, **28**, 54–64 (1936).

19. Haaland, M. Spontaneous tumors in mice. *Fourth Sci. Rep. Imp. Cancer Res. Fund*, 1–111 (1911).
20. Heston, W. E., Vlahakis, G., and Tsubura, Y. Strain DD, a new high mammary tumor strain, and comparison of DD with strain C3H. *J. Natl. Cancer Inst.*, **32**, 237–251 (1964).
21. Huesby, R. A., and Bittner, J. J. A comparative morphological study of the mammary glands with reference to the known factors influencing the development of mammary carcinoma in mice. *Cancer Res.*, **6**, 240–255 (1946).
22. Ida, N., Fukuhara, A., and Ohba, Y. Several aspects of vertical transmission of Moloney virus. *Natl. Cancer Inst. Monograph*, **22**, 287–311 (1966).
23. Kaplan, H. S. On the etiology and pathogenesis of leukemia: A review. *Cancer Res.*, **14**, 535–548 (1954).
24. Law, L. W. Radiation carcinogenesis. *Advan. Biol. Med. Phys.*, **7**, 295–342 (1960).
25. Lee, A. E. Genetic and viral influences on mammary tumors in BR_6 mice. *Brit. J. Cancer*, **22**, 77–82 (1968).
26. Lee, A. E. Mammary tumor development in BR_6 mice: Ovarian influences and 5-hydroxyptamine. *Brit. J. Cancer*, **24**, 561–567 (1970).
27. Matsuzawa, A., Suzuki, K., and Yamamoto, T. Studies on DDD mouse with special reference to mammary gland tumors. *Japan. J. Exp. Med.*, **40**, 159–181 (1970).
28. Matsuzawa, A. Unpublished data.
29. Medina, D., and DeOme, K. B. Influence of mammary tumor virus on the tumor-producing capacities of nodule outgrowth free of mammary tumor virus. *J. Natl. Cancer Inst.*, **39**, 551–555 (1967).
30. Mühlbock, O. Hormonal genesis of mammary cancer. *Advan. Cancer Res.*, **4**, 371-392 (1956)).
31. Mühlbock, O., and Bentvelzen, P. The transmission of the mammary tumor viruses. *Perspect. Virol.*, **6**, 75–81 (1969).
32. Nandi, S. Effect of hormones on mammary-tumor development from transplanted hyperplastic alveolar nodules in hypophysectomized-ovariectomized-adrenalectomized C3H/Crgl mice. *J. Natl. Cancer Inst.*, **27**, 173–185 (1961).
33. Nandi, S. Effect of hormones on maintenance of hyperplastic alveolar nodules in mammary gland of various strains of mice. *J. Natl. Cancer Inst.*, **27**, 187–201 (1961).
34. Nandi, S. The histocompatibility-2 locus and susceptibility to bittner virus borne by red blood cells in mice. *Proc. Natl. Acad. Sci. U.S.*, **58**, 485–492 (1967).
35. Nandi, S. Host-virus interactions in mouse mammary tumor system. *In* "Carcinogenesis: A broad critique," Williams and Wilkins Co., Baltimore, pp. 295-314 (1967).
36. Nandi, S., and DeOme, K. B. An interference phenomenon associated with resistance to infection with mouse mammary tumor virus. *J. Natl. Cancer Inst.*, **35**, 299–308 (1965).
37. Nandi, S., and DeOme, K. B. Mammary tumor virus activity in blood and mammary tissues of C3H and BALB/cfC3H strains of mice. *J. Natl. Cancer Inst.*, **35**, 309–318 (1965).
38. Nandi, S., Handin, M., and Young, L. Strain-specific mammary tumor virus activity in blood of C3H and BALB/cfC3H mice. *J. Natl. Cancer Inst.*, **36**, 803–808 (1966).

39. Nandi, S., Knox, D., DeOme, K. B., Handin, M., Finster, V. V., and Pickett, P. B. Mammary tumor virus activity in red blood cells of BALB/cfC3H mice. *J. Natl. Cancer Inst.*, **36**, 806–815 (1966).
40. Pitelka, D. R., Bern, H. A., DeOme, K. B., Schooley, C. N., and Wellings, S. R. Virus-like particles in hyperplastic alveolar nodules of the mammary gland of the C3H/HeCrgl mouse. *J. Natl. Cancer Inst.*, **20**, 541–553 (1958).
41. Pitelka, D. R., DeOme, K. B., and Bern, H. A. Virus-like particles in precancerous hyperplastic mammary tissues of C3H and C3Hf mice. *J. Natl. Cancer Inst.*, **25**, 753–777 (1960).
42. Pullinger, B. D. and Iversen, S. Mammary tumor incidence in relation to age and number of litters in C3Hf RIII mice. *Brit. J. Cancer*, **14**, 267–278 (1960).
43. Rich, M. A. Virus-induced murine leukemia. *In* " Experimental Leukemia," ed. by M. A. Rich, North-Holland Publishing Co., Amsterdam, pp. 15–49 (1968).
44. Ritter, R. I., and Nandi, S. Time of appearance of viral activity in red blood cells of mice infected naturally or artificially with mammary tumor virus. *J. Natl. Cancer Inst.*, **40**, 1313–1317 (1968).
45. Smith, G. H. Role of the milk agent in disappearance of mammary cancer in C3H/StWi mice. *J. Natl. Cancer Inst.*, **36**, 685–701 (1966).
46. Squartini, F. Progress report to USPHS Research Grant C–3844 Path.: A study of mammary cancer. *Lavori Inst. anat. isol. patol. Univ. Perugia*, **22**, 97–145 (1962).
47. Squartini, F. Responsiveness and progression of mammary tumors in high-cancer-strain mice. *J. Natl. Cancer Inst.*, **28**, 911–926 (1962).
48. Squartini, F. Reciprocal interference between mouse mammary tumor virus and leukemia virus. *Nature*, **214**, 730–732 (1967).
49. Squartini, F., and Rossi, G. Detection of a leukemogenic agent in BALB/c mice foster-nursed by RIII. *Lavori Inst. anat. istol. patol. Univ. Perugia*, **22**, 185–188 (1962).
50. Squartini, F., and Rossi, G. "Alta incidenza di leucemia nei topi BALB/c allattati da RIII." Atti di un Simposio Internazionale su I Virus nelle Leucemie dei Mammiferi. Accademia Nazionale dei Lincei, Roma, pp. 129–148 (1964).
51. Staats, J. Standardized nomenclature for inbred strains of mice, fourth listing. *Cancer Res.*, **28**, 391–420 (1968).
52. Van Nie, R., and Thung, P. J. Responsiveness of mouse mammary tumors to pregnancy. *Eur. J. Cancer*, **1**, 41–47 (1965).
53. Zeilmaker, G. H. Transmission of mammary tumor virus by female GR mice: Results of egg transplantation. *Int. J. Cancer*, **4**, 261–266 (1969).

RECOVERY OF ROUS SARCOMA VIRUS FROM NON-VIRUS-PRODUCING ROUS SARCOMA CELLS

Nobuo YAMAGUCHI, Mieko TAKEUCHI, Shigeo HINO, and Tadashi YAMAMOTO
Institute of Medical Science, University of Tokyo*

The induction of Rous sarcoma virus (RSV) production in mixed cultures of mammalian Rous sarcoma cells and chick embryo cells was investigated. A high frequency of induction was observed when the cells had been subjected to cell fusion reaction using ultraviolet inactivated hemagglutinating virus of Japan (UV-HVJ) and when the UV-HVJ had been treated with an appropriate dilution of anti-HVJ serum, indicating that induction occurred in heterokaryons of mammalian Rous sarcoma cells and chick embryo cells. However, the number of infective centers in the mixed cultures was as small as 1% of the heterokaryons. Virus induction was not inhibited by 20 mM thymidine, an inhibitor of DNA synthesis.

Mammalian Rous sarcoma cells arising after infection with RSV do not release infectious virus, as a general rule. Such sarcoma cells carry the genome of RSV and can be activated to release infectious RSV progeny when inoculated into young chickens or cultivated with chick embryo cells (see *25*). Since intimate cell to cell contact seems to facilitate the recovery of RSV, several investigators have used the improved cell fusion technique described by Okada *et al.* (*10*) and Harris and Watkins (*4*) to increase the recovery (*6*, *8*, *15–19*, *24*, *27*, *28*). The cell fusion technique has also been used to recover infectious virus from simian virus 40 (SV40) or polyoma virus transformed cells (*2*, *3*, *7*, *26*). The present paper deals with some aspects of the " induction " of RSV production in mixed cultures of mammalian Rous sarcoma cells and chick embryo cells.

Characteristics of Rous Sarcoma Cell Lines

An ascites sarcoma strain, SR-C3H/He ascites, transplantable in C3H/He mice, was established in our laboratory from a sarcoma which arose after inoculation of chicken Rous sarcoma cells into a newborn mouse (*29*). No infectious RSV was demonstrated in the sarcoma cells. However, when more than 10^5 of these mouse sarcoma cells were inoculated into young chickens, typical chicken sarcomas could be induced which released infectious RSV. Cell-free extract of more than 10^6 mouse sarcoma cells never produced such a chicken sarcoma.

* Shirokanedai 4-6-1, Minato-ku, Tokyo 108 (山口宣生, 竹内美恵子, 日野茂男, 山本　正).

To investigate the process of the recovery of RSV, a cultured cell line, SR-C3H-2127, was established from SR-C3H/He ascites and cloned 3 times by the method described by Puck *et al.* (*14*). SR-C3H-2127 cells grew in an agar medium composed of Eagle's minimum essential medium with 20% calf serum, 10% Bactotryptose phosphate broth (Difco), and 0.45% Bacto-agar (Difco). The plating efficiency was 70–80%. The cells were first tested for the RSV genome by cultivating them with virus-susceptible chicken cells. But infectious RSV was not detected during 48 days' observation (*27*). Because the number of SR-C3H-2127 cells co-cultivated with chicken cells was limited, they were then tested for the genome *in vivo*. They induced tumors in 10–15% of chickens with 10^7 cells and no tumors in chickens with 10^6 cells. On the other hand, an ascites sarcoma subline of SR-C3H/He ascites, Th-62 (*20*), induced tumors in chicken with a higher frequency; tumors developed in all the chickens inoculated with 2×10^6 cells and in 40% inoculated with 2×10^5 cells (Table I). The low frequency of RSV induction in the cultured cell line was common among cultured cell lines of Rous sarcomas, in contrast to the high frequency in ascites sarcoma cell lines (Table II). This difference in the frequency of RSV induction may be due not to the difference in the state of the RSV genome in cells, but to the difference in the frequency of spontaneous cell fusion between sarcoma cells and chick embryo

TABLE I. Induction of Tumors in Chicken by Rous Sarcoma Cells

Expt. No.	Cell lines[a]	Cell number inoculated					
		10^7	2×10^6	10^6	2×10^5	10^5	2×10^4
1	SR-C3H-2127	0/4[b]		0/12		0/11	
2	SR-C3H-2127	3/18		0/18		0/8	
3	Th-62		4/4		2/5		0/5

[a] Th-62 was a subline of an ascites sarcoma, SR-C3H/He ascites, from which the cultured cell line SR-C3H-2127 was derived.

[b] No. of chickens that produced tumor(s) / No. of chickens inoculated.

TABLE II. Production of RSV in Mixed Cultures of Irradiated Rous Sarcoma and Chick Embryo Cells in the Absence or Presence of UV-HVJ[a]

Cell lines	Species and strains	Days of *in vitro* cultivation before test	Presence of UV-HVJ	Production of RSV[b]
SR-C3H-2127	C3H/He mouse	350–800	±	±
SR-C57B-3	C57BL/6 mouse	140–530	±	±
SR-H-312	Syrian hamster	150–290	±	±
Th-62	C3H/He mouse	0	±	+ +
2008	C57BL/6 mouse	0	±	+ +
SR-DDD	DDD mouse	0	±	+ +

[a] Gamma-irradiated 2×10^5 Rous sarcoma and nonirradiated 6×10^5 chick embryo cells were co-cultivated after being shaken at 37° in the presence or absence of UV-HVJ. After 3 transfers, the cell suspensions were frozen and thawed, then tested for RSV production.

[b] A plus sign indicates presence of RSV production in the mixed culture; minus sign indicates absence of RSV production in the mixed culture.

cells in mixed culture, because not only the ascites sarcoma cells but also the cultured cells could induce RSV with a similar frequency when UV-HVJ was added to the mixed cultures to fuse them with chick embryo cells.

Cell Fusion as a Prerequisite for RSV Induction

Since cell fusion seems to be required for the induction of RSV production, the correlation between cell fusion and RSV induction was examined. The procedures used for cell fusion followed those described by Okada (*11*), with some modifications. Rous sarcoma cells and chick embryo cells were each suspended in modified Hanks' solution, inoculated into a test tube, and then UV-HVJ was added. The cells clumped immediately and the size of the clumps was roughly proportional to the amount of virus added. The tube was kept in an ice water bath for 20 min and was shaken for an additional 20 min at 37°. During this time the cells in the clumps were observed to undergo various degrees of cell fusion (*11*). The time course of the acquisition of RSV-inducing ability of SR-C3H-2127 cells during cell fusion reaction is shown in Fig. 1. The number of cells that produced RSV and became infective centers was proportional to the degree of cell fusion during the time of the reaction. This finding indicates that infectious RSV may be produced in heterokaryons of Rous sarcoma and chick embryo cells.

Okada *et al.* (*12*) and Okada and Murayama (*13*) have reported that the aggre-

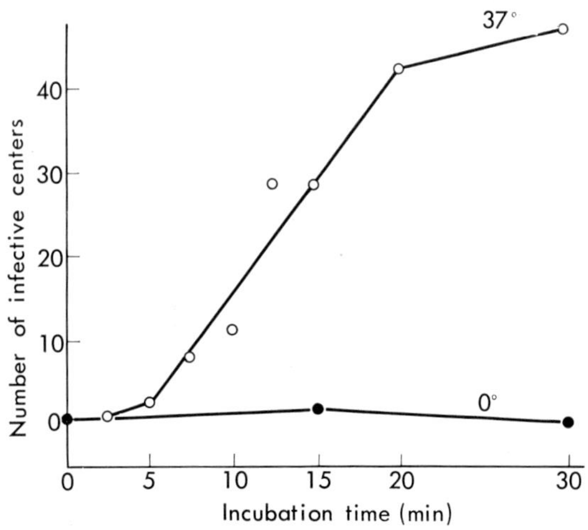

FIG. 1. Time course of RSV induction during incubation with shaking at 37°

Samples of 0.3 ml of γ-irradiated SR-C3H-2127 cell suspension (2.7×10^6 cells / ml), 0.3 ml of chick embryo cell suspension (8.0×10^6 / ml), and 0.4 ml of HVJ-antiserum mixture (prepared with equal volumes of 5,000 HAU / ml of HVJ and 20 HIU / ml of antiserum), were mixed in 2 series of test tubes. After keeping the tubes at 0° for 20 min they were incubated at 37° with shaking. At a certain interval, incubation was stopped by adding 3 ml of cold 1 mM EDTA solution to the samples. Aliquots of one-fourth of the sample were distributed into petri dishes and the number of infective centers was counted after incubation for 7 days at 40° under agar medium (○). ● control, kept at 0°, without shaking at 37°.

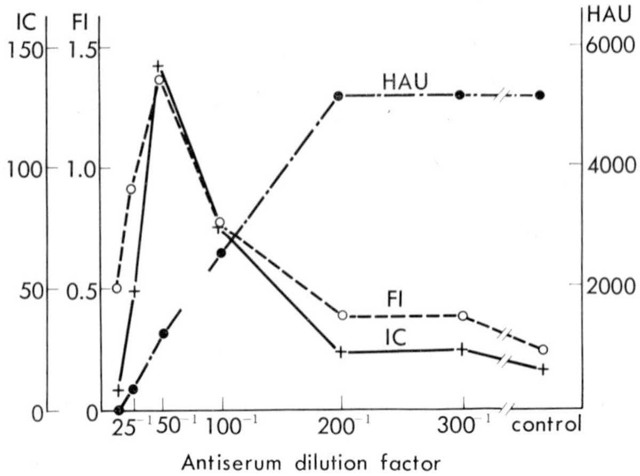

FIG. 2. The effect of anti-HVJ serum on HA titers, cell fusion activity, and RSV-inducing activity of HVJ

An HVJ suspension (5,000 HAU / ml) and a serially diluted anti-HVJ serum were mixed in equal volumes. After incubation for 60 min at room temperature and overnight at 4°, each sample was determined for its HA titers, cell fusion activity, and RSV-inducing activity. The cell fusion activity of each sample was expressed as a fusion index (FI), calculated after the cell fusion reaction using SR-C3H-2127 cells. RSV-inducing activity was estimated by infective center (IC) assay: After the cell fusion reaction had taken place in the presence of HVJ treated with anti-HVJ serum, the mixed cultures were prepared with 2×10^5 or 2×10^4 γ-irradiated SR-C3H-2127 cells and 6×10^5 chick embryo cells per plate, and the number of infective centers (IC) was counted after 7 days' incubation. ○ FI; ● HAU / ml; + number of IC per 2.0×10^5 SR-C3H-2127 cells.

gates of HVJ formed by the addition of anti-HVJ serum had a higher cell fusion activity than that of untreated HVJ. The RSV-inducing activity of UV-HVJ was also affected by anti-HVJ serum. The RSV-inducing activity decreased when an excess of anti-HVJ serum was used but increased when appropriately diluted anti-HVJ serum was used. The HVJ-anti-HVJ mixture with a higher RSV-inducing activity also had a higher cell fusion activity, despite the fact that its hemagglutinating activity was lower than that of the untreated HVJ (Fig. 2). These findings also suggest that Rous sarcoma cells are induced to produce RSV, not by contact or aggregation with chick embryo cells, but by fusion with them.

Since it was suggested that initiation of virus multiplication occurred in heterokaryons, the number of heterokaryons was compared with that of infective centers (Table III). The results indicated that only 1% of heterokaryons were giving rise to infective centers. The RSV induced from SR-C3H-2127 cells belongs to subgroup D of RSV (*5*), and the low susceptibility of chick embryo cells to infection by RSV of this subgroup has been reported previously (*23*). It was, therefore, suggested that the low ratio of infective centers to heterokaryons may be due to the less efficient transmission of RSV from heterokaryons to neighboring chick embryo cells, and some RSV-producing heterokaryons may fail to be registered as infective centers. Svoboda and Dourmashkin have reported that 10–100%

TABLE III. Foci in Mixed Cultures in Relation to Numbers of Heterokaryons[a]

Expt. No.	Presence of UV-HVJ	Ratios of heterokaryons to labeled nuclei	Ratios of labeled nuclei to chick embryo nuclei	No. of chick embryo nuclei per dish ($\times 10^4$)	Calculated No. of heterokaryons per dish ($\times 10^3$)	No. of foci per dish	Foci as percentage of hetero-karyons
1	+	210/1544	406/2533	42.3±3.5[b]	9.2	93.0±5.2[b]	1.01
	–	1/1387				0	0
2	+	233/1439	451/2862	33.6±2.7	8.6	84.0±2.0	0.97
	–	0/1500				0	0

[a] The cell fusion reaction was performed with SR-C3H-2127 cells that had been prelabeled with ^{3}H-thymidine, and chick embryo cells using UV-HVJ. The reaction mixture was inoculated into petri dishes; one of the dishes contained coverslips. After incubation for 16 hr, the cultures were overlaid with agar medium to allow development of foci. Coverslips were fixed and the portion of heterokaryons was determined by autoradiography. The number of chick embryo nuclei attached to a petri dish was determined by enumeration of nuclei at 16 hr after cell fusion reaction.

[b] Standard deviation of mean.

of heterokaryons of RSV-transformed Chinese hamster cells and chick embryo cells formed infective centers (*19*), and recently Machala *et al.* (*8*) showed that all heterokaryons produced RSV coat antigen. There may be some difference in the state of the viral genome in various mammalian Rous sarcoma cells. In SV40-transformed cells, 1 to 20% of the heterokaryons were reported to produce infectious virus (*7*, *26*).

Effect of Excess Thymidine on RSV Induction

Replication of RSV in chick embryo cells can be divided into at least 2 stages. The initiation of RSV infection is blocked by a low concentration of actinomycin D, an inhibitor of transcription, and by inhibitors of DNA synthesis such as amethopterin, fluorodeoxyuridine, 5-fluorouracil, bromo- and iodo-deoxyuridine, cytocine arabinoside, and high concentrations of thymidine. After RSV infection is established, however, the inhibitors of DNA synthesis no longer interfere with RSV production. On the other hand, RSV production remains sensitive to actinomycin D (see *25*). Although the interpretation of these effects leaves much room for speculat.on, the recent discovery of RNA-dependent DNA polymerase in virus particles (*1*, *22*) favors Temin's hypothesis that the replication of RSV RNA involves DNA " provirus " (*21*).

Synthesis of DNA in chick embryo cells can be suppressed effectively and specifically by 20 mM thymidine (*9*). The concentration of thymidine also blocked DNA synthesis in SR-C3H-2127 cells. The effect in SR-C3H-2127 cells was irreversible and the continuous exposure of this compound for 20 hr resulted in death of the cells. Since the effect of thymidine is reversible in chick embryo cells (*9*), the requirement for DNA synthesis in RSV induction was examined using thymidine.

The frequency of RSV-induction in the mixed cultures assayed by infective

TABLE IV. Effect of Excess Thymidine on RSV Induction[a]

Expt. No.	Treatment with thymidine after cell fusion (hr)	Foci/dish
1	0	111 ± 7.1[b]
	0–12	114 ± 29.8
2	0	78 ± 11.0
	0–48	80 ± 10.2

[a] Chick embryo and irradiated SR-C3H–2127 cells were fused with UV-HVJ and seeded in petri dishes with normal or thymidine-containing media. In experiment 2, chick embryo cells were also irradiated with 7,000 R to inhibit restoration of DNA synthesis after thymidine removal. After the treatment with thymidine, the cells were overlaid with normal agar medium and the number of infective centers was counted after 9 days of incubation at 38°. The number of irradiated SR-C3H-2127 cells per petri dish was 2×10^5 (expt. 1) and 10^5 (expt. 2).

[b] Standard deviation of mean.

centers showed no change with thymidine treatment (Table IV). Although the RSV yield in the mixed cultures was slightly reduced by thymidine treatment (Fig. 3), this slight decrease in RSV production may not be significant and may be due to the toxic effect of thymidine on SR-2127 cells, because even pretreatment of the cells with thymidine before cell fusion also caused some decrease in RSV yield.

These findings show that the initiation of RSV production in heterokaryons does not require DNA synthesis, in contrast to RSV infection in chick embryo

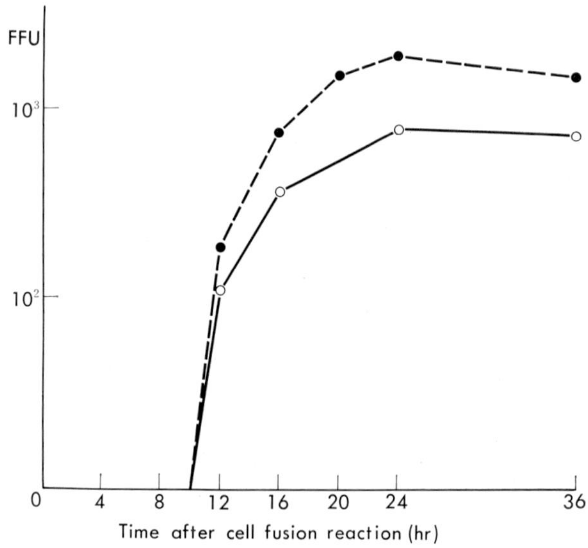

FIG. 3. Effect of excess thymidine on RSV-induction

Chick embryo and SR-C3H-2127 cells were incubated for 8 hr in medium containing thymidine (20 mM) and they were mixed, fused with UV-HVJ, washed to remove thymidine, and seeded in petri dishes (1.2×10^6 chick embryo and 6×10^5 SR-C3H-2127 cells per dish) with normal (●) or thymidine-containing (○) medium. The media were replaced by fresh media at 4-hour intervals, frozen and later assayed for RSV.

cells which does require it, and further suggest that RSV has completed its first stage of replication in mammalian Rous sarcoma cells. The factor(s) responsible for the induction of RSV in heterokaryons provided by chick embryo cells is not known. Chick embryo cells may derepress the RSV genome or supply some factor(s) needed for viral maturation. At present it is difficult to conclude which of these alternatives is operative.

REFERENCES

1. Baltimore, D. RNA-dependent DNA polymerase in virion of RNA tumor viruses. *Nature*, **226**, 1209–1211 (1970).
2. Fogel, M., and Sachs, L. The activation of virus synthesis in polyoma-transformed cells. *Virology*, **37**, 327–334 (1969).
3. Gerber, P. Studies on the transfer of subviral infectivity from SV40-induced hamster tumor cells to indicator cells. *Virology*, **28**, 501–509 (1966).
4. Harris, H., and Watkins, J. F. Hybrid cells derived from mouse and man: Artificial heterokaryons of mammalian cells from different species. *Nature*, **205**, 640–646 (1965).
5. Kawai, S., and Yamamoto, T. Isolation of different kinds of non-virus-producing chick cells transformed by Schmidt-Ruppin strain (subgroup A) of Rous sarcoma virus. *Japan. J. Exp. Med.*, **40**, 243–256 (1970).
6. Koprowski, H., and Jensen, F. Transmission of tumor viruses in heterokaryons. *Federation Proc.*, **26**, 313 (1967).
7. Koprowski, H., Jensen, F. C., and Steplewski, Z. Activation of production of infectious tumor virus SV40 in heterokaryon cultures. *Proc. Natl. Acad. Sci. U.S.*, **58**, 127–133 (1967).
8. Machala, O., Donner, L., and Svoboda, J. A full expression of the genome of Rous sarcoma virus in heterokaryons formed after fusion of virogenic mammalian cells and chicken fibroblasts. *J. Gen. Virol.*, **8**, 219–229 (1970).
9. Nakata, Y., and Bader, J. P. Studies on the fixation and development of cellular transformation by Rous sarcoma virus. *Virology*, **36**, 401–410 (1968).
10. Okada, Y., Suzuki, T., and Hosaka, Y. Interaction between influenza virus and Ehrlich's tumor cells. III. Fusion phenomenon of Ehrlich's tumor cells by the action of HVJ Z strain. *Med. J. Osaka Univ.*, **7**, 709–717 (1957).
11. Okada, Y. Analysis of giant polynuclear cell formation caused by HVJ virus from Ehrlich's ascites tumor cells. I. Microscopic observation of giant polynuclear cell formation. *Exp. Cell Res.*, **26**, 98–107 (1962).
12. Okada, Y., Yamada, K., and Tadokoro, J. Effect of antiserum on the cell fusion reaction caused by HVJ. *Virology*, **22**, 397–409 (1964).
13. Okada, Y., and Murayama, F. Fusion of cells by HVJ: Requirement of concentration of virus particles at the site of contact of two cells for fusion. *Exp. Cell Res.*, **52**, 34–42 (1968).
14. Puck, T. T., Marcus, P. I., and Cieciura, S. J. Clonal growth of mammalian cells *in vitro*: Growth characteristics of colonies from single HeLa cells with and without a " feeder " layer. *J. Exp. Med.*, **103**, 273–284 (1956).
15. Shevliaghyn, V. J., Biryulina, T. I., Tikhonova, Z. N., and Karazas, N. V. Activation of Rous virus in the transplanted golden hamster tumor with the aid of artificial heterokaryon formation. *Int. J. Cancer*, **4**, 42–46 (1969).
16. Svoboda, J., Machala, O., and Hlozánek, I. Influence of Sendai virus on RSV

formation in mixed culture of virogenic mammalian cells and chicken fibroblasts. *Folia Biol.* (*Praha*), **13**, 155–157 (1967).

17. Svoboda, J., Hlozánek, T., and Machala, O. Rescue of Rous sarcoma virus in mixed cultures of virogenic mammalian and chicken cells, treated and untreated with Sendai virus and detected by focus assay. *J. Gen. Virol.*, **2**, 461–464 (1968).
18. Svoboda, J., and Machala, O. Early steps in Sendai virus-mediated rescue of Rous sarcoma virus from virogenic mammalian cells. *J. Virol.*, **2**, 951–952 (1968).
19. Svoboda, J., and Dourmashkin, R. Rescue of Rous sarcoma virus from virogenic mammalian cells associated with chick embryo cells and treated with Sendai virus. *J. Gen. Virol.*, **4**, 523–529 (1969).
20. Takeuchi, M., Hino, S., and Yamamoto, T. Studies on Rous sarcoma virus in mice. II. Clonal analysis of cell populations of the SR-RSV-induced mouse ascites sarcoma (SR-C3H/He ascites . *Japan. J. Exp. Med.*, **37**, 107–120 (1967).
21. Temin, H. M. Carcinogenesis by avian sarcoma viruses. *Cancer Res.*, **28**, 1835–1838 (1968).
22. Temin, H. M., and Mizutani, S. RNA-dependent DNA polymerase in virions of Rous sarcoma virus. *Nature*, **226**, 1211–1213 (1970).
23. Toyoshima, K., and Vogt, P. K. Enhancement and inhibition of avian sarcoma viruses by polycations and polyanions. *Virology*, **38**, 414–426 (1969).
24. Vigier, P. Persistence du genome du virus de Rous dans des cellules du hamster converties *in vitro*, et action du virus Sendai inactivé sur sa transmission aux cellules de poule. *Compt. Rend.*, **264**, 422–425 (1967).
25. Vogt, P. K. Avian tumor viruses. *In* " Advances in Virus Research," ed. by K. H. Smith and M. A. Laufer, Academic Press, New York, Vol. 11, pp. 293–385 (1965).
26. Watkins, J. F., and Dulbecco, R. Production of SV40 virus in heterokaryons of transformed and susceptible cells. *Proc. Natl. Acad. Sci. U.S.*, **58**, 1396–1403 (1967).
27. Yamaguchi, N., Takeuchi, M., and Yamamoto, T. Rous sarcoma virus production in mixed culture of mouse tumor cells and chicken embryo fibroblasts by the addition of UV-irradiated HVJ. *Japan. J. Exp. Med.*, **37**, 83–86 (1967).
28. Yamaguchi, N., Takeuchi, M., and Yamamoto, T. Rous sarcoma virus production in mixed cultures of mammalian Rous sarcoma cells and chick embryo cells. *Int. J. Cancer*, **4**, 678–689 (1969).
29. Yamamoto, T., and Takeuchi, M. Studies on Rous sarcoma virus in mice. I. Establishment of an ascites sarcoma induced by Schmidt-Ruppin strain of Rous sarcoma virus in C3H/He mouse. *Japan. J. Exp. Med.*, **37**, 37–50 (1967).

ROLE OF AN AVIAN SARCOMA VIRUS GENOME IN CELL TRANSFORMATION*

Kumao TOYOSHIMA†

*Department of Microbiology, University of Washington***

Many mutants isolated after UV irradiation had lost the capacity to transform cells, though the capacity to replicate was fully maintained. Two temperature-sensitive mutants tested showed temperature-sensitive regulation of cell transformation. These results suggest that a) some function(s) of the viral genome is required for the initiation of cell transformation as well as for its maintenance (this supports the third postulate in the introduction); b) certain steps of virus replication are needed for the fixation of the tumor-producing capacity of the virus; and c) the transforming function does not directly affect virus reproduction.

In this paper, I would like to discuss the function of the viral genome in cells transformed by an avian sarcoma virus. At the beginning of my studies, my colleagues and I postulated the role of this virus in cell transformation as one of the following: 1) the enhancement of natural transformation by nongenetic damage in cells, for example, by effecting membrane changes which release cells from contact inhibition; 2) modification of the cell genome as a result of virus infection as may occur during the process of integration of the viral DNA into the cell DNA; or 3) transformation of the cell by the action of a principle encoded in the viral genome. In order to test these possibilities, two different approaches were employed. One was modification of the viral genome by ultraviolet (UV) irradiation and the other was the analysis of temperature-sensitive (ts) mutants. Detailed data were described elsewhere (*5*, *13*, *14*).

An avian sarcoma virus, Bratislava 77 (*12*) was used for this experiment. This virus was chosen because of its wide host range (*2*, *7*), and because of the simplicity of its mode of infection (*2*).

Modification of the Viral Genome by UV Irradiation

The response of avian sarcoma viruses to UV irradiation has been extensively studied by Rubin and his co-workers (*4*, *8*, *10*, *11*). For the most part our results were consistent with their findings: namely, avian tumor viruses are much more resistant to inactivation by UV irradiation than ordinary myxoviruses, and radio-

* Supported by United States Public Health Service Research Grant No. CA 10569 from the National Cancer Institute, National Institutes of Health.

** Seattle, Washington 98105, U.S.A. (豊島久真男).

† Present address: Research Institute for Microbial Diseases, Osaka University, Osaka.

induced damages are not rescuable by co-infection with Rous-associated virus (RAV). In our experiment, foci produced by UV-irradiated B77 virus were isolated onto feeder cells by the techniques of Duff and Vogt (*2*), and were tested for their capacity to maintain the transformed state as well as the capacity to produce progeny virus. Unexpectedly, transformed cells disappeared from some cultures after several transfers. The percentage of cultures that lost their transformed cells increased with increasing doses of UV irradiation (Fig. 1). These cultures were not synthesizing sarcoma virus during the course of the regression of transformation. Other cultures, in which the number of transformed cells was increasing, produced various amounts of sarcoma virus. Cultures that had regressing foci were tested for resistance to superinfection by the original B77 virus. The majority of such cultures, 32 out of 37, were resistant and were found to produce viruses that could not transform fibroblasts but could induce interference with B77 virus. In the second series of UV experiments, foci produced by UV-irradiated B77 virus were planted onto feeder cells and observed for 5 days under agar overlay. Twenty foci were selected as nonproducers on the basis of the fact that they did not induce rapid transformation of feeder cells. These foci were placed into microplate wells and cultivated for 4 to 5 days without feeder cells. Supernatant fluids were tested for transforming and interfering capacities (Table I). Fifteen out of 20 foci released nontransforming virus which was detectable by interference tests. Five of these produced B77 virus simultaneously with nontransforming virus. These nontransforming viruses were serologically indistinguishable from B77 virus and had the same host range as B77. These viruses were designated as nontransforming B77 (NT-B77).

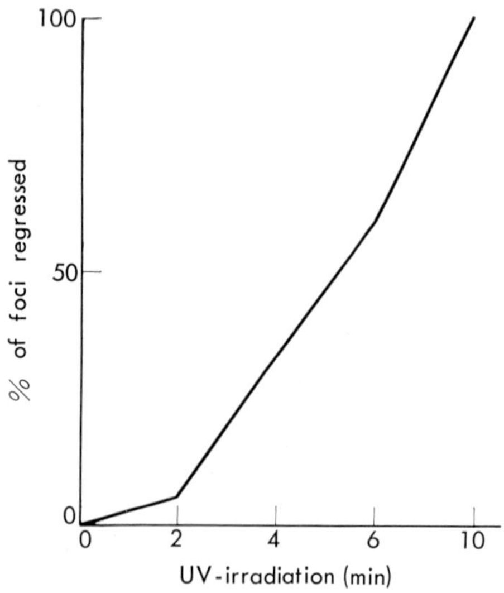

FIG. 1. Rate of regression of foci induced by UV-irradiated B77
This figure is based on Table I in Toyoshima *et al.* (*14*). Foci produced in chick embryo fibroblast cultures under agar were transferred more than 5 times at 3-day intervals.

TABLE I. Analysis of Virus Production by "Less-Progressive" Foci Induced by UV-irradiated B77 Virus at the Second Transfer

Production of virus		No. of samples
B77	NT-B77	
+	−	5
+	+	5
−	+	10
−	−	0
Total		20

Origin of NT-B77 and the Meaning of UV Experiments

Since the starting pools of B77 virus were made from a stock cloned twice in the absence of associated virus in excess of the sarcoma virus titer, NT-B77 isolates are likely to be radio-induced mutants of B77 virus. The possibility has not been excluded, however, that this cloned virus segregated small amounts of associated virus which were less sensitive to UV-radiation. The NT-B77 isolates are probably the direct descendants of B77 viruses.

The mechanism of regression of transformation induced by UV-irradiated viruses is unclear, although the correlation between regression of transformation and absence of transforming virus was clear.

Similar findings were reported by Goldé (*6*), with the radio-induced NT-mutants of the Schmidt-Ruppin strain of Rous sarcoma virus (SR-RSV). She described NP cells as being still cancerous. However, the tumorigenic doses of $1.2–6\times10^5$ were very high, considering her belief that one-third of the cultured cells were transformed. This may also suggest partial regression of cell transformation. The NT-mutants retain complete information for replication and these results indicate that the reproducing capacity of the viruses is completely separable from the transforming capacity. The capacity to transform cells, however, seems to be dependent on virus-reproducing capacity to a considerable extent because the occurrence of the transformed foci not producing any virus is quite rare.

Requirements for Sarcoma Virus Genome Functions to Cause and Maintain the Transformation of Cells

In transformation induced by avian sarcoma viruses, some expression(s) of viral function has been maintained. In DNA viruses many ts-mutants have been isolated, but none of them so far has shown temperature-sensitive regulation of cell transformation (*1*, *3*). This observation does not support the requirement for continuous expression of the viral genome in the maintenance of transformation.

Attempts were made to isolate temperature-sensitive mutants of B77 virus in order to study the genetic function of a sarcoma virus in cell transformation. Since the efficiency of transformation is very high with avian sarcoma viruses, cell-transforming capacity could be employed as the marker to select ts-mutants. The physiological characteristics of the initial 2 mutants isolated have been studied.

1. Temperature-sensitive regulation of transformation by ts-mutants

The 2 mutants (ts-75 and ts-149) produced foci at 35° (permissive temperature), but not at 41° (nonpermissive temperature). In addition to this temperature sensitivity, the foci produced by these mutants at 35° became unrecognizable when the culture were shifted to 41°, while foci roduced by wild-type B77 virus increased in size regardless of the temperature (Photos 1–3). This morphological reversion of transformed cells was discernible as early as 4 hr after shifting to 41°. When these cultures were shifted to permissive temperature again, the foci reappeared (Table II). Reappearance of foci usually began about 6 hr after shift down and was completed 2 days later. At this time, all the foci marked before shifting up had reappeared. These results indicate that the function of the viral genome is continuously required for maintenance of the transformed state as well as for the induction of transformation.

TABLE II. Effect of Temperature-shift on the Foci Produced by ts-75 and ts-149

Virus clone	Plate sign	No. of foci per plate		
		35° 7 days	Shift up[a] 2 days	Shift down[b] 1 days
ts–75	L–0	660	0	165
	L–1	37	0	11
ts–149	L–0	2000	±[c]	TNTC[d]
	L–1	210	0	41
wt–141[e]	L–1	265	265	240
	L–2	nc[f]	20	nc

[a] After counting the foci produced at 35°, cultures were shifted to 40.5°.
[b] Cultures incubated for 2 days at 40.5° were shifted again to 35°.
[c] Could not count, but not completely negative. [d] Too numerous to count.
[e] Wild-type B77 clone. [f] Not counted.

2. Temperature sensitivity of 2 ts-mutants with respect to replication

The mutants ts-75 and ts-149 were also temperature sensitive in their replication, but at different steps. Mutant ts-75 had a temperature-sensitive function in a late replication step. Virus production of the cells infected with ts-75 stopped quickly by shifting to 41° even after transfers at 35°, but these cells retained the capacity of virus production if shifted to 35° again. If the cells were infected at 41°, group-specific (gs) antigen and virus RNA were synthesized and accumulated in the cells, although production of viruses or noninfectious particles was not observed. Maturation of the virus occurred almost instantaneously after shifting the culture to 35°. Mutant ts-149 was sensitive in an early function. When the cells infected with this virus at 35° were shifted to 41°, the cells continued to synthesize virus although transformation disappeared several hours after shifting. Cells infected with ts-149 at 41° did not produce virus or any virus component tested. After 3 days of incubation at 41° these cells did not fully recover their virus-producing capacity. Early shift experiments from 35° to 41° suggested that the temperature-sensitive step of ts-149 replication had already begun 6 hr after infection and was completed within 18 hr after infection.

3. *Fixation of the transforming capacity*

Cultures infected with ts-75 at 41° fully retained the capacity to produce foci if they were shifted to 35° as late as 7 days after infection. On the other hand, cultures infected with ts-149 at 41° gradually lost the transforming capacity if they were shifted to 35°C after 3 days. These facts, together with the temperature sensitivities in virus replication, suggest that an early function in virus replication is needed, not only for the fixation of the virus-reproducing capacity, but also for fixation of the cell-transforming capacity.

Recently, Martin reported the isolation of ts-mutants from SR-RSV A (*9*). The representative strain of his isolates, T 1, was temperature sensitive only in transforming ability and not in virus replication. This strain grew well at 41° and progeny made at this temperature retained full potential for transformation. The foci produced by this strain were also reversible by shifting the temperature to 41°. All these results are compatible with our findings.

4. *Behavior of the ts-mutants in soft agar and* in vivo

Cells infected with wild-type B77 produced compact colonies in soft agar both at 35° and at 41°. Those infected with ts-mutants produced compact colonies at 35° and flat colonies at 41° in soft agar, whereas noninfected cells did not grow in agar. This means that some modifications of cells by ts-mutants were recognizable even at 41°.

These ts-mutants failed to produce sarcomas when inoculated into chicks, although a focus-forming unit of wild-type B77 roughly corresponds to a tumor-producing dose. This is not surprising, because the body temperature of the chick is 41°. Further autologous transplantation experiments were conducted. Fibroblasts transformed *in vitro* at 35° were inoculated into wing webs of the

TABLE III. Autologous Transplantation of Chick Fibroblasts Transformed *in Vitro* by ts-Mutants at Permissive Temperature

Virus	No. of chicks	Tumor		Inoculum	
		+ or − No.	Days P. I.	$\times 10^5$ Cells	$\times 10^3$ FFU
ts-75	8	+4	11–16	5.6–18	3.2–84
		−4	—	2.0–12	4.0–44
ts-149	8	+1	14	4.4	3.6
		−7	—	1.6–10	1.6–74
wt-141†	4	+4	5–10	1.0–10	4.6–80
		−0	—	—	—

Adaptation of Table IV from Friis *et al.* (*5*). † A wild-type clone.

birds from which the fibroblast cultures had been prepared, and tumor production was observed (Table III). Tumors appeared rapidly in all birds inoculated with cells transformed by wild-type B77. However, the tumor production of the cells transformed by ts-mutants was slow and had a lower frequency. Most of the tumors produced by cells transformed with ts-mutants might be explained by leakiness of the mutants.

CONCLUSIONS

From our results (*5*, *13*, *14*), together with the results reported by Martin (*9*) and Goldé (*6*), we may tentatively conclude that a) some function(s) of the viral genome is required for the initiation of cell transformation as well as for its maintenance (this supports the third postulation in the introduction); b) certain steps of virus replication are needed for the fixation of the tumor-producing capacity of the virus; and c) the transforming function does not directly affect virus reproduction.

Acknowledgments

I would like to thank Dr. P. K. Vogt and Dr. R. R. Friis for discussing the manuscript and Susan Norwood, Sally Olson, and Christel Allgaier for excellent technical assistance.

REFERENCES

1. Di Mayorca, G., Callender, J., Marin, G., and Giordano, R. Temperature-sensitive mutants of polyoma virus. *Virology*, **38**, 126–133 (1969).
2. Duff, R. G., and Vogt, P. K. Characteristics of two new avian tumor virus subgroups. *Virology*, **39**, 18–30 (1969).
3. Eckhart, W. Complementation and transformation by temperature-sensitive mutants of polyoma virus. *Virology*, **38**, 120–125 (1969).
4. Friesen, B., and Rubin, H. Some physicochemical and immunological properties of an avian leukosis virus (RIF). *Virology*, **15**, 387–396 (1961).
5. Friis, R. R., Toyoshima, K., and Vogt, P. K. Conditional lethal mutants of avian sarcoma viruses. I. Physiology of ts 75 and ts 149. *Virology*, **43**, 375–389 (1971).
6. Goldé, A. Radio-induced mutants of the Schmidt-Ruppin strain of Rous sarcoma virus. *Virology*, **40**, 1022–1029 (1970).
7. Hlavayová, E., Smida, J., Altaner, C., and Svec, F. Pathogenicity of virus B77 in rats. *Folia Biol.* (*Praha*), **10**, 301–306 (1964).
8. Levinson, W., and Rubin, H. Radiation studies of avian tumor viruses and of Newcastle disease virus. *Virology*, **28**, 533–542 (1966).
9. Martin, G. S. Rous sarcoma virus: A function required for the maintenance of the transformed state. *Nature*, **227**, 1021–1023 (1970).
10. Rubin, H. Growth of Rous sarcoma virus in chick embryo cells following irradiation of host cells or free virus. *Virology*, **11**, 28–47 (1960).
11. Rubin, H., and Temin, H. M. A radiological study of cell-virus interaction in the Rous sarcoma. *Virology*, **7**, 75–91 (1959).
12. Thurzo, V., Smida, J., Smidova-Kovarova, V., and Simkovic, D. Some properties

of the fowl virus tumor B77. *Acta Int. Union Against Cancer*, **19**, 304–305 (1963).
13. Toyoshima, K., and Vogt, P. K. Temperature-sensitive mutants of an avian sarcoma virus. *Virology*, **39**, 930–931 (1969).
14. Toyoshima, K., Friis, R. R., and Vogt, P. K. The reproductive and cell-transforming capacities of avian sarcoma virus B77: Inactivation with UV light. *Virology*, **42**, 163–170 (1970).

EXPLANATION OF PHOTOS

PHOTO 1. Morphological change in a focus produced by ts-75 after temperature shift. a: A focus of ts-75 after 5 days at 36°. b: The same focus, 66 hr after shift to 41°.

PHOTO 2. Morphological change of a focus produced by ts-149 after temperature shift. a: A focus of ts-149 after 5 days at 36°. b: The same focus, 60 hr after shift to 41°.

PHOTO 3. A focus produced by a wild-type 577 (wt-140). a: After five days at 36°. b: The same focus, 66 hr after shift to 41°.

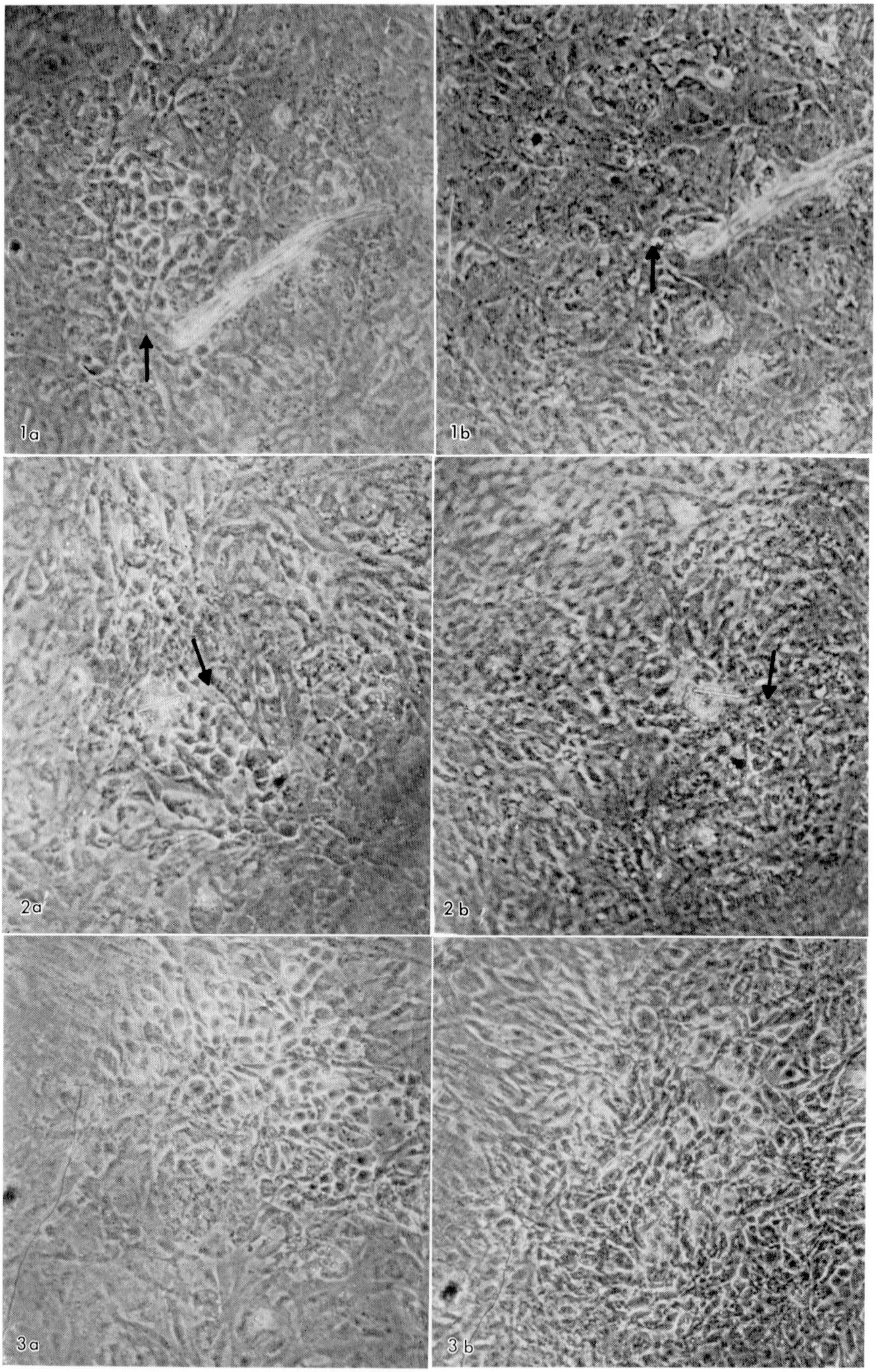
1a
1b
2a
2b
3a
3b

GANN Monograph on Cancer Research 12, 1972

SYNTHESIS OF MURINE LEUKEMIA VIRUS: ELECTRON MICROSCOPIC AUTORADIOGRAPHY

Hiromitsu OKANO and Marvin A. RICH
Department of Pathology, Cancer Research Institute, Faculty of Medicine, Kyushu University and*
*Department of Cell Biology, Albert Einstein Medical Center***

Synthesis of murine leukemia virus (Rich), particularly in the terminal phase of maturation, was studied by a high-resolution technique of electron microscopic autoradiography. The results obtained suggest (1) that the interval between RNA synthesis and assembly of complete virions is brief (less than 1 hr); (2) that the enveloped or budding A particles, representing an early virion stage, may be subsequently transformed into C-type virions; and (3) that there is no extensive lag between cellular and viral RNA labeling.

While the viral etiology of murine leukemia and mammary tumor has been extensively documented, relatively little is known of the specific mechanisms involved. Our direct knowledge of the specific events that occur during infection and viral proliferation is limited to the electron microscopic visualization of viral materials during the terminal phase of their maturation at cell surfaces (*3*, *4*, *6*, *11*, *13*). Knowledge concerning the modes, site, and duration of the intracellular events following infection is at present lacking. The sequence of events that occur during the assembling of viral components is similarly unknown.

It is generally assumed, however, that the C-type virions in mouse leukemia and the B-type virions in mouse mammary tumor represent later stages of virion maturation than such virions as enveloped A or budding A. But there has been little evidence to support this hypothesis. The techniques of high-resolution electron microscopic autoradiography can be used to elucidate the intracellular components of the terminal phase of viral synthesis. In a preliminary study, Okano and Rich reported the time parameter for viral synthesis following the exposure of infected cells to tritiated uridine (*9*). The time parameter for viral proliferation and the mode of viral maturation can be estimated, using virus proliferating mouse (ICR/Ha Swiss) embryo fibroblasts which had been infected, in culture, with murine leukemia virus (Rich, ref. *12*), and labeling the virus with tritiated uridine. The specific labelings of virus with tritiated uridine have been demonstrated by Duesberg and Robinson on murine leukemia virus (*5*), and by Cardiff *et al.* on mammary tumor virus (*2*).

Virions and developed silver grains can be counted under the electron microscope. In our experiments, all virions with characteristic A- and C-type

* Katakasu 1,276, Fukuoka 812 (岡野博光).
** Philadelphia, Pennsylvania 19141, U.S.A.

morphologies in each 15 to 20 grid squares, chosen at random, at each time interval, were examined for the presence of overlying silver grains.

Photographs 1a and 1b show typical silver grain deposition on the virions of A and C types. The two electron micrographs designated 1a and 1b show the same area in each consecutive section, indicating clearly the same pattern of silver deposition on the area of virion localization. This shows that the grain deposition indicates the specific radioactivity from the labeled virions. Photographs 2 and 3 show silver grain deposition after 1-hr exposure and continuous exposure, respectively.

Despite the short exposure and incubation period, the first appearance of labeled virions occurred as early as 1 hr after the start of exposure. The proportion of labeled virions increased during the first 7 hr after the 1-hr exposure and reached a plateau at approximately 13%.

Over the time period from 30 min to 24 hr of continuous exposure to ^{3}H-uridine, the proportion of labeled virions rose to 30%. The labeling patterns following continuous and pulse exposure to tritiated uridine are compared in Fig. 1.

Using the proportion of labeled virions from the continuous exposure data, a logistic equation could be expected (*8*) from the rate curve (when the time scale is transformed by logarithm (Fig. 1)). According to Morisita's theory (*8*) on the logistic equation, an asymptote value was calculated from this curve to be 30.79%. This is the theoretical maximal value, shortly after 24 hr of incubation with ^{3}H-uridine. As was shown in this study, the actual labeling rate (30.0%) of virions was very close to this theoretical rate (30.79%). This suggests that the ^{3}H-uridine added to the culture media had been depleted and that the synthesis of labeled RNA had terminated at this time.

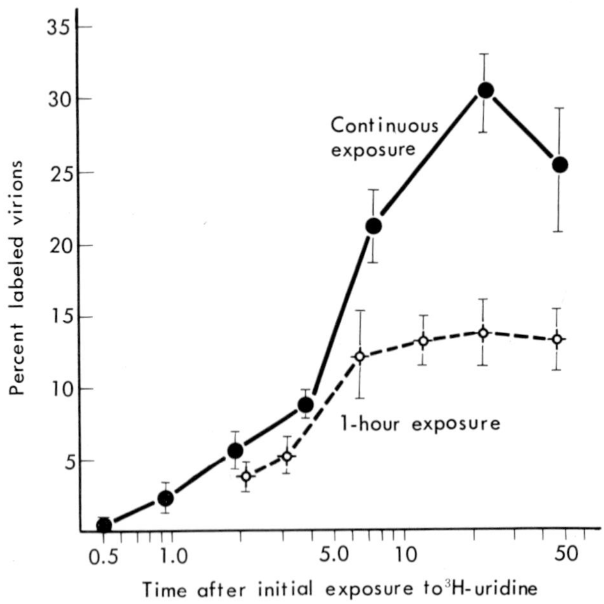

FIG. 1. Patterns of total virion labeling in both pulse (broken line) and continuous exposure experiments (solid line)

To compare cellular and viral incorporation of RNA precursors, the cells chosen randomly from each of 10 grid squares at each time interval were examined by autoradiography. The counts were performed on a 1 μ^2 area of nucleoplasm, nucleolus, and adjacent cytoplasm. The results clearly showed that the site of the first appearance of silver grains after exposure to ^{3}H-uridine was the nucleolus. On the nucleus and on the cytoplasm, in both pulse and continuous exposure groups, the silver grains that developed were few in number in the early period of incubation. Following this period, the silver grains deposited on the cytoplasmic area rapidly increased in number, reaching a maximum at 24 hr of incubation and decreased at 48 hr in both experimental groups. In contrast to the increasing density of silver grains on the cytoplasm, the labeling of the nucleus and nucleolus decreased gradually (pulse exposure) or remained constant (continuous exposure).

A comparison of the labeling patterns of various cell components indicated that the pattern of cytoplasmic labeling was quite similar to that observed on virions. This similarity suggests that the synthesis of viral RNA occurs quite rapidly, paralleling the synthesis of cytoplasmic RNA. The minimum time from the administration of ^{3}H-uridine to the appearance of morphologically distinct, labeled virions represents the maximum time required for viral synthesis. The data presented here suggest that this time period does not exceed 1 hr. Rabotti *et al.* (*10*) and Michelson-Fiske *et al.* (*7*), using autoradiographic techniques, reported similar time values for the synthesis of Rous sarcoma virus. Bader, using direct chemical analysis, found labeled RNA in avian and murine leukemia virions within 2 hr of addition of radioactive uridine to the infected cultures (*1*).

In the continuous exposure experiment, the proportion of labeled A-type and C-type virions was determined separately at each time interval. The rate of labeling observed for A-type virions was greater than that of C-type virions. This is more clearly compatible with the hypothesis that C-type virions arise from A-type virions. This is supported by the ratio of A-type to C-type particles as a function of time exposure to tritiated uridine. The ratio of labeled A-type to C-type virions was 1: 1 at the shortest exposure (1 hr), reflecting the approximate equalness in number of labeled A- to C-type virions after this period of exposure. This A/C ratio decreased with longer exposure to ^{3}H-uridine, as the number of labeled C-type virions increased. The temporal relationship and relative rates of labeling for A- and C-type virions presented in this study suggest that C-type virions arise from A-type virions, and that this conversion occurs at a somewhat slower rate than does the synthesis of A-type virions.

The A/C ratio was estimated by de Harven to be around 2 to 5% in Friend leukemia virus from culture fluid (*3*). Since the counting was done in his study on the virions within the culture fluid, and the budding virions were not included, the resultant A/C ratio was lower than that of our study.

In conclusion, the results suggest that (1) the interval between RNA synthesis and assembly of complete virions is brief (less than 1 hr); (2) the enveloped or budding A particles, representing an early virion stage, may be subsequently transformed into C-type particles; and (3) there is no extensive lag between cellular and viral RNA labeling.

REFERENCES

1. Bader, J. P. Synthesis of the RNA of RNA-containing tumor viruses. I. The interval between synthesis and envelopment. *Virology*, **40**, 494–504 (1970).
2. Cardiff, R. D., Blair, P., and Nakayama, P. *In vitro* cultivation of mouse mammary tumor virus: Detection of MTV production by radioisotope labeling and identification by immune precipitation. *Proc. Natl. Acad. Sci. U.S.*, **59**, 895–902 (1968).
3. De Harven, E. Viremia in Friend murine leukemia: The electron microscope approach to the problem. *Pathol. Biol.*, **13**, 125–134 (1965).
4. De Harven, E. Morphology of murine leukemia viruses. *In* " Experimental Leukemia," ed. by Marvin A. Rich, Appleton-Century-Crofts, New York, pp. 97–129 (1968).
5. Duesberg, P. H., and Robinson, W. S. Nucleic acid and proteins isolated from the Rauscher mouse leukemia virus (MLV). *Proc. Natl. Acad. Sci. U.S.*, **55**, 219–227 (1966).
6. Imai, T., Okano, H., Matsumoto, A., and Horie, A. The mode of virus elaboration in C3H mouse mammary carcinoma as observed by electron microscopy in serial thin sections. *Cancer Res.*, **26**, 443–453 (1966).
7. Michelson-Fiske, S., Haguenau, F., and Rabotti, G. F. Cinétique du dévelopment du virus du sarcome de Rous (souche Schmidt-Ruppin). Estimation du temps d'incorporation d'arginine dans les protéines virales. Etude par autoradiographie au microscope électronique. *Comp. Rend., Ser. D*, **269**, 2475–2478 (1969).
8. Morisita, M. The fitting of logistic equation to the rate of increase of population density. *Res. Popul. Ecol.*, **7**, 52–55 (1965).
9. Okano, H., and Rich, M. A. Time cycle for intracellular synthesis of murine leukemia virus. *Nature*, **224**, 77–78 (1969).
10. Rabotti, G. F., Fiske, S., and Haguenau, F. Cinétique du dévelopment du virus de sarcome de Rous (souche Schmidt-Ruppin). Estimation du temps de maturation par autoradiographie au microscope électronique. *Comp. Rend, Ser. D*, **267**, 2243–2246 (1968).
11. Rich, M. A. Virus-induced murine leukemia. *In* " Experimental Leukemia," ed. by Marvin A. Rich, Appleton-Century-Crofts, New York, pp. 15–49 (1968).
12. Rich, M. A., Geldner, J., and Meyers, P. Studies on murine leukemia. *J. Natl. Cancer Inst.*, **35**, 523–536 (1965).
13. Rich, M. A., and Johns, L. W. Quantitative distribution of virions in virus-induced murine leukemia. *J. Natl. Cancer Inst.*, **41**, 1463–1475 (1968).

EXPLANATION OF PHOTOS

PHOTOS 1a and 1b. The developed silver grains on the virions as well as on the cytoplasm. Note the consecutive sections showing the same distribution pattern of grain deposition, which indicates a specificity of grain deposition. The culture was exposed to ^{3}H-uridine for 6 hr after unlabeled uridine for 26 hr.

PHOTO 2. Deposition of silver grains on the virions and cytoplasm after 1-hr pulse exposure to ^{3}H-uridine. Incubated for 47 hr after the exposure.

PHOTO 3. Deposition of silver grains on the virions and cytoplasm after 4-hr continuous exposure to ^{3}H-uridine.

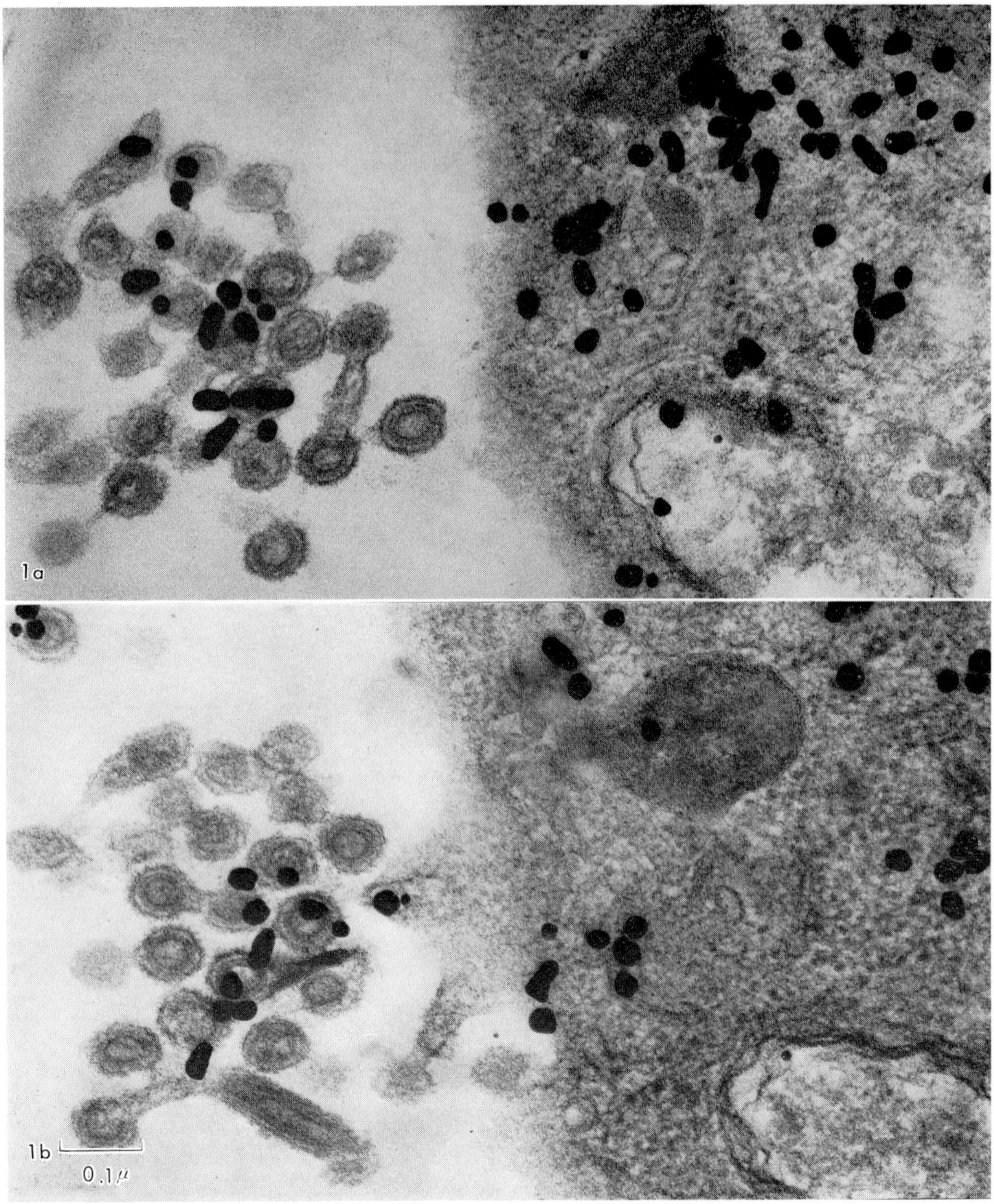
1a
1b
0.1μ

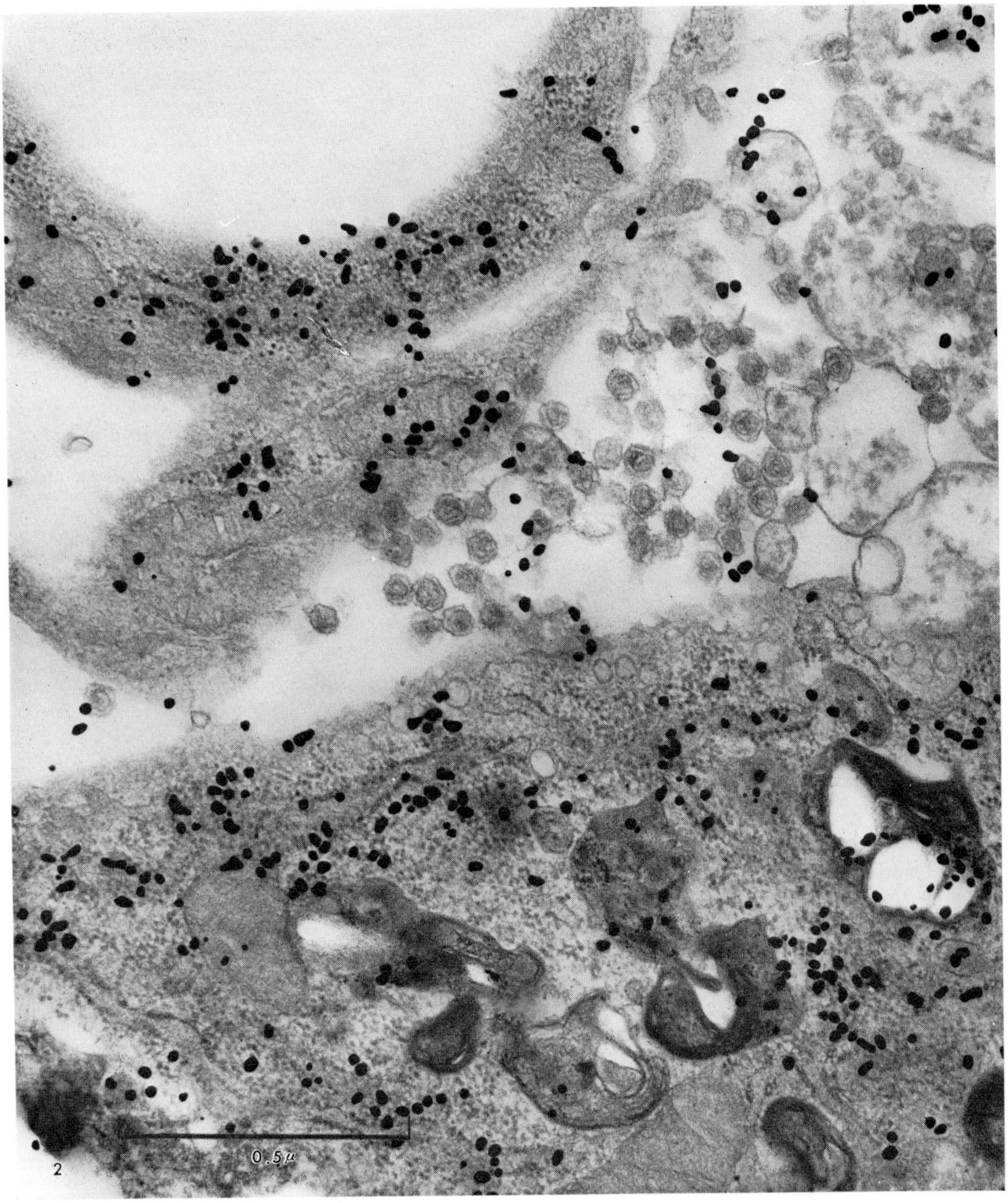
0.5μ
2

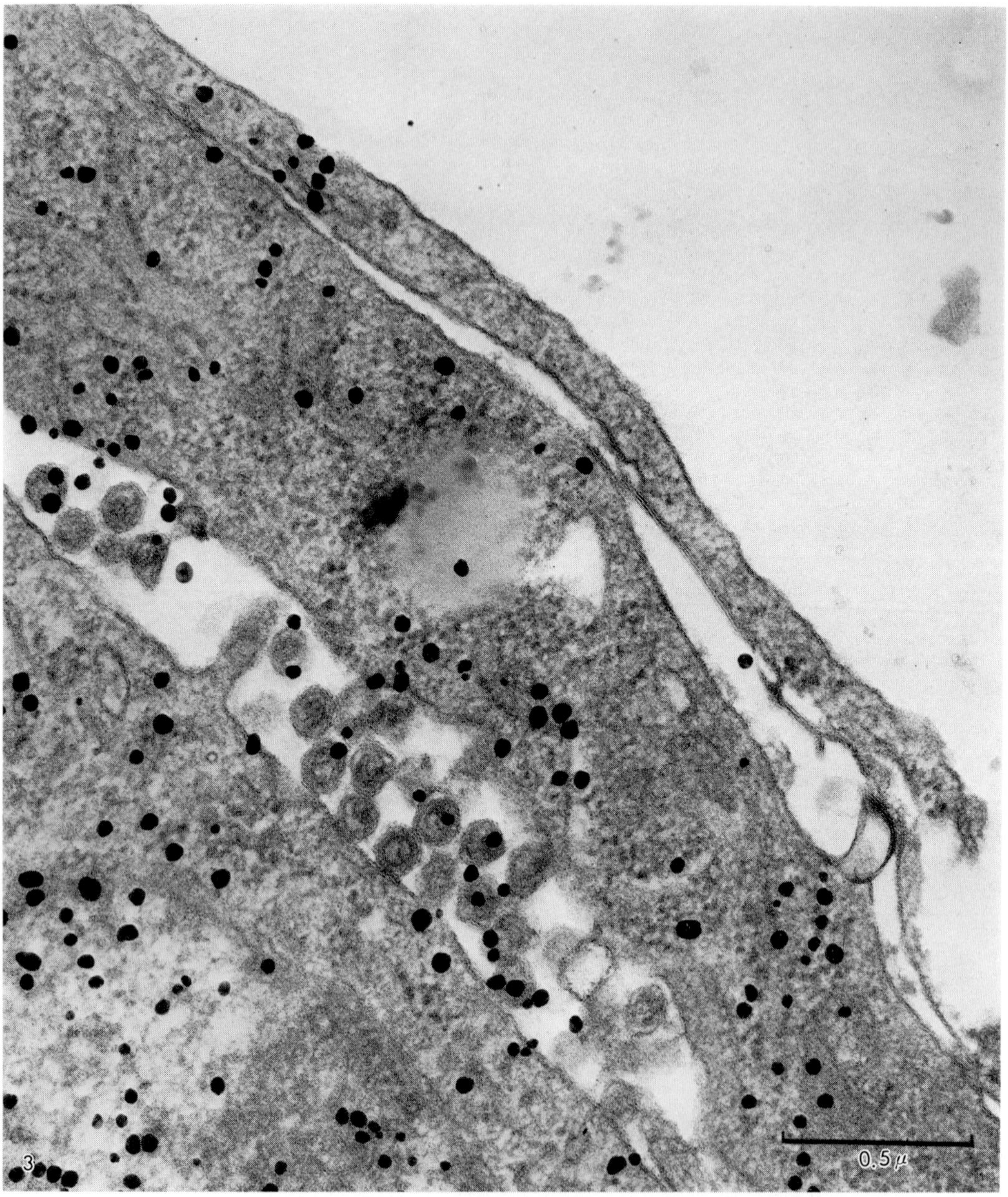
3
0.5 μ

PRESENCE OF AN RNA TUMOR VIRUS GENOME IN NORMAL CELLS*

Tsutomu MIYAMOTO

*Department of Bacteriology, Nagasaki University School of Medicine***

A new mode of presence of an RNA tumor virus genome in normal cells is described. Although known avian leukovirus particles never appeared in normal chick embryo cells, it was found that a genetic factor, similar to the genome of this virus group, was present in cells derived from the majority of these embryos. This genetic factor was designated as chick cell-associated helper factor (chf). Following infection of these " normal " cells with avian leukoviruses except for the α-type of Bryan high titer strain of Rous sarcoma virus (RSV), chf was recovered by maturation into a complete infectious virus. The newly isolated virus, designated as RAV-60, does not belong to any known subgroup of avian tumor viruses in biological activities. The mechanism of rescue of chf to RAV-60 might consist of a genetic recombination between chf and avian leukovirus.

From the data accumulated to date, it was suggested that chf exists in a cellular chromosome as an integrated form and that it is defective in its ability to mature into the complete virus. Both chf and RAV-60 serve as a helper for RSV. Thus, it has become apparent that the infectiousness of RSVβ(O) is acquired by phenotypic mixing as a form of RSVβ(chf) or RSVβ(RAV-60). Alpha-type RSV, however, cannot rescue chf to RAV-60, indicating that some of the defects of α-type RSV, which is deficient in DNA polymerase activity, are common to chf.

Classification of Chick Embryo and Rous Sarcoma Virus

Chick embryos have been classified into several types on the basis of their genetic susceptibility to the subgroups of avian leukoviruses (*2, 19*). For example, C/A- and C/B-type chick embryo cells are resistant to subgroups A and B, respectively; C/O-type chick embryo cells are susceptible to all known subgroups.

Recently, we found that a genetic factor, which is called " chick cell-associated helper factor (chf)," similar to the genome of avian leukosis virus (ALV) in some biological functions, was present in apparently normal cells derived from a majority of C/O-type embryos (*10*) and in these cells both group-specific internal

* This work was carried out at The Department of Viral Oncology, The Public Health Research Institute of The City of New York, Inc., New York, N.Y. U.S.A.

** Sakamoto-machi, Nagasaki 852 (宮本 勉).

and viral envelope antigens were regularly synthesized, although mature viruses never appeared (unpublished data). The C/O-type embryos which are free of chf are now designated as the C/O′ type. Infection of chf-containing C/O cells with the Bryan high titer strain of Rous sarcoma virus (RSV) results in the formation of infectious RSV known as RSVβ(O), free from any known ALVs. On the other hand, infection of the chf-negative C/O′ cells leads to the formation of noninfectious particles called RSVβ'(O) (*9, 10*). Except for the properties described above, no significant difference is found between C/O and C/O′ cells in susceptibility to known subgroups of avian leukoviruses and in the capacity to support their multiplication. RSVβ(O) is infectious for Japanese quail cells, C/A, and some C/O or C/O' chick embryos (*6, 10, 17, 21, 22*); C/O and C/O′ embryos susceptible or resistant to RSVβ(O) can be expressed by addition of the prefixes s- and r-, respectively.

Therefore, the so-called C/O-type chick embryo cells are differentiated into 4 subtypes based on their susceptibility to RSVβ(O) and their capacity to produce RSVβ(O) after transformation by low doses of RSVβ(ALV) or RSVβ(O). The characteristics of these subtypes are summarized in Table I.

As described above, the infectiousness of RSV(O) is conditioned by the type of host cells in which the RSV(O) was produced. There is another type of noninfectious RSV(O) known as RSVα(O) which is conditioned by the genetic character of the virus. Noninfectious RSVβ'(O) differs from infectious RSVβ(O) only in its phenotype, but noninfectious RSVα(O) produced from C/O cells transformed by α-type RSV is different from β-type* in genotype. The clearest evidence for the difference between α- and β-type RSV(O) is the following. The type of RSV progeny derived from the transformed cells depends on the type of RSV used for transforming cells. A majority of transformed cell lines obtained from the infection of RSV produce the same type of RSV as the parent RSV. Each type is a stable genotype with fixed characteristics throughout a large number

TABLE I. Characteristics of Host Cells

Subtypes of embryo		Presence of chf[a]	Susceptibility to		Form of β-type RSV produced after transformation
			RSVβ(O)	RSV(ALV)	
C/O	r-C/O	Yes	r[b]	s	RSVβ(O)[c]
	s-C/O	Yes	s[b]	s	RSVβ(O)
C/O′	r-C/O′	No	r	s	RSVβ'(O)
	s-C/O′	No	s	s	RSVβ'(O)
Japanese quail cells		No	s	s or r[d]	RSVβ'(O)

[a] chf: chick cell-associated helper factor.

[b] r: resistant; s: susceptible. 10^6 FFU of RSVβ(O) from 10^5 to 10^6 foci on the susceptible cultures and no foci on the resistant ones.

[c] RSVβ(O) is infectious for quail, C/A, s-C/O, and s-C/O′ cells, while RSVβ'(O) is not infectious for any cell thus far tested.

[d] Quail cells are susceptible to subgroups A, C, and D but not to subgroup B.

* All RSVβ(O) and RSVβ'(O), and their pseudotypes, should be described "β-type" RSV, and the description of "α-type" RSV parallels this.

TABLE II. Various Types of Transformed Cells

Transformed cell	Characteristics of RSV(O) produced				Recovery of RSV(ALV) by superinfection of ALV[c]	Predominant type of RSV(ALV) recovered[d]
	Type of RSV(O)	Infectiousness for quail cells[a]	Transforming ability[b]	Type of variant		
β-Type, C/O	RSVβ(O)	Yes	Yes	phenotypic	Yes	β
β-Type, C/O′	RSVβ′(O)	No	Yes	↓ genotypic ↑	Yes	β
α-Type, C/O	RSVα(O)	No	No	phenotypic	Yes	α
α-Type, C/O′	RSVα′(O)	No	No		Yes	α

[a] And for C/A, s-C/O, and s-C/O′ cells.

[b] Tested by using ultraviolet-irradiated Sendai virus; 1×10^7 cells were suspended in 1 ml of freshly prepared RSV (10^6 or more particles) and 1 ml of UV-Sendai virus (2000–5000 hemagglutinating units) was added with DEAE-dextran (50 μg / ml). The mixture was incubated in an ice-bath for 25 min, then at 37° for 20 min with occasional gentle rocking, and then was seeded into plates. Transformation of cells overlayed by agar about 15 hr after seeding was observed microscopically on the 7th day.

[c] RSV(ALV) was obtained by superinfection of the transformed cells listed in the first column with ALV.

[d] The method used for typing RSV is essentially the same as that described in ref. *6*.

of host cell passages, and the type does not depend on the cell type used. In addition, RSVα(O) lacks the cell-transforming ability. Both RSVβ(O) and RSVβ'(O) can transform even r-C/O or r-C/O′ cells with the aid of ultraviolet-irradiated (UV-) Sendai virus. On the other hand, RSVα(O) and RSVα′(O) are incapable of transforming chick or quail cells even in the presence of UV-Sendai virus. Only RSVα (ALV) can transform cells (*6*, *8*, *9*).

Thus, we can differentiate 2 genotypic variants of RSV and 2 phenotypic ones in each variant in genotype. Table II shows various types of transformed cells which produce the variants described above. The reason why RSVα(O) is noninfectious may be due to the lack of RNA-dependent DNA polymerase activity in the virion (*7*). The differences in infectiousness between RSVβ(O) and RSVβ′(O) are described in the following sections. Briefly, like another pseudotype of RSV, the infectiousness of RSVβ(O) is given by an envelope component derived from a new helper virus which is rescued from chf-containing C/O cells by infection with RSV itself or ALV.

Evidence for the Presence of chf in Normal C/O Cells and Its Function (*10*, *11*)

The clearest evidence for the presence of chf in normal C/O cells is that infection by RSV or ALV grown in C/O cells converts C/O′ cells into producers of infectious RSVβ(O). In other words, chf in a dormant form in C/O cells is turned into a " transmissible form " of chf by infection with avian leukoviruses, and transmissible chf enables RSV to mature into infectious virus in the recipient C/O′ cells after its introduction together with the leukovirus used for rescue. The transmissible form of chf has some similarity to ALV as a helper for RSV, since it appears to determine both the antigenicity and the host range specificity of RSVβ(O), and then it interferes with RSVβ(O).

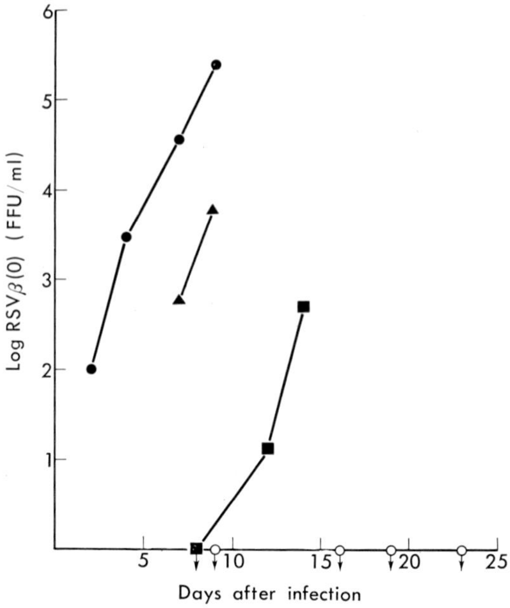

FIG. 1. Production of RSVβ(O) from s-C/O′ cultures infected with RSVβ(O) s-C/ O′cells (1.2×10^6) were infected with serial 10-fold dilutions of 5×10^4 FFU of RSVβ(O) (● undiluted ; ▲ 10^{-1} ; ■ 10^{-2} ; ○ 10^{-3}). The number of transformed cells in each culture reached more than 10^6 by the day the last titration was done. The titer of RSVβ(O) in culture fluid was assayed on quail cells. Points with arrows indicate that RSVβ(O) was undetectable, but RSVβ′(O) was produced.

The presence of transmissible chf was first demonstrated by the production of infectious RSVβ(O) in s-C/O′ cells transformed with RSVβ(O). The s-C/O′ cells were infected with serial dilutions of RSVβ(O) and the yield of RSVβ(O) from the cultures at various times after infection was determined. As shown in Fig. 1, although the cell transformation occurred in all cultures, RSVβ(O) was synthesized only in cultures infected with lower dilutions of RSVβ(O). On the contrary, only RSVβ′(O) was produced in cultures infected with high dilutions. Moreover, the time required for the appearance of RSVβ(O) in the cultures was highly dependent on the input virus concentration. One explanation for this phenomenon may be the presence in RSVβ(O) preparation of a small amount of a mutant which is capable of growing in C/O′ cells. This possibility was ruled out, however, by the fact that the RSV(O) obtained from C/O′-transformed cells induced by RSVβ(O), which is harvested from s-C/O′ cells transformed by large amounts of RSVβ(O), was β′-type. Finally, these results lead to the hypothesis that there is a factor, chf, present in normal C/O cells and essential for the formation of infectious RSVβ(O). The chf is rescued by β-type RSV in a transmissible form and is transmitted from C/O to C/O′ cells by being carried by a minor fraction of RSVβ(O), resulting in formation of RSVβ(O) which is dependent on the spread or growth of transmissible chf. Also, the transmissible chf itself must multiply at least in the presence of the RSV genome.

Results supporting this idea were obtained by using RAV-2 grown in C/O cells (RAV-2•C/O). RAV-2•C/O was obtained by inoculating serial dilutions of RAV-2 into r-C/O. Stocks of RAV-2•C/O were harvested from the terminal dilution of the infected cultures. Serial dilutions of RAV-2•C/O were inoculated into β-type C/O′-transformed cells which were obtained from C/O′ cells infected with low doses of RSVβ(ALV) and were producing RSVβ′(O). Infection by low dilutions of RAV-2•C/O resulted in the formation of both RSV(RAV-2) and RSVβ(O). Infection by high dilutions of RAV-2•C/O and by RAV-2•C/O′ resulted in formation of only RSV(RAV-2). This experiment clearly demonstrates the presence of chf in C/O cells which can be picked up and transmitted to C/O′ cells, not only by RSV but also by RAV-2 and possibly by all known ALVs.

What is the role of chf? It is apparent that chf is essential for the formation of infectious RSV(O). We have found that RSVβ′(O) lacks the capacity to absorb the antibody against RSVβ(O) (unpublished data), suggesting that the structure of their surface antigens is not identical. If chf is directly involved in the synthesis of the surface antigen or determinant component essential for the infectiousness of RSVβ(O), then avian leukovirus grown in C/O cells may contain particles with the same coat antigen as RSVβ(O).

RAV-2•C/O and RAV-2•C/O′ were treated with anti-RAV-2 alone or with both anti-RAV-2 and anti-RSVβ(O). Serial dilutions of the treated and untreated viruses were inoculated into r-C/O and s-C/O cells and the recovery of RAV-2 in these cultures was examined. The results are summarized in Table III. The complete neutralization of RAV-2•C/O′ by anti-RAV-2 is demonstrated, indicating that RAV-2•C/O′ consists of a phenotypically homogeneous population of viruses with RAV-2 antigenicity. RAV-2•C/O treated with anti-RAV-2 loses its infectivity for r-C/O cells but still retains it for s-C/O. This residual infectivity is, however, neutralized by anti-RSVβ(O). This result shows that RAV-2•C/O consists of phenotypically heterogeneous RAV-2; one with

TABLE III. Demonstration of RSVβ(O)-Phenotypic Characteristics in RAV-2

Virus	Treated with	Recovery[a] of RAV-2 from: r-C/O, Dilution ($-\log_{10}$) 0	1	2	3	4	5	6	7	s-C/O, Dilution ($-\log_{10}$) 0	1	2	3	4	5	6	7
RAV-2•C/O	Untreated	+	+	+	+	+	+	+	−[b]	+	+	+	+	+	+	+	−
RAV-2•C/O	Anti-RAV-2	−	−	−	−	−	−	−	−	+	+	−	−	−	−	−	−
RAV-2•C/O	Anti-RAV-2+ Anti-RSVβ(O)	−	−	−	−	−	−	−	−	−	−	−	−	−	−	−	−
RAV-2•C/O′	Untreated	+	+	+	+	+	+	+	−	+	+	+	+	+	+	+	−
RAV-2•C/O′	Anti-RAV-2	−	−	−	−	−	−	−	−	−	−	−	−	−	−	−	−

[a] RAV-2•C/O or RAV-2•C/O′ was mixed with anti-RAV-2 or anti-RAV-2 plus anti-RSVβ(O). Then, serial 10-fold dilutions of the treated and untreated viruses were made and 0.1 ml of each dilution was inoculated into both r-C/O and s-C/O cells. The production of RAV-2 in each culture was examined both by interference with RSV(RAV-2) infection and by the ability of culture fluid to synthesize RSV(RAV-2) in transformed cells free from ALV.

[b] + positive recovery of RAV-2; − no recovery.

its own envelope, the other with an envelope specific for RSVβ(O) characterized both by host range and surface antigen. From this it is concluded that chf in C/O cells is responsible for formation of an envelope component of RSVβ(O), which is probably essential for the infectiousness of RSVβ(O), and that chf is also able to modify the phenotype of ALV with its envelope component.

From the results of interfering experiments between ALV and RSV(ALV) (*4*, *12*, *20*), the transmissible form of chf would be expected to induce interference with RSVβ(O), since chf seems to specify the envelope of RSVβ(O). Cultures of both s-C/O and s-C/O′ cells were infected with RAV-1•C/O and RAV-1•C/O′. The infected and uninfected control cultures were transferred every 3 or 4 days and challenged with RSV(RAV-1) and RSVβ(O) at each transfer. The results are shown in Fig. 2. All infected cultures became resistant to RSV(RAV-1) at the first transfer. On the other hand, except for s-C/O′ cells infected with RAV-1•C/O′ which are completely free from chf, all 3 cultures showed slowly developed but distinct resistance to RSVβ(O), indicating that transmissible chf in the preparation of RAV-1•C/O or in s-C/O cells spread to the entire population of

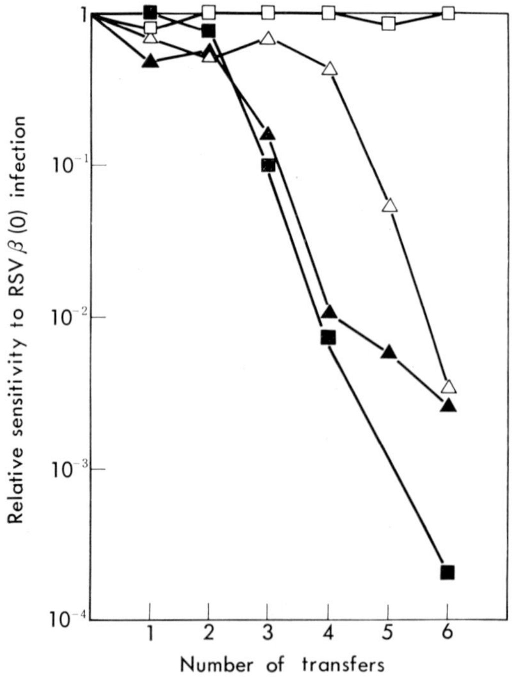

FIG. 2. Establishment of resistance to RSVβ(O) infection in cultures infected with RAV-1•C/O or RAV-1•C/O′

The s-C/O and s-C/O′ cells were infected with undiluted RAV-1•C/O or RAV-1•C/O′ and transferred every 3 or 4 days. RSV focus formation on the infected cells was compared with that on the respective control cells by challenging with RSVβ(O) after each transfer. ■ s-C/O′ cells infected with RAV-1•C/O; □ s-C/O′ cells infected with RAV-1•C/O′; ▲ s-C/O cells infected with RAV-1•C/O; △ s-C/O cells infected with RAV-1•C/O′.

cells in each culture following multiplication of RAV-1 and interfered with RSVβ(O).

The Absence of Complete Virus in Normal C/O Cells (10, 11)

Normal C/O cells are fully susceptible to all known subgroups (A to D) of avian leukoviruses, indicating the absence of known ALV. We have also failed to isolate any ALV from C/O cells. The fact that there is chf in C/O cells, and the transmissible form of chf in preparations of ALV grown in C/O cells raised the possibility of spontaneous formation from normal C/O cells of an unknown ALV. This was, however, ruled out by the following experiments.

First, no radioactive virus was observed in the sucrose gradient centrifugation of culture fluid and in the trypsin fraction (*5*, *6*) obtained from normal C/O cells incubated with ^{3}H-uridine-containing media. Second, the formation of infectious RSVβ(O) in β-type s-C/O′-transformed cells was not induced by inoculating the concentrated culture fluid, trypsin fraction, and the homogenate or sonicate of normal C/O cells, even together with UV-Sendai virus.

Isolation and Characterization of a New Virus from "Normal" C/O Cells (11)

As described above, the transmissible form of chf behaves as a complete helper virus. It establishes complete resistance to RSVβ(O), indicating the multiplication of its genome in infected cells and the spread of the genome over the entire population of cells by reinfection.

An attempt was made, therefore, to isolate such a new virus free from known ALV. RAV-1·C/O was incubated with anti-RAV-1, and then the serial dilutions of this antibody-treated virus were inoculated into quail cells. After 9 transfers the cultures infected by the 10^5 dilution became resistant to RSVβ(O) but remained fully susceptible to RSV(RAV-1). A new virus was obtained from the culture fluid of this dilution. The same virus has also been isolated from C/O cells infected with RAV-1·C/O′ and RAV-2·C/O′, but not from C/O′ cells infected with RAV-1·C/O′ or RAV-2·C/O′. The virus was designated as RAV-60 and characterization of this newly isolated virus was carried out.

The following are the properties of RAV-60 thus far tested. a) Function as helper virus: like other ALV, RAV-60 served as a helper for RSV. RSVβ(RAV-60) obtained from β-type s-C/O′-transformed cells superinfected with RAV-60 was indistinguishable from RSVβ(O). b) Host range: the host range of RAV-60 is the same as that of RSVβ(O), *i.e.*, s-C/O, s-C/O′, s-C/A, and quail cells. c) Multiplication: RAV-60 grows in those susceptible cells without any cytopathogenic effect and does not require the presence or assistance of other RSV or ALV for its replication. d) Antigenicity: RAV-60 is antigenically identical to RSVβ (O). On the other hand, no cross-antigenicity was found between RAV-60 and 3 other known subgroups (Table IV). e) Interference: the relationship of RAV-60 to other ALV was studied by interference and the results are summarized in Table V. RSV(RAV-60) had the same specificity as RSVβ(O) in its sensitivity to interference induced by ALVs. RAV-60 was unrelated to subgroups A and C

TABLE IV. Antigenic Relationship between RAV-60 and Other Subgroups

Subgroup	Virus	Surviving fraction of RSV† after incubation with Anti-RAV-1	Anti-RAV-2	Anti-RAV-50	Anti-RSVβ(O)
—	RSV(RAV-60)	0.95	1.0	1.0	<0.0001
—	RSVβ(O)	0.98	0.95	1.0	<0.0001
A	RSV(RAV-1)	<0.0001	0.82	0.84	0.95
B	RSV(RAV-2)	0.93	<0.00001	0.12	0.95
D	RSV(RAV-50)	0.82	0.066	0.00028	1.0

† 0.1 ml of antisera for various strains of avian leukovirus was mixed with 0.9 ml of the various RSV (about 10^5 FFU) and incubated at 37° for 30 min. The surviving fraction of RSV was assayed by focus formation on s-C/O′ cells.

TABLE V. Interfering Patterns between RAV-60 and Other ALVs

Subgroup	Challenge virus	Efficiency of RSV infection[a] on cells previously infected with None	RAV-1 (A)	RAV-2 (B)	RAV-50 (D)	RAV-60 —
—	RSV(RAV-60)	1.0	1.0	<0.0001	<0.0001	<0.0001
—	RSVβ(O)	1.0	1.0	<0.0001	<0.0001	<0.0001
A	RSV(RAV-1)	1.0	0.00025	0.56	0.50	0.90
B	RSV(RAV-2)	1.0	0.80	<0.0002	0.0075	0.75
C	PR-RSV[b]	1.0	0.90	0.60	0.70	0.90
C	B-77	1.0	1.0	0.75	0.55	0.70
D	RSV(RAV-50)	1.0	0.96	0.046	<0.0001	0.01-0.001
D	CZ-RSV[c]	1.0	1.0	0.001	<0.0001	0.001

[a] The s-C/O′ cell cultures were infected with 2×10^6 infectious units of each ALV and transferred more than 3 times. The infectivity of the various RSVs on the infected cultures was compared with that on uninfected s-C / O′ cells.

[b] Prague strain of RSV. [c] Carr-Zilber strain of RSV.

but appeared to be related to subgroups B and D by interference patterns, despite the lack of antigenic similarity with those latter 2 subgroups (Table IV). Although ALVs of subgroups B and D induced strong interference with RSV(RAV-60), RAV-60 induced only weak interference with subgroup D and none with subgroup B. f) Physicochemical properties: both RAV-60 and RSV(RAV-60) had a buoyant density of 1.16 in sucrose solutions, which is identical to other known ALV. The RNA extracted from RAV-60 sedimented at 69–71S.

Failure to Isolate RAV-60 from C/O Cells Transformed with α-type RSV

As described in the preceding sections, RAV-1, RAV-2, and β-type RSV can rescue chf to RAV-60. However, this fact did not support the suggestion that all known avian leukoviruses may rescue chf to RAV-60. From the following results, it was found that RSVα(O) grown in C/O cells transformed with α-type RSV did not contain RAV-60 (*11*).

The culture fluid of more than 10 different isolates of α-type C/O-transformed cells was tested for the presence of the new virus by checking its ability to induce resistance to RSVβ(O) in quail and s-C/O′ cells. No resistance was detected in any of the cultures. Then, the inoculation of RSVα(O) with UV-Sendai virus into β′-type s-C/O′-transformed cells did not result in RSVβ(O) production.

Moreover, RAV-60 was not induced from C/O cells by inoculating RSVα(O) together with UV-Sendai virus, indicating that RSVα(O) is unable to rescue chf to the complete virus.

DISCUSSION

The chick embryos used here were supplied as C/O type from leukosis-free flocks; more than 70 percent of the embryos contained chf, but they contained no demonstrable amount of complete virus. However, a new helper virus, RAV-60, was isolated from the chf-containing " normal " chick cells by infection with avian leukoviruses except for α-type RSV. Although pathogenic activity has not yet been established, RAV-60 is similar to ALV in all other biological and physicochemical properties. The facts described above suggest that chf is present in normal C/O cells as a functionally or genetically defective viral genome and requires the assistance of a complete avian leukovirus for its maturation into infectious RAV-60. However, the defectiveness of chf genome is only partial since chf seems to code for viral internal and/or envelope antigens even in normal C/O cells (unpublished data). Recently, a new virus, designated as RAV-O, was also isolated from some C/A chick embryo cell cultures (*18*). Although the main properties of RAV-O are quite similar to those of RAV-60, further investigation is necessary to clarify the relationship between them.

The fact that RAV-60, once rescued, does not require any assistance from another virus for its replication suggests that the mode of rescue of chf by ALV to a complete virus might be genetic recombination between these two. There is evidence suggesting that the genetic information of chf exists in the cellular chromosomes (*10*, *13*), probably in a form similar to the provirus proposed by Temin (*15*). Recent demonstrations of DNA polymerase activity in the virions of RNA tumor viruses (*1*, *3*, *14*, *16*) strongly supports the idea that the genetic information of RNA tumor viruses may persist as DNA integrated into the host cell genome. If the genetic information of chf is DNA type and the genome of RAV-60 is RNA type, it is of interest to know whether the rescue of chf to RAV-60 involves genetic recombination of chf and active leukovirus at the RNA level or at the DNA level.

Together with rescue of chf to a mature virus by β-type RSV, chf, or RAV-60 also serves as a helper for RSV, *i.e.*, the infectiousness of RSVβ(O) is determined by an envelope component which is mediated by the function of chf and is not synthesized by the RSV genome. The functional cooperation between chf and β-type RSV is essentially different from that in the formation of RSV(ALV) from RSV-transformed cells by ALV. As stated already, once rescued, RAV-60 behaves as a complete virus and can grow without any assistance from another virus for its replication. On the other hand, the acquisition of infectiousness of RSVβ (O) is formed by phenotypic mixing between RSV and chf or RAV-60 as a form of

RSV(ALV). Therefore, RSVβ(O) could be expressed as RSVβ(chf) or RSVβ (RAV-60).

Because of their unique characteristics as described above, RAV-60 and RSV (RAV-60) could be classified into a new subgroup, E, of avian leukovirus.

Alpha-type transformed cells produce physically intact RSV particles, and superinfection of these cells with ALV forms infectious RSVα(ALV) (*6, 8*). However, RSVα(O) derived from α-type C/O transformed cells is a noninfectious particle incapable of transforming cells even in the presence of UV-Sendai virus (*9*). Moreover, the preparation of RSVα(O) does not contain RAV-60. Thus, α-type RSV fails to rescue chf to RAV-60, but in a preliminary experiment, RAV-60 served as helper for α-type RSV to make infectious RSVα (RAV-60). From these results, it is conceivable that, in addition to the defect in the formation of an envelope component, the α-type RSV has another defect common to chf. This might be the genetic information essential for the establishment of infection, *i.e.*, information concerning an enzymatic activity, probably DNA polymerase activity, required at the time of infection, since the α-type RSV genome itself has the genetic information for both transformation of cells and virus assembly.

Here, chf represents a new type of cell-associated tumor virus genome. It could be present in " normal " cells as an integrated gene and is transferred from cell to cell, or chf could be a cellular gene which has acquired some degree of autonomy in the course of its long evolution.

Acknowledgments

I am grateful to Dr. H. Hanafusa for discussions during the preparation of the manuscript.

REFERENCES

1. Baltimore, D. RNA-dependent DNA polymerase in virions of RNA tumor viruses. *Nature*, **226**, 1209–1211 (1970).
2. Duff, R. G., and Vogt, P. K. Characteristics of two new avian tumor virus subgroups. *Virology*, **39**, 18–30 (1969).
3. Fujinaga, K., Parsons, J. T., Beard, J. W., Beard, D., and Green, M. Mechanism of carcinogenesis by RNA tumor viruses. III. Formation of RNA·DNA complex and duplex DNA molecules by the DNA polymerase(s) of avian myeloblastosis virus. *Proc. Natl. Acad. Sci. U.S.*, **67**, 1432–1439 (1970).
4. Hanafusa, H. Analysis of the defectiveness of Rous sarcoma virus. III. Determining influence of a new helper virus on the host range and susceptibility to interference of RSV. *Virology*, **25**, 248–255 (1965).
5. Hanafusa, T., and Hanafusa, H. Interaction among avian tumor viruses giving enhanced infectivity. *Proc. Natl. Acad. Sci. U.S.*, **58**, 818–825 (1967).
6. Hanafusa, H., and Hanafusa, T. Further studies on RSV production from transformed cells. *Virology*, **34**, 630–636 (1968).
7. Hanafusa, H., and Hanafusa, T. Non-infectious RSV deficient in DNA polymerase. *Virology*, **43**, 313–316 (1971).
8. Hanafusa, H., Hanafusa, T., and Miyamoto, T. Two origins for formation of non-infectious virus from Rous sarcoma cells. *In* " Defectiveness, Rescue and Stimu-

lation of Oncogenic Viruses (2nd International Symposium on Tumor Viruses, Royaumont, 1969)," Centre Natl. de la Res., Sci., Paris, pp. 195–199 (1970).

9. Hanafusa, T., Miyamoto, T., and Hanafusa, H. A type of chick embryo cell that fails to support formation of infectious RSV. *Virology*, **40**, 55–64 (1970).
10. Hanafusa, H., Miyamoto, T., and Hanafusa, T. A cell-associated factor essential for formation of an infectious form of Rous sarcoma virus. *Proc. Natl. Acad. Sci. U.S.*, **66**, 314–321 (1970).
11. Hanafusa, T., Hanafusa, H., and Miyamoto, T. Recovery of a new virus from apparently normal chick cells by infection with avian tumor viruses. *Proc. Natl. Acad. Sci. U.S.*, **67**, 1797–1803 (1970).
12. Hanafusa, T., Hanafusa, H., and Rubin, H. Differential responsiveness of Rous sarcoma virus stocks to specific cellular resistance induced by avian leukosis viruses. *Virology*, **22**, 643–645 (1964).
13. Payne, L. N., and Chubb, R. C. Studies on the nature and genetic control of an antigen in normal chick embryos which reacts in the COFAL test. *J. Gen. Virol.*, **3**, 379–391 (1968).
14. Spiegelman, S., Burney, A., Das, M. R., Keydar, J., Schlom, J., Travinicek, M., and Watson, K. Characterization of the products of RNA-directed DNA polymerases in oncogenic RNA viruses. *Nature*, **227**, 563–567 (1970).
15. Temin, H. M. The participation of DNA in Rous sarcoma virus production. *Virology*, **23**, 486–494 (1964).
16. Temin, H. M., and Mizutani, S. RNA-dependent DNA polymerase in virions of Rous sarcoma virus. *Nature*, **226**, 1211–1213 (1970).
17. Vogt, P. K. A virus released by " non-producing " Rous sarcoma cells. *Proc. Natl. Acad. Sci. U.S.*, **58**, 801–808 (1967).
18. Vogt, P. K., and Friis, R. R. An avian leukosis virus related to RSV(O): Properties and evidence for helper activity. *Virology*, **43**, 223–234 (1971).
19. Vogt, P. K., and Ishizaki, R. Reciprocal patterns of genetic resistance to avian tumor viruses in two lines of chickens. *Virology*, **26**, 664–672 (1965).
20. Vogt, P. K., and Ishizaki, R. Patterns of viral interference in the avian leukosis and sarcoma complex. *Virology*, **30**, 368–374 (1966).
21. Weiss, R. Spontaneous virus production from "nonvirus producing" Rous sarcoma cells. *Virology*, **32**, 719–723 (1967).
22. Weiss, R. A. The host range of Bryan strain Rous sarcoma virus synthesized in the absence of helper virus. *J. Gen. Virol.*, **5**, 511–528 (1969).

GANN Monograph on Cancer Research 12, 1972

FIXATION AND DEVELOPMENT OF GENOMES OF RNA TUMOR VIRUSES

Yozo Nakata†

*National Cancer Institute, National Institutes of Health**

The research reported herein clearly demonstrated that there are at least 2 steps before expression of the genome of RNA tumor viruses, *i.e.*, fixation and development. For fixation of the viral genome, a transitory DNA synthesis alone is required. Activity of nucleic acid polymerases has been demonstrated, although the molecular significance of this activity in carcinogenesis is still unclear. For the development of the fixed viral genome, intactness of DNA and synthesis of RNA and protein were required. However, DNA synthesis was no longer required. Cellular conditions, such as the degree of cell crowding, also influence the successful infection of RNA tumor viruses.

It is well known that infection by RNA tumor viruses results in the production of viruses and the malignant transformation of cells with natural host cell systems, although only malignant transformation would be seen in trans-species infection and viral production alone would be caused in embryonic cells infected by leukemia viruses. The existence of the viral genome in nonproducing malignant transformed cells has been demonstrated by genome rescue experiments. The most remarkable characteristic of infection by RNA tumor viruses is that viruses are produced by budding from the cell surface (Photo 1) and thus the parent cell survives and makes its progeny. On the other hand, DNA tumor viruses are produced by the bursting of the infected cell and thus result in death of the parent cell, as is the case in most viral infections (Fig. 1). A second major characteristic of RNA tumor virus infections is the malignant transformation of infected cells. The fact that a different morphology of focus is seen when a different strain (type) of a virus group is used (Photo 2) seems to suggest that the viral genome itself is responsible for the malignant transformation (carcinogenesis) of the infected cell.

Biological studies have demonstrated the occurrence of the eclipse phase before the expression of viral genomes. In order to elucidate the mechanisms of carcinogenesis, biochemical studies on the eclipse phase in terms of these two characteristics of RNA tumor viral infection, *i.e.*, viral production and malignant transformation, have been conducted in our laboratory. It has been shown that there are at least 2 steps before expression of the viral genome, *i.e.*, fixation and development (*7–12*).

* Bethesda, Maryland, 20014, U.S.A.

† Present address: Institute for Cancer Research, Osaka University Medical School, Osaka 553 (中田陽造).

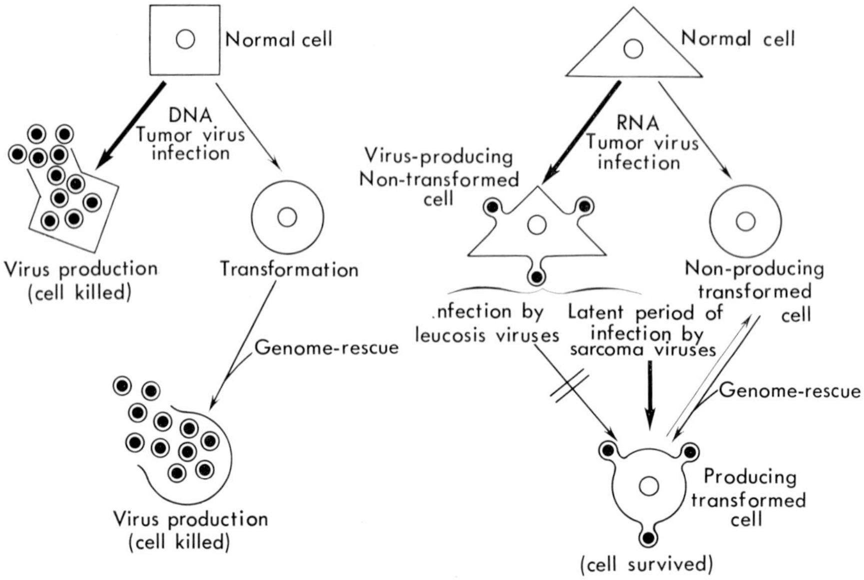

FIG. 1. Mode of infection of tumor viruses

Fixation of the Viral Genome into the Cell

It has been shown that DNA synthesis is a transitory requirement for successful transformation of cells by RNA tumor viruses (*1*, *9*, *10*, *15*). Specific inhibition of DNA synthesis by thymidine, cytosine arabinoside, or X-ray irradiation prevented malignant transformation when applied for a 12-hr period immediately after infection. The DNA requirement is known to be transitory, because inhibition of DNA synthesis before infection or after a 12-hr delay had little effect on the subsequent transformation (Table I). The requirement of transitory DNA synthesis is reflected in the results of experiments examining the relationship between the cell cycle and viral infection. In order to examine this, cells were synchronized with respect to the cell cycle using thymidine. Cells in

TABLE I. Effect of Transitory DNA Synthesis on Malignant Transformation

Exposure to thymidine (hr)	RSV (RAV–1)	MSV (Moloney-MLV)
None	470,000	61,000
−12 to 0	530,000	67,000
0 to 12	3,800	300
12 to 24	480,000	60,000

Cells were seeded 1 day before the experiment. Thymidine (20 mM)-containing medium was added to cultures for a 12-hr interval prior to, immediately after, or 12 hr after addition of the RNA tumor virus, and was replaced with growth medium at appropriate period. The number of foci on either chick (RSV) or rat (MSV) embryo cell monolayer was counted 5 days after infection.

TABLE II. The Cell Cycle and Viral Infection

Time of exposure (hr after thymidine treatment)	Foci	
	RSV (RAV-1)	MSV (Moloney-MLV)
0	460,000	78,000
8	7,200	270
16	9,800	290

Embryo cells were synchronized by exposure to and release from thymidine (20 mM) on 2 consecutive days. After the second exposure to thymidine, monolayers were exposed to viruses at the given times for 1 hr. Mitoses were observed microscopically between 8 and 16 hr after being released from thymidine. The number of foci was counted 5 days after infection.

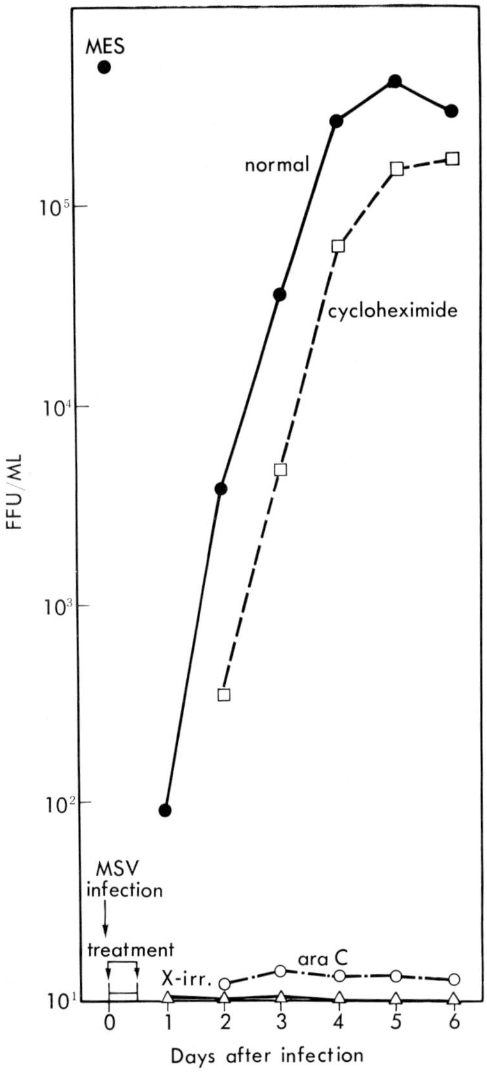

FIG. 2. Production of MSV(Moloney-MLV) Approximately 10^6 cells of NIH-Swiss mouse embryo secondary culture were seeded on a 100-mm plastic petri dish 1 day before infection. After washing with TBS, the monolayers were exposed to MSV (*ca.* 10^6 FFU of MSV in 1 ml growth medium) for 1 hr at 37° in a CO_2 incubator. Then, 10 ml of medium with or without inhibitors (10^{-4} M cytosine arabinoside or 0.5 μg / ml cycloheximide) was added. X-Irradiation (5,000 R) was carried out 6 hr before infection. The media were harvested at 24-hr intervals. Virus production was determined by the focus assay (*9*).

TABLE III. Effect of Transitory RNA Synthesis on Malignant Transformation

Exposure to actinomycin D (hr)	RSV (RAV–1)	MSV (Moloney-MLV)
None	490,000	74,000
−12 to 0	270,000	36,000
0 to 12	210,000	30,000
12 to 24	320,000	48,000

Experimental procedure was the same as in Table I, except for the inhibitor (2 μg/ml actinomycin D). Actinomycin D is toxic and *ca.* 50% of cells were damaged.

TABLE IV. Effect of Transitory Protein Synthesis on Malignant Transformation

Exposure to cycloheximide (hr)	RSV (RAV–1)	MSV (Moloney-MLV)
None	450,000	69,000
−12 to 0	420,000	61,000
0 to 12	370,000	54,000
12 to 24	390,000	68,000

Experimental procedure was the same as in Table I, except for the inhibitor (0.5 μg/ml cycloheximide).

different phases were exposed to RNA tumor viruses. Results indicated the high efficiency of malignant transformation during or just prior to the S phase of cells synchronized in the mitotic cycle (Table II). It was also shown that a single round of DNA synthesis (S phase) is sufficient for subsequent transformation (*9*, *10*).

This is also true of the subsequent production of RNA tumor viruses (Fig. 2). Therefore, it is suggested that as an early event the transitory DNA synthesis is required for the successful infection of RNA tumor viruses.

For fixation of the viral genome, synthesis of RNA and protein was not required (Tables III and IV). Therefore, it was suggested that no brand-new protein (enzyme) is required to be synthesized in order for successful infection to occur (*11*). Thus, the participation of some factor(s) of the virion or of the cell in fixation of the viral genome was suggested (*11*).

In this connection, it should be noted that the enzymic activities of DNA polymerase and RNA polymerase have been elucidated (*2*, *4*, *6*, *7*, *12–14*, *16–19*, Nakata *et al.*, in preparation). Virions of avian and murine tumor viruses contain enzymic activity of viral RNA-dependent DNA polymerase (Table V). However, the size of the reaction products has been shown to be relatively small (*4–5* S). Furthermore, experiments on DNA-RNA homology have shown that there is always relatively high homology between viral RNA and normal cell DNA (*3*, *5*, *7*, *12*, *20*). Therefore, there are still many problems to be solved before the newly synthesized polydeoxyribonucleotide(s) can be identified as the new gene(s) for viral carcinogenesis. Besides the activity of DNA polymerase, RNA-dependent RNA replicase activity was also shown (*6*, *17–19*). However, because there are 4 enzymes that are responsible respectively for the independent incorporation of 4 ribonucleoside triphosphates into the acid-insoluble polyribonucleotide

TABLE V. Nucleic Acid Polymerases in Virions

Reaction system	RSV (RAV-1)	MSV (Moloney-MLV)
^{3}HdATP+dGTP+dCTP+dTTP	0.128	0.130
RNase+[^{3}HdATP+dGTP+dCTP+dTTP]	0.025	0.020
^{3}HATP	0.13	0.11
^{3}HGTP	1.22	1.06
^{3}HCTP	1.41	1.46
^{3}HUTP	0.25	0.30
^{3}HGTP+ATP+CTP+UTP	1.23	1.06

Enzyme preparations were obtained by treating purified virions with Nonidet or Triton X 100. The reaction mixture contained 20 μmoles of potassium phosphate buffer (pH 8.0), 2 μmoles $MnCl_2$(DNA) or $MgCl_2$(RNA), 500 nmoles of nucleoside triphosphate(s), and 0.18–0.21 mg protein of virions. Total volume was adjusted to 0.5 ml. Specific activities of radio-labeled substrates were *ca.* 5,000 cpm/nmole each. Values are expressed as nmoles/mg protein/30 min.

(Table V), the proposed existence of RNA-dependent RNA " replicase " has to be studied more carefully in terms of the replication of viral RNAs (*7*, *8*). Thus, although there are some enzymic activities in virions, it is very important to accumulate more data in order to determine the precise molecular mechanisms of viral carcinogenesis (fixation of the viral genome into the cell).

Development of the Viral Genome

The existence of the eclipse phase before the phenotypic manifestation (virus production and malignant transformation) suggests that the fixation of the viral genome alone is not sufficient for the phenotypic manifestation. Indeed, the following experiments (see Table VI) show the existence of a second step, the development of the viral genome, which leads to the phenotypic manifestation of the fixed genome (*7– 9*, *12*, Nakata *et al.*, in preparation).

Sparse and confluent cell cultures were exposed to RNA tumor viruses, *i.e.*, RSV(RAV-1) or MSV(Moloney-MLV). Cells from both groups were then washed, dispersed with trypsin, and replated in order to remove the restraints of cell crowding and thus to allow macromolecular syntheses to proceed at their maximal level. Trypsinization is known to remove superficially adsorbed RNA tumor viruses and hence it may preclude complicated results caused by late infections. When foci were allowed to develop in the confluent cultures without dispersal of the cells, few foci were found compared with those originating in the sparse cultures (see square #1, Table VI). This was not caused by the failure of the initial events like adsorption or penetration of viruses but was the result of a failure of the fixation of the viral genome, because focus-forming centers were obtained after early trypsinization (see square #2, Table VI). Over 70% of the infected cells of sparse cultures were recoverable as focus-forming centers after trypsinization (the plating efficiency). The number of focus-forming centers on the confluent cultures was much greater than that on the sparse cultures. One of the reasons for this seems to be the greater probability of virus-cell contacts in the former. Delay

TABLE VI. Effect of Cell Crowding and Medium on Malignant Transformation by RSV (RAV–1)

Monolayer	Medium after infection		Foci without transfer	Foci after transfer at	
	0–24 hr	24–48 hr		0 hr	24 hr
Sparse	Fresh	Fresh	470,000 (#1)	330,000 (#2)	670,000 (#3)
Confluent	Conditioned	Conditioned	62		
Confluent	Conditioned	Fresh	87	440,000	139
Confluent	Fresh	Conditioned	630 (#4)		
Confluent	Fresh	Fresh	8,600	430,000	79,000 (#5)

Sparse and confluent cultures of chick embryo secondary culture cells were exposed to various dilutions of RSV (RAV–1). Fresh or conditioned medium (*9*) was added for a 24-hr interval immediately after infection and the media were replaced for a subsequent 24-hr interval as noted. Cell transfers were performed by dispersing with trypsin (*9*). On the second day after infection, fresh agar medium was added to all cultures. Foci were counted 6 days after infection.

of trypsinization for 24 hr resulted in failure of the rescue of the viral gene expression, focus formation (see square #3, Table VI). In the meantime, the number of centers doubled in the control sparse cultures, as would be expected in a culture of dividing cells. These results can be explained by the failure of confluent cultures in conditioned medium to provide the DNA synthesis required for successful infection. The addition of fresh medium to nondispersed confluent cultures for early 24 hr after infection resulted in the increase of the number of foci compared with the number of foci in the cultures under conditioned medium (see square #4, Table VI). The cultures that were maintained with fresh medium for 24 to 48 hr developed many more foci than those maintained with conditioned medium for that period. Since the extent of DNA synthesis as an early event in infection is at the same level in both cases, this result shows the existence of at least one more step before the manifestation of the viral genome after its fixation. Fewer than 2% of the foci appearing in sparse cultures developed in confluent cultures with fresh medium for 0 to 48 hr. This fact must be explained by the difference of cell crowding. This also appears to be true on the basis of a comparison of the number of focus-forming centers developed by the transfer of confluent monolayers 24 hr after infection (see square #5, Table VI) and the number of foci developed in the cultures maintained in the fresh medium for 0 to 48 hr without the transfer (see square #4, Table VI). The marked reduction must be due to the difference in the degree of cell crowding, because the freshness of the medium was the same. Thus, the existence of the process of the development of viral genetic information was demonstrated, in addition to the process of fixation of the viral genome. Also, the development of malignant transformation after initial fixation of the viral genome was shown to be dependent on the culture medium and on cell crowding, *i.e.*, on the metabolic conditions and perhaps the state of the cell membrane.

Virus production is one of the phenotypic manifestations of carcinogenesis by RNA tumor virus infection. Although DNA synthesis was not required (Table

TABLE VII. Inhibition of DNA Synthesis and Production of Viruses

Treatment	Virus production (FFU/ml)	
	RSV (RAV-1)	MSV (Moloney-MLV)
None	950,000	180,000
Cytosine arabinoside	830,000	140,000
Thymidine	920,000	180,000
X-Irradiation	920,000	160,000

Five-day-old infected monolayers on 100-mm petri dishes were exposed as noted (10^{-4} M cytosine arabinoside, 20 mM thymidine, or 5,000 R of X-ray) and the production of viruses for 8 hr in 5 ml medium was examined.

TABLE VIII. Effect of UV-Irradiation on Production of Viruses

Time of exposure (min)	Virus production (FFU/ml)	
	RSV (RAV-1)	MSV (Moloney-MLV)
0	920,000	230,000
20	3,900	1,600

Five-day-old infected monolayers on 100-mm petri dishes were exposed to ultraviolet ray (G.E. germicidal mercury vapor lamp having a peak at 2537 Å, and providing 10 ergs/mm²/sec at a distance of 25 cm) under 1 ml of TBS. After washing the monolayers with growth medium, a 5-ml growth medium was added and the cultures were incubated for 8 hr.

TABLE IX. Effect of Actinomycin D on Production of Viruses

Addition (μg/ml)	Virus production (FFU/ml)	
	RSV (RAV-1)	MSV (Moloney-MLV)
0	940,000	160,000
2	0	0

Experimental procedures were the same as in Table VII, except for the inhibitor.

TABLE X. Effect of Cycloheximide on Production of Viruses

Addition (μg/ml)	Virus production (FFU/ml)	
	RSV (RAV-1)	MSV (Moloney-MLV)
0	940,000	170,000
0.5	4,800	550

Experimental procedures were the same as in Table VII, except for the inhibitor.

VII), the intactness of DNA (Table VIII) and the synthesis of RNA (Table IX) and protein (Table X) were required for virus production, *i.e.*, the development of fixed viral genetic information (*12*).

The fixation and development of carcinogenic genome(s), in similar fashions, would be possible in *in vivo* systems. Many of the tissues of adult vertebrates are composed of crowded cells in states of repressed growth. A genotypic change, either spontaneous or induced, may become fixed in relation to sporadic cell division (S phase of the cell cycle) and thus convert a cell to a potential malignant cell. The failure to express the genetic change phenotypically could prevent the cell from developing the characteristics of the malignancy. The results presented here provide experimental confirmation of such a possibility with RNA tumor viruses in a cell culture system.

REFERENCES

1. Bader, J. P. Transformation by RSV: A requirement for DNA synthesis. *Science*, **149**, 757–758 (1965).
2. Baltimore, D. RNA-dependent DNA polymerase in virions of RNA tumor viruses. *Nature*, **226**, 1209–1211 (1970).
3. Baluda, M. A., and Nayak, D. P. DNA complementary to viral RNA in leukemic cells induced by AMV. *Proc. Natl. Acad. Sci. U.S.*, **66**, 329–336 (1970).
4. Garapin, A. C., McDonnell, J. P., Levinson, W. E., Quintrell, N., Fanshier, L., and Bishop, J. M. DNA polymerase associated with RSV and AMV: Properties of the enzyme and its product. *J. Virol.*, **6**, 589–598 (1970).
5. Harel, L., Harel, J., and Huppert, J., Partial homology between RNA from Rauscher mouse leukemia virus and cellular DNA. *Biochem. Biophys. Res. Commun.*, **28**, 44–49 (1967).
6. Haruna, I., Watanabe, I., and Ohno, T. Studies on RNA-dependent RNA polymerase from leukemia and ascites tumor cells. *Proc. Int. Cancer Congr.*, **10**, 389 (1970).
7. Nakata, Y. Malignant tumors: Carcinogenesis by RNA tumor viruses. *Metabolism and Diseases*, **7**, 910–920 (1970).
8. Nakata, Y. RNA tumor viruses and carcinogenesis by them. *In* "Gan to Kakusan (Cancer and Nucleic Acids)," ed. by M. Muramatsu, Nankodo Co. Ltd., Tokyo, in press.
9. Nakata, Y., and Bader, J. P. Transformation by murine sarcoma virus: Fixation (DNA synthesis) and development. *J. Virol.*, **2**, 1255–1261 (1968).
10. Nakata, Y., and Bader, J. P. Studies on the fixation and development of cellular transformation by RSV. *Virology*, **36**, 401–410 (1968).
11. Nakata, Y., and Bader, J. P. Nucleic acid synthesis and oncogenic RNA virus infection. *Proc. Int. Cancer Congr.*, **10**, 146 (1970).
12. Nakata, Y., Nakata, K., and Sakamoto, Y. Carcinogenesis by murine sarcoma virus. *Proc. Japan. Cancer Assoc.*, **29**, 83 (1970).
13. Rokutanda, M., Rokutanda, H., Green, M., Fujinaga, K., Ray, R. K., and Gurgo, C. Formation of viral RNA-DNA hybrid molecules by DNA polymerase of sarcoma-leukemia viruses. *Nature*, **227**, 1026–1028 (1970).
14. Spiegelman, S., Burny, A., Das, M. R., Keydar, J., Schlom, J., Travnicek, M., and Watson, K. Characterization of the products of RNA-directed DNA polymerases in oncogenic RNA viruses. *Nature*, **227**, 563–567 (1970).
15. Temin, H. Studies on carcinogenesis by avian sarcoma viruses. V. Requirement for new DNA synthesis and for cell division. *J. Cell. Physiol.*, **69**, 53–64 (1967).
16. Temin, H., and Mizutani, S. RNA-dependent DNA polymerase in virions of RSV. *Nature*, **226**, 1211–1213 (1970).
17. Watanabe, I., Haruna, I., Ohno, T., Yamada, Y., and Nagaka, K. Specific

inhibitor for RNA-dependent RNA polymerase (RNA replicase). *Proc. Int. Cancer Congr.*, **10**, 389 (1970).
18. Watson, K. F., and Beaudreau, G. S. Isolation of RNA-dependent RNA polymerase from virus infected myeloblasts. *Biochem. Biophys. Res. Commun.*, **37**, 925–932 (1969).
19. Watson, K. F., Haruna, I., and Beaudreau, G. S. Purification of RNA-dependent RNA polymerase from leukemic cells. *Proc. Am. Assoc. Cancer Res.*, **8**, 71 (1967).
20. Yoshikawa-Fukada, M., and Ebert, J. D. Hybridization of RNA from RSV with cellular and viral DNA's. *Proc. Natl. Acad. Sci. U.S.*, **64**, 870–877 (1969).

EXPLANATION OF PHOTOS

PHOTO 1. Budding of MSV(Moloney-MLV).

PHOTO 2. Focus formation on a cultured monolayer by RSV. 2a: Early focus. Focus by Schmidt-Ruppin RSV proceeds as 2b and 2c (diffuse type), although that by Bryan high-titer RSV(RAV-1) proceeds as 2d, 2e, and 2f (compact tumor type). In 2f, the tumor was lost into the culture medium.

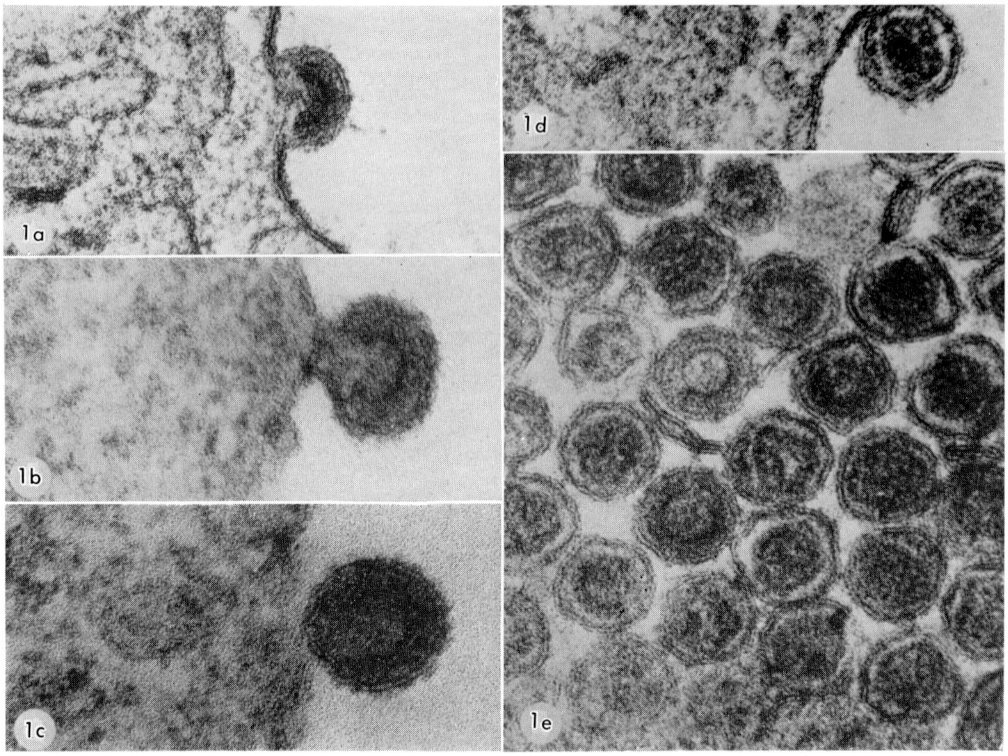
1a
1b
1c
1d
1e

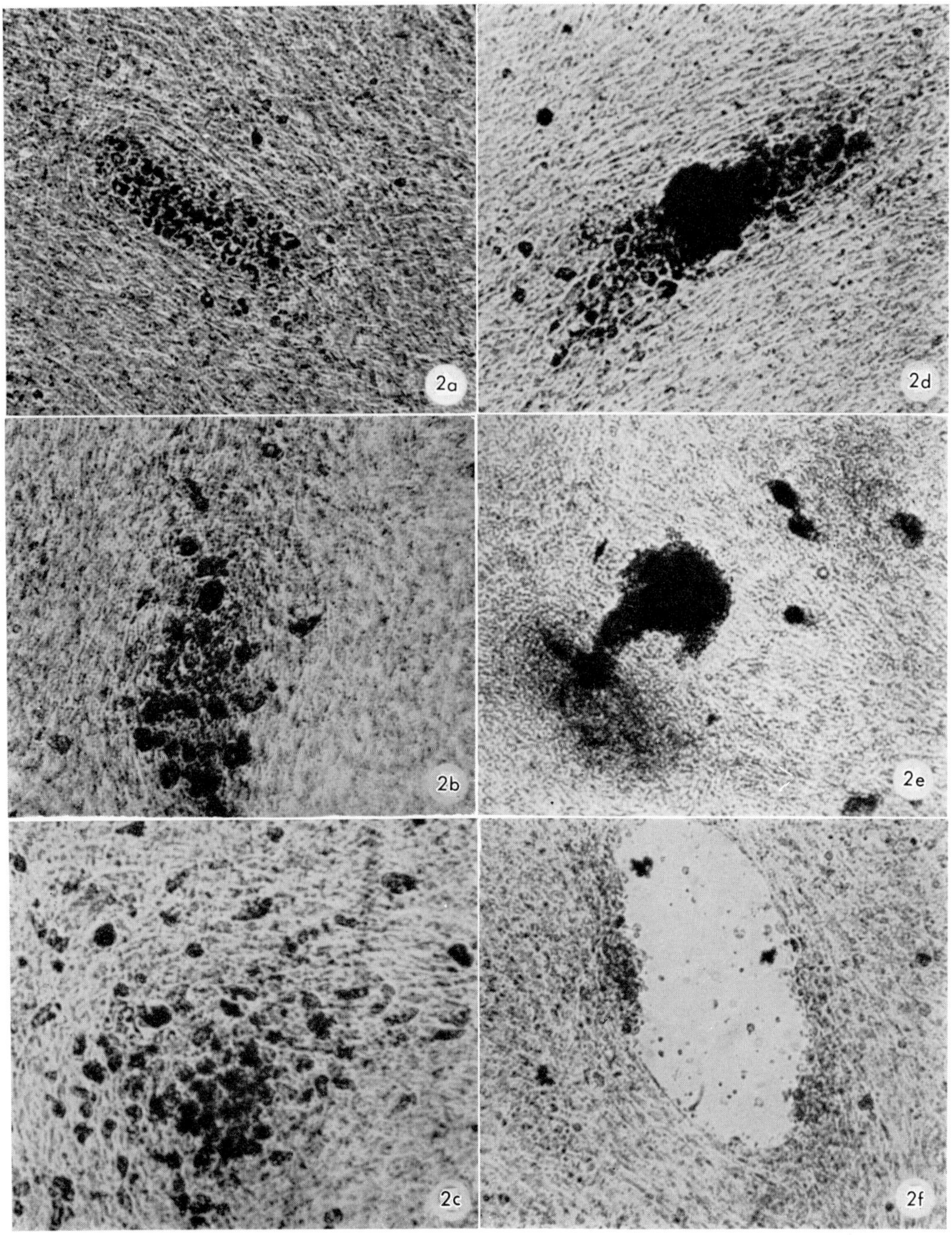
2a
2d
2b
2e
2c
2f

GANN Monograph on Cancer Research 12, 1972

RNA-DEPENDENT AND DNA-DEPENDENT DNA POLYMERASE REACTIONS INDUCED BY AVIAN MYELOBLASTOSIS VIRUS AND FELINE SARCOMA VIRUS

Kei FUJINAGA† and Maurice GREEN

Laboratory of Viral Oncology, Aichi Cancer Center Research Institute and Institute for Molecular Virology, St. Louis University School of Medicine***

RNA-dependent and DNA-dependent DNA polymerase(s) of avian myeloblastosis virus (AMV) and feline sarcoma virus (FeSV) are unmasked by treatment with the nonionic detergent Nonidet P-40. Native calf thymus DNA and adenovirus DNA stimulate DNA synthesis by detergent-disrupted virions. DNA-synthesizing reactions by AMV and FeSV virions are extremely rapid and show 2-phase kinetics, the rapid formation of RNA–DNA hybrid intermediates followed by free DNA. More than half of *in vitro* synthesized DNA is double stranded. The DNA product sediments at 5 to 7S, corresponding to the average molecular weight of 150,000 daltons, and has buoyant densities of 1.721 to 1.725.

Virions of several RNA-containing leukemia and sarcoma viruses possess DNA polymerase activities, first shown independently by Temin and Mizutani (*14*) and by Baltimore (*1*), followed by findings in several other laboratories (*2–5*, *11–13*). Viral RNA-DNA hybrid molecules were formed as intermediates with DNA base sequences complementary to those of viral RNA. Thus, these virions contain a unique enzyme, an RNA-dependent DNA polymerase, which catalizes the transcription of DNA from a viral RNA template (*4*, *12*). In addition to RNA-dependent DNA polymerase activity, virions of RNA tumor viruses possess DNA-dependent DNA polymerase activity as shown by the synthesis of duplex DNA molecules in the absence of added DNA template (*2*, *3*) and by the stimulated DNA synthesis in the presence of added duplex DNA template (*2*, *3*, *9*, *13*).

In this review, we describe the DNA polymerase reactions of the virions of avian myeloblastosis (AMV) (*2*) and feline sarcoma viruses (FeSV) (*3*). These involve rapid 2-step DNA synthesis reactions in which the initial formation of RNA-DNA hybrid intermediates is followed by the synthesis of duplex DNA molecules. Added duplex DNA templates stimulate the synthesis of DNA by the virion. Some of the properties of synthesized viral DNA are described. The

† Present address : Cancer Research Institute, Sapporo Medical College, Sapporo 060.
* Kanokoden 81, Tashiro-cho, Chikusa-ku, Nagoya 464 (藤永　蕙).
** 3681 Park Ave., St. Louis, Missouri, U.S.A.

work was done at the Institute for Molecular Virology, St. Louis University School of Medicine, St. Louis, Missouri.

DNA Polymerase Reaction Induced by Purified Virions

As shown in Table I, treatment of purified virions with the non-ionic detergent Nonidet P-40 (NP40) is required for the detection of DNA polymerase, RNA-dependent, and DNA-dependent polymerase activities. In the presence of NP40, purified virions incorporated ^{3}H-dTTP into an acid-insoluble, alkali-stable form

TABLE I. RNA-dependent and DNA-dependent DNA Polymerase Activity of AMV (*2*)

Virus treatment	Added DNA 10 μg	Incorporation of ^{3}H-dTTP (cpm)[a]
None	None	70
	Adenovirus type 2 DNA	80
	Calf thymus DNA	79
0.02% NP40	None	2,804
	Adenovirus type 2 DNA	12,189
	Calf thymus DNA	45,722
0.02% NP40 + 100 μg/ml RNase[b]	None	231
	Adenovirus type 2 DNA	8,535
	Calf thymus DNA	30,356

[a] Average of duplicate enzyme assays.
[b] Virus was preincubated with 100 μg/ml of pancreatic RNase for 30 min in the presence of 0.02% Nonidet P-40 prior to the DNA polymerase assay.

TABLE II. Effect of NP40 on AMV DNA Polymerase Activity

Expt. No.	NP40 concentration (%)		Time of incubation at 37° (min)	Incorporation of ^{3}H-dTTP (cpm)[a]
	Preincubation mixture	Incubation mixture		
1[b]	0.50	0.10	0	58
	None	None	60	70
	0.10	0.020	60	4,494
	0.50	0.10	60	4,211
2[c]	—	0.020	0	73
	—	None	60	68
	—	0.010	60	42
	—	0.020	60	7,017
	—	0.040	60	4,200
	—	0.10	60	3,254

[a] Average of duplicate enzyme assays under standard conditions (*2*) with 10 μCi of ^{3}H-dTTP (11.4 Ci/mmole).
[b] Purified virus (4.1 μg of viral protein) was incubated with NP40 for 15 min at 0°, diluted 5-fold in substrate mixture, and incubated further at 37°.
[c] Purified virus (4.3 μg of viral protein) was incubated at 37° in substrate mixture containing NP40.

TABLE III. Effect of Preincubation with NP40 on AMV DNA Polymerase Activity

(°)	Preincubation temperature time (min)	Time of incubation at 37° (min)	Incorporation of ^{3}H-dTTP (cpm)[a]
0°[b]	15	0	64
	5	60	2,255
	10	60	2,606
	15	60	2,141
	20	60	2,641
	30	60	2,582
37°[c]	5	60	3,054
	10	60	2,081
	15	60	2,794
	20	60	2,711
	30	60	2,928

[a] Average of duplicate enzyme assays under standard conditions (*2*) with 10 μCi of ^{3}H-dTTP (11.4 Ci/mmole).

[b] Purified virus (2.1 μg of viral protein) was incubated with NP40 at 0°, diluted 5-fold in substrate mixture, and incubated further at 37°.

[c] Purified virus (2.1 μg of viral protein) was incubated with NP40 at 37°, diluted 5-fold in substrate mixture, and incubated further at 37°.

and the addition of native adenovirus or calf thymus DNA markedly stimulated the incorporation. RNase treatment of virions in the presence of NP40 abolished RNA-dependent DNA polymerase activity, but the addition of adenovirus or calf thymus DNA to RNase-treated virions resulted in remarkable incorporation of ^{3}H-dTTP.

Maximum incorporation was obtained after preincubation of the virion with 0.1% of NP40 (final NP40 concentration of 0.02%) or by inclusion of 0.02% NP40 in the reaction mixture (Table II). Little dependence on either temperature or time of preincubation with NP40 was observed for the unmasking of viral DNA polymerase activity (Table III).

The virion polymerase has an optimum pH of 8.0 and requires Mg^{2+} (optimal 2.5 mM) or Mn^{2+} (optimal 1.0 mM) for activity (*2*). The omission of a single deoxyribonucleoside triphosphate reduced the incorporation into the acid-insoluble, alkali-stable form by approximately 90% (*2*).

The reaction kinetics of AMV DNA polymerase is shown in Fig. 1. In contrast to DNA polymerase reactions reported previously, DNA-synthesizing reactions by AMV and FeSV virions are extremely rapid and show two distinct rates of polymerization, the initial rapid reaction for 4 min at 37° and the less rapid reaction for 20 to 60 min. A minimum polymerization rate of 10 to 20 nucleotides/sec was calculated on the initial reaction by AMV virions (*2*), a value comparable to the *in vivo* rate of DNA replication in mammalian cells (*6*).

Formation of RNA-DNA Hybrid Molecules as Reaction Intermediates

Equilibrium centrifugation of the reaction mixture in Cs_2SO_4 density gradi-

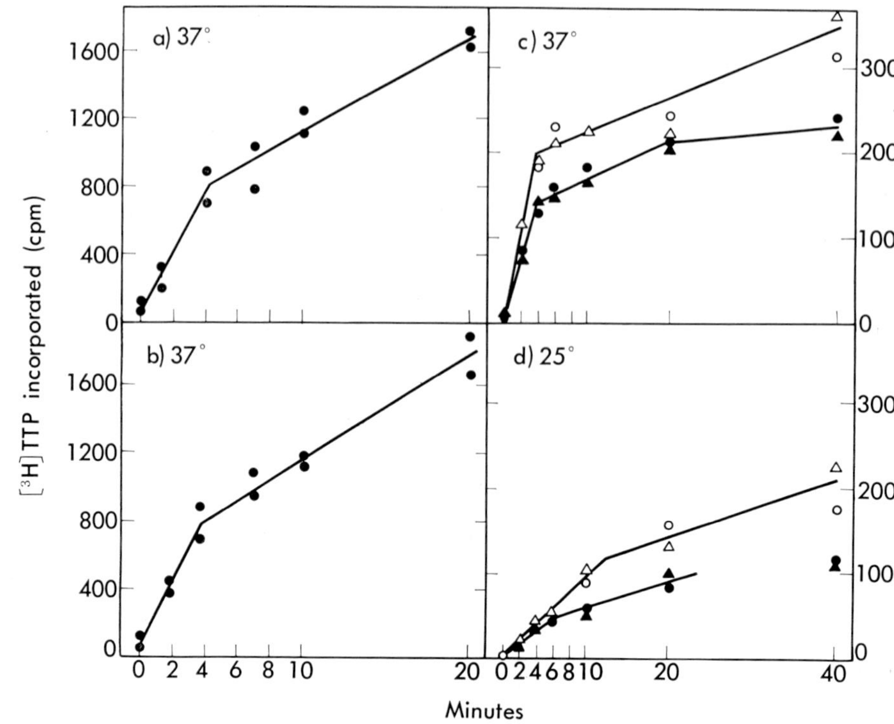

FIG. 1. Reaction kinetics of the AMV polymerase reaction (*2*)

AMV (0.2 volume) was incubated with 0.2% NP40 (a, b), 0.1% NP40 (c, d, lower curve), or 0.02% NP40 (c, d, upper curve) in the absence of substrate for at least 5 min at the individual temperature, and mixed with 0.8 volume substrate mixture at the individual temperature without NP40 (a, b, c, d, lower curve) or with 0.02% NP40 (c, d, upper curve). Acid-insoluble, alkali-stable radioactivities of duplicate 50 μl aliquots of the reaction mixture were determined after stopping the reaction at the indicated times by the addition of 0.1 volume of 0.1 M EDTA (a, b) or 150 μl of 1 N $HClO_4$ (c, d). Each aliquot contained 2.1 μg (a, b) or 3.2 μg (c, d) of viral protein and 5 μCi of ^{3}H-dTTP (11.4 Ci / mmole). Experiments a and b are duplicate enzyme reactions with the same AMV preparations; c and d used different AMV preparations.

ents was performed (Fig. 2). The " RNA-rich " hybrids banding close to free RNA were detected early at 30 sec (AMV) and 12 sec (FeSV) after the reaction began (*2*). The " intermediate hybrid " containing increased amounts of DNA was observed between RNA and DNA (Fig. 2). This indicates the formation of RNA-DNA hybrid molecules as reaction intermediates. At later periods of reaction, most of the ^{3}H-DNA molecules synthesized are free of viral RNA templates and band at the position of free DNA (Fig. 2). The formation of an " intermediate hybrid " suggests that most of the viral RNA base sequences are transcribed into ^{3}H-DNA (*2*). Hybridization between viral RNA and saturating levels of the DNA product has shown that most of the viral RNA is transcribed into DNA (Duesberg, personal communication; Green, unpublished data).

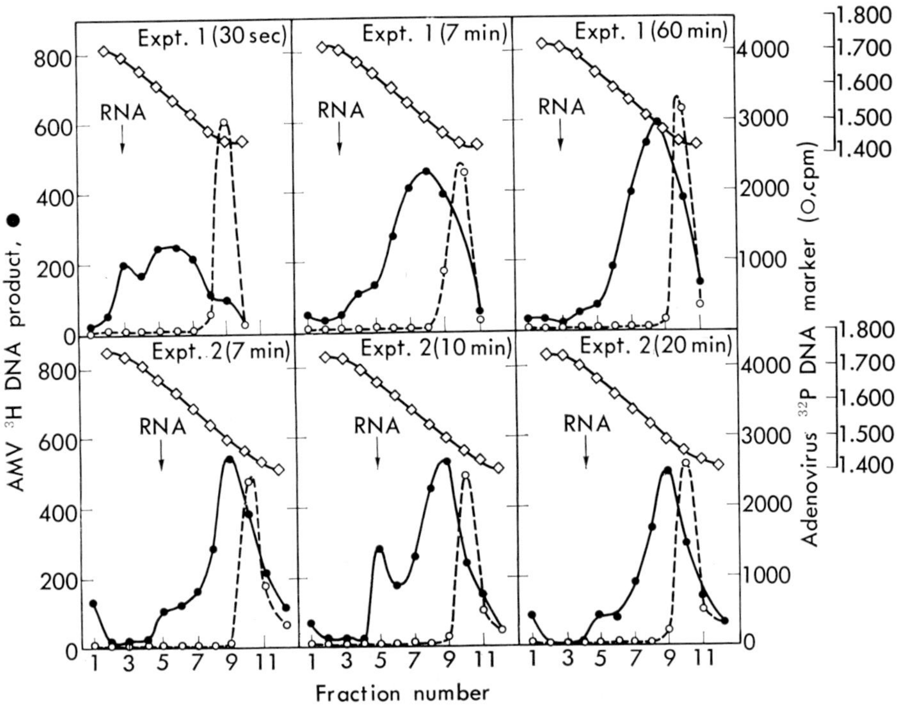

FIG. 2. Analysis of the AMV DNA product by equilibrium centrifugation in Cs_2SO_4 density gradient (*2*)

The DNA polymerase reaction was carried out as described in the legend to Fig. 1 (c, upper curve), and the reaction was stopped by adding 0.1 volume of 0.1 M EDTA. For Expt. 2, an aliquot of the reaction product of Fig. 1 (b) was used. The reaction product was purified and centrifuged to equilibrium with human KB cell RNA and adenovirus type 7 ^{32}P-DNA added as markers in Cs_2SO_4 density gradient. Fractions were collected and the refractive index, optical density, and acid-insoluble radioactivity were determined.

Synthesis of Duplex DNA Molecules

The strand characteristics of the DNA products, which consist mainly of template-free DNA, were analyzed by hydroxyapatite column chromatography and exonuclease I digestion. Single-strand DNA was eluted with 0.12 M phosphate buffer (PB) pH 6.8 while duplex DNA was eluted with 0.4 M PB, as shown by control experiments using native and denatured adenovirus and cellular DNAs (Fig. 3). Fifty to seventy percent of the FeSV and AMV DNAs synthesized eluted with 0.4 M PB, and 30 to 50% with 0.12 M PB (Fig. 3), indicating that more than half of the synthesized DNA was double stranded. However, 20 to 30% of the alkali-treated AMV DNA was not eluted by 0.12 M PB, indicating that a portion of the AMV DNA is duplex even after alkali denaturation. This may reflect the presence of cross-linking or a hairpin structure in AMV DNA products.

Escherichia coli exonuclease I digests single-strand DNA molecules from the 3′-OH end but does not convert duplex DNA molecules into an acid-soluble form,

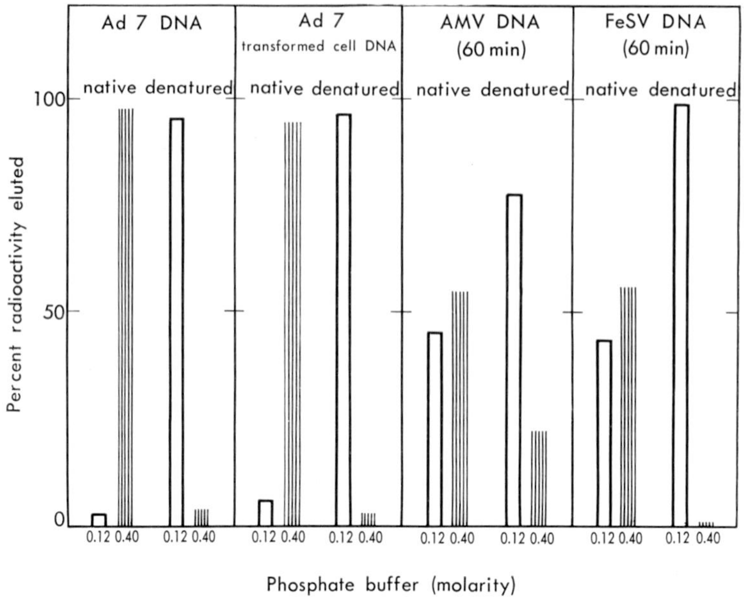

FIG. 3. Hydroxylapatite chromatography of product DNA (*2, 3*)

The ^{3}H-DNA product was purified, and a portion denatured with 0.2 N NaOH at 80° for 20 min, and neutralized. After sonication, native or denatured DNA in 4 ml of 0.12 M phosphate buffer (PB), pH 6.8, containing 0.4% sodium dodecyl sulfate was passed through a hydroxylapatite column maintained at 60°. The column was eluted with three 4-ml portions of 0.12 M PB containing 0.4% sodium dodecyl sulfate and with three 4-ml portions of 0.40 M PB. The acid-insoluble radioactivity of each fraction was determined.

TABLE IV. Action of Exonuclease I on the DNA Product of the Avian Myeloblastosis and Feline Sarcoma Virus DNA Polymerase (*2, 3*)[a]

DNA	Time of incubation at 37° (min)	Acid-insoluble DNA			
		Before denaturation		After denaturation[b]	
		cpm	%	cpm	%
AMV ^{3}H-DNA (60-min product)	0	1,239	100	1,208	100
	40	871	70	417	35
FeSV ^{3}H-DNA (30-min product)	0	786	100	780	100
	40	428	54	89	11
Adenovirus ^{32}P-DNA	0	2,669	100	2,248	100
	40	2,592	97	112	5

[a] Treatment with exonuclease I was carried out by incubating purified DNA product in 0.067 M glycine-NaOH buffer, pH 9.5, 6.7 mM $MgCl_2$, 10 mM 2-mercaptoethanol at 37° for 40 min with 10 units of exonuclease I.

[b] DNA was treated with 0.2 N NaOH at 80° for 20 min and neutralized prior to treatment with exonuclease I.

as was demonstrated by control experiments with native and denatured adenovirus and cellular DNAs (Table IV). The results of exonuclease I digestion of AMV and FeSV DNA products agreed with those obtained by hydroxyapatite column chromatography analysis (Fig. 3). We conclude that 50 to 70% of FeSV and AMV DNA products have a duplex DNA character.

There are 3 types of reactions catalyzed by RNA tumor virions: the initial formation of an RNA-DNA hybrid, the subsequent synthesis of a duplex DNA molecule in the absence of added template, and the synthesis of DNA molecules stimulated by the addition of duplex DNA. Whether the same or different protein molecules have these enzyme activities is not yet known. The characterization of purified DNA polymerase(s), their template specificity, and further analysis of the mechanism of polymerase reaction will be of great importance.

Properties of Synthesized DNA, and the Significance of the DNA Polymerase Reaction

Equilibrium density gradient centrifugation of alkali-denatured DNA product in CsCl resulted in a broad distribution of ^{3}H-DNA with mean buoyant densities

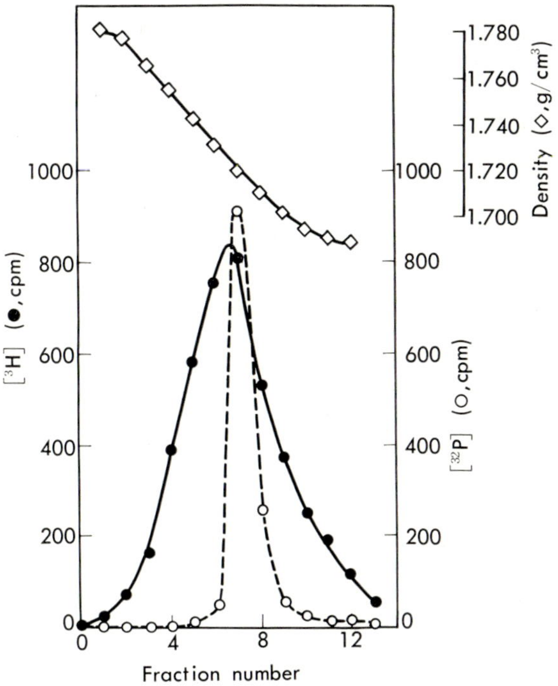

FIG. 4. Buoyant density of the AMV DNA product in CsCl density gradient (*2*)
An aliquot of purified AMV ^{3}H-DNA (Fig. 2, Expt. 1, 60 min) was denatured, neutralized, and centrifuged for 72 hr at 42,000 rpm to equilibrium in CsCl density gradient, with adenovirus type 7 ^{32}P-DNA added as a marker. Fractions were collected, and the refractive index and acid-insoluble radioactivities were determined.

of 1.721 for AMV-DNA and 1.725 for FeSV-DNA (Fig. 4). The broad distribution of ^{3}H-DNA product in CsCl density gradient compared to that of marker Ad 7 DNA is probably due to the low molecular weight of synthesized DNA and to the heterogeneity in base composition among DNA molecules.

The size of denatured single-strand ^{3}H-DNA was estimated by zone sedimentation in alkaline sucrose gradients (Fig. 5). Sedimentation values of 5 to 7S were obtained based on the 34S adenovirus ^{14}C-DNA marker (*2, 3*), corresponding to an average molecular weight of 150,000 daltons (*2, 3*). The size of single-strand ^{3}H-DNA molecules synthesized was 2 to 7% of that of viral RNA. Viral DNA

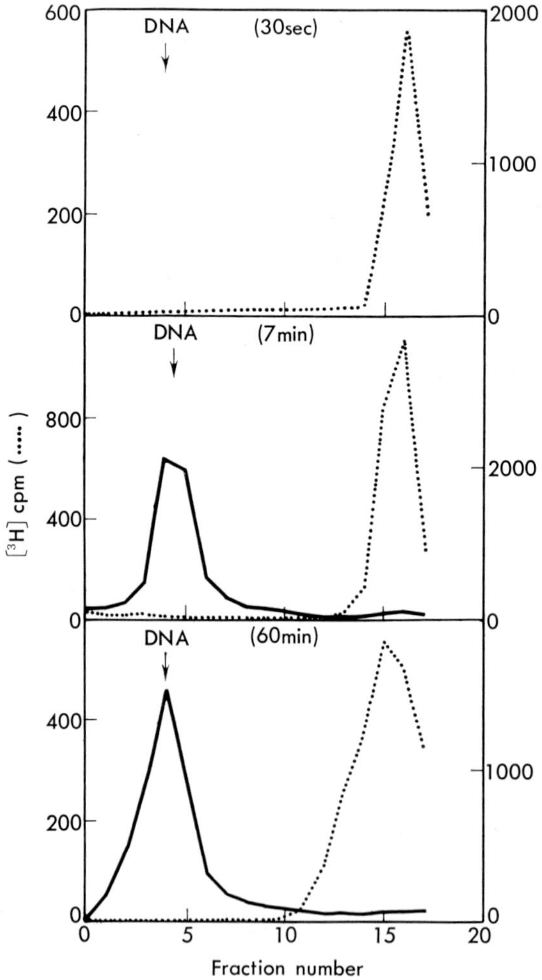

FIG. 5. Zone sedimentation of the AMV DNA product in alkaline sucrose density gradients

An aliquot of AMV ^{3}H-DNA (Fig. 2, Expt. 1) was denatured and centrifuged with a marker of ^{14}C-thymidine labeled adenovirus type 7 for 9 hr at 36,000 rpm at 4° through linear 5 to 20% sucrose gradient in 0.3 N NaOH, 0.7 M NaCl, and 0.001 M EDTA. Fractions were collected and the acid-insoluble, alkali-stable radioactivity was determined (*2*).

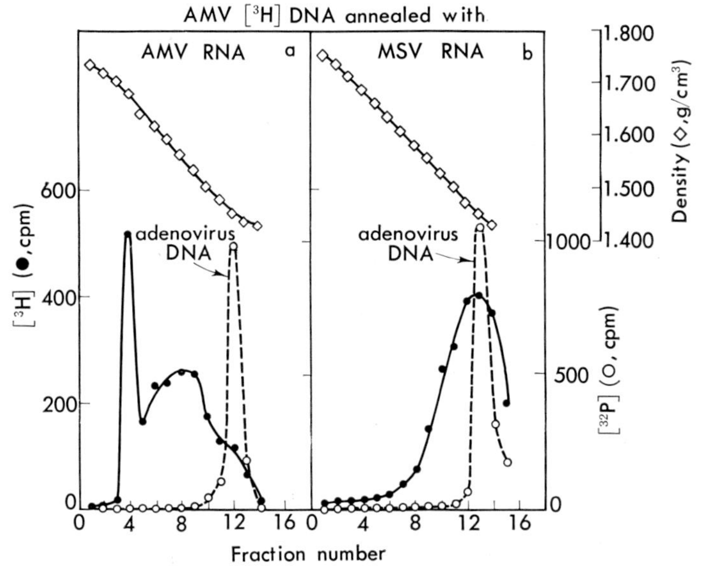

FIG. 6. Hybridization of AMV DNA with viral RNA (*2*)

A 60-min AMV ^{3}H-DNA (Fig. 2, Expt. 1) was purified, denatured, and hybridized with 2 μg of AMV RNA (a) or MSV RNA (b) in 2 × SSC for 24 hr at 66°. The products were analyzed by equilibrium centrifugation in Cs_2SO_4 density gradient using adenovirus type 7 ^{32}P-DNA as a marker, as described in Fig. 2.

molecules are synthesized probably as short fragments (*10*) of the entire viral genome. The possible synthesis of large viral DNA molecules *in vivo*, with the aid of other enzymes such as ligases, remains to be established.

Hybridization between viral RNA and the denatured product DNA was performed and the DNA-RNA hybrid was analyzed by Cs_2SO_4 equilibrium density gradient centrifugation. As shown in Fig. 6, 60 to 70% of AMV ^{3}H-DNA banded at the " RNA-rich " and intermediate hybrid positions in the gradient when the hybridization was carried out between AMV RNA and denatured AMV ^{3}H-DNA. The 30 to 40% of ^{3}H-DNA that does not hybridize may represent in part " positive " DNA strands which cannot hybridize with viral RNA-" positive " strands. No detectable DNA-RNA hybrid was formed between MSV (murine sarcoma virus) RNA and denatured AMV ^{3}H-DNA. These results clearly show that virions have a unique enzyme, an RNA-dependent DNA polymerase, and that they synthesize viral DNA sequences complementary to RNA viral genome.

The flow of genetic information from viral RNA to DNA may play an important role in virus replication and cell transformation. Further *in vivo* studies on the synthesis of viral DNA from the RNA viral genome, the formation of duplex DNA molecules, the biological functions of the viral DNA product, and the transcription of viral DNA will provide a basic understanding of the mechanisms of virus replication and cell transformation by RNA tumor viruses.

Huebner and Todaro (7) proposed that normal cellular genes contain RNA tumor virus genetic information and that the expression of the " oncogene," a part of the viral genome, is required for carcinogenesis. The expression of some of the RNA tumor virus genome during embryonic development in the mouse was reported recently (*8*). The information flow from RNA to DNA may possibly be involved in normal cellular gene expression during embryonic development, differentiation, and other normal cell functions. Future studies along these lines are sure to be exciting and informative.

Acknowledgments

This investigation was supported by contract PH43–67–692 from the Etiology Area, Viral Carcinogenesis Branch, National Cancer Institute, National Institutes of Health, Bethesda, Maryland, U.S.A.

REFERENCES

1. Baltimore, D. RNA-dependent DNA-polymerase in virions of RNA tumor viruses. *Nature*, **226**, 1209 (1970).
2. Fujinaga, K., Parsons, J. T., Beard, J., Beard, D., and Green, M. Mechanism of carcinogenesis by RNA tumor viruses. III. Formation of RNA-DNA complex and duplex molecules by the DNA polymerase(s) of avian myeloblastosis virus. *Proc. Natl. Acad. Sci. U.S.*, **67**, 1432 (1970).
3. Fujinaga, K., and Green, M. Mechanism of carcinogenesis by RNA tumor viruses. V. Analysis of the RNA and DNA dependent DNA polymerase activities of the teline sarcinoma virus. *J. Gen. Virol.*, **12**, 85 (1971).
4. Green, M., Rokutanda, K., Fujinaga, K., Ray, R. K., Rokutanda, H., and Gurgo, C. Mechanism of carcinogenesis by RNA tumor viruses. I. An RNA dependent DNA polymerase in murine sarcoma viruses. *Proc. Natl. Acad. Sci. U.S.*, **67**, 385 (1970).
5. Hatanaka, M., Huebner, R. J., and Gilden, R. V. DNA polymerase activity associated with RNA tumor viruses. *Proc. Natl. Acad. Sci. U.S.*, **67**, 143 (1970).
6. Huberman, J. A., and Riggs, A. D. On the mechanism of DNA replication in mammalian chromosomes. *J. Mol. Biol.*, **32**, 327 (1968).
7. Huebner, R. J., and Todaro, G. J. Oncogenes of RNA tumor viruses as determinants of cancer. *Proc. Natl. Acad. Sci. U.S.*, **64**, 1087 (1969).
8. Huebner, R. J., Kelloff, G. J., Sarma, P. S., Lane, W. T., Turner, H. C., Gilden, R. V., Oroszland, S., Meier, H., Nyers, D. D., and Peters, R. L. Group-specific (gs) antigen expression of the C-type RNA tumor virus genome during embryogenesis: Implications for ontogenesis and oncogenesis. *Proc. Natl. Acad. Sci. U.S.*, **67**, 366 (1970).
9. Mizutani, S., and Temin, H. M. *Nature*, **228**, 424 (1970).
10. Okazaki, R., Okazaki, T., Sakabe, K., Sugimoto, K., Kainuma, R., Sugino, A., and Iwatsuki, N. *In vivo* mechanism of DNA chain growth. *Cold Spring Harbor Symp. Quant. Biol.*, **33**, 129 (1968).
11. Rokutanda, M., Rokutanda, H., Green, M., Fujinaga, K., Ray, R. K., and Gurgo, C. Formation of viral RNA-DNA hybrid molecules by the DNA polymerase of sarcoma-leukemia viruses. *Nature*, **227**, 1026 (1970).
12. Spiegelman, S., Burny, A., Das, M. R., Keydar, J., Schlom, J., Travnicek, M.,

and Watson, K. Characterization of the products of RNA-directed DNA polymerase in oncogenic RNA viruses. *Nature*, **227**, 563 (1970).
13. Spiegelman, S., Burny, A., Das, M. R., Keydar, J., Scholm, J., Travnicek, M., and Watson, K. DNA-directed DNA polymerase activity in oncogenic RNA viruses. *Nature*, **227**, 1029 (1970).
14. Temin, H. M., and Mizutani, S. RNA-dependent DNA polymerase in virion of Rous sarcoma virus. *Nature*, **226**, 1211 (1970).

GANN Monograph on Cancer Research 12, 1972

CHANGES IN ENZYMES IN THE MOUSE SPLEEN AFTER FRIEND VIRUS INFECTION

Takahiko TAGUCHI and Tetsuo ONO

Department of Physiology, Zoological Institute, Faculty of Science, Tokyo Kyoiku University and Department of Biochemistry, Cancer Institute***

The quantitative as well as qualitative changes in enzymes involved in the synthesis of nucleic acids in the mouse spleen in the course of infection with Friend virus were examined.

The activity of thymidine kinase, uridine kinase, and DNA polymerase in the spleen was found to increase with infection by Friend virus. However, virus infection produced no qualitative alteration in the enzyme forms of thymidine kinase and uridine kinase that was ascertainable in examinations using DEAE-cellulose column chromatography and starch zone electrophoresis.

Using phosphocellulose column chromatography of DNA polymerase, a peak of enzyme activity which was not found in the extract from normal mouse spleen was detected in that from mouse spleen infected with Friend virus. This peak was evident in the extract of mouse spleen 4 days after infection, and the activity increased thereafter. However, this form of DNA polymerase was found also in extract from a mouse spleen with exaggerated hematopoiesis induced by the injection of acetylphenylhydrazine. On histological examination, an increase of erythroblasts was observed in the spleens of mice infected with Friend virus as well as those treated with acetylphenylhydrazine. From these facts, it seems likely that the appearance of this abnormal peak of DNA polymerase activity after infection should be attributable to the proliferation of erythroblasts in the spleen.

The intracellular distribution of RNA-dependent DNA polymerase in the spleens of mice infected with Friend virus was also investigated.

A number of RNA viruses that are oncogenic in many species of animals have been reported, but the mechanism of carcinogenesis by these viruses is not as clear as in the case of DNA viruses. For example, it is well known that virus-specific thymidine kinase (*12*, *15*) and DNA-dependent DNA polymerase (*4*, *14*, *16*) are induced by infection with DNA viruses. As for RNA viruses, however, specific enzymes coded in RNA virus genome and involved in the synthesis of nucleic acid needed for multiplication of RNA virus and its target cells have not been known,

* Otsuka 3-29-1, Bunkyo-ku, Tokyo 112 (田口隆彦).
** Kami-Ikebukuro 1-37-1, Toshima-ku, Tokyo 170 (小野哲生).

with the exception of phage RNA replicase (*3*, *10*, *19*) and RNA-dependent DNA polymerase in viral particles, reported quite recently.

Friend virus (7) is an oncogenic RNA viruses, and in mice it causes Friend disease, which is characterized by marked splenomegaly. Therefore, we examined the quantitative changes in enzymes involved in the synthesis of nucleic acid in the mouse spleen in the course of infection with Friend virus and further searched for Friend virus-specific enzymes.

In these experiments, thymidine kinase, uridine kinase, DNA-dependent DNA polymerase, and RNA-dependent DNA polymerase were chosen as enzymes involved in the synthesis of nucleic acid; their activities in the spleen were determined, and they were fractionated by starch zone electrophoresis, DEAE-cellulose column chromatography, and phosphocellulose column chromatography.

Quantitative Changes in Enzymes

Figure 1A shows the enlargement of mouse spleen after injection by Friend virus; the infected mouse spleen was about 5 times heavier than a normal uninfected one.

Thymidine kinase activity in the mouse spleen increased after infection with Friend virus and its activity in mouse spleen 20 days after infection was about twice that in uninfected spleen.

Uridine kinase activity in mouse spleen infected with Friend virus exhibited much fluctuation in the course of infection.

As shown in Fig. 1B, DNA polymerase activity primed by calf thymus native DNA in mouse spleen 20 days after infection was about 1.5 times as high as that from an uninfected mouse. On the other hand, DNA polymerase activity primed by heat-denatured DNA from calf thymus in mouse spleen 20 days after infection was about 3 times as high as that from an uninfected one.

However, the activity of thymidine kinase, uridine kinase, and DNA polymerase primed by both native DNA and heat-denatured DNA in mouse liver did not increase after Friend virus infection (Figs. 2 C and D).

Qualitative Changes in Enzymes

Furthermore, we tested whether or not the changes in enzyme activity in mouse spleen were due to the induction of new enzymes.

1. Thymidine kinase and uridine kinase

In the first place, crude enzyme extracts from spleen were fractionated by starch zone electrophoresis. During electrophoresis, thymidine kinase and DNA polymerase were inactivated almost completely. As for uridine kinase, one active peak was shown after electrophoresis of crude extract from mouse spleen infected with Friend virus, and one small peak was also detected in the fractions from uninfected mouse spleen.

This procedure showed that the active peak of uridine kinase fractionated from

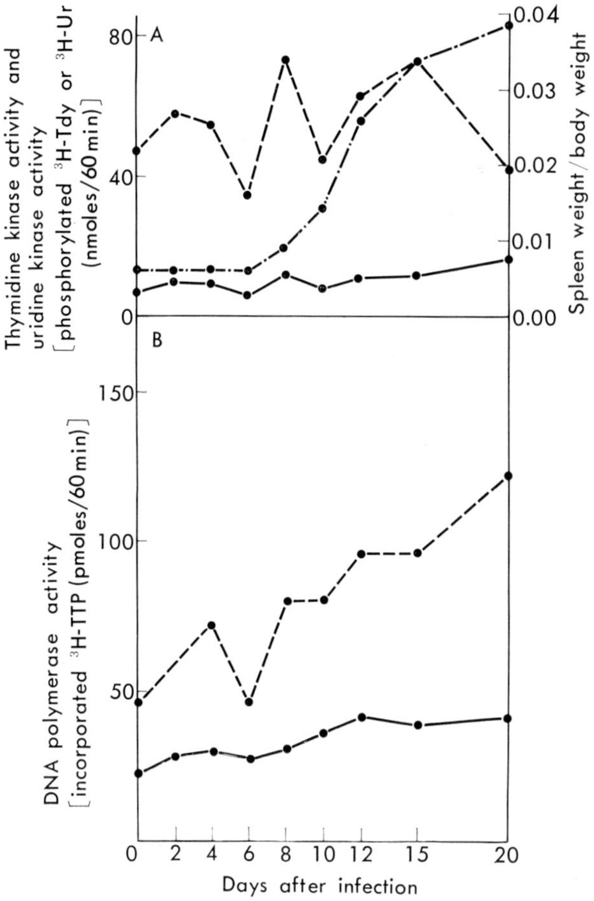

FIG. 1. Changes in spleen weight and the activity of thymidine kinase, uridine kinase, and DNA polymerase in mouse spleen after infection with Friend virus

Mice of dd strain (20–25 g body weight) were inoculated intraperitoneally with 0.1 ml of 10% (w / v) homogenate of spleens from mice with Friend disease. Thymidine kinase, uridine kinase, and DNA polymerase were assayed using the crude extract (supernatant of high-speed (105,000 $\times g$) centrifugation of 20% homogenate of spleens). Thymidine kinase activity was measured by a procedure analogous to that described by Bresnick and Karjala (*6*). Uridine kinase activity was measured by a method similar to that used for the assay of thymidine kinase, except that ^{3}H-uridine was used instead of ^{3}H-thymidine in the reaction mixture. DNA polymerase activity was measured by a procedure similar to that described by Bollum (*5*).

A. Thymidine kinase activity (●——●) and uridine kinase activity (●- - -●) were expressed by nmoles of phosphorylated ^{3}H-thymidine or ^{3}H-uridine in the reaction mixture after 60 min at 37° by 0.1 ml of enzyme extract. (●–·–●) changes in spleen weight/body weight.

B. DNA polymerase activity using native DNA (●——●) and heat-denatured DNA (●- - -●) as the template were expressed by pmoles of ^{3}H-TTP incorporated into DNA in the reaction mixture by 0.05 ml of enzyme extract for 60 min at 37°.

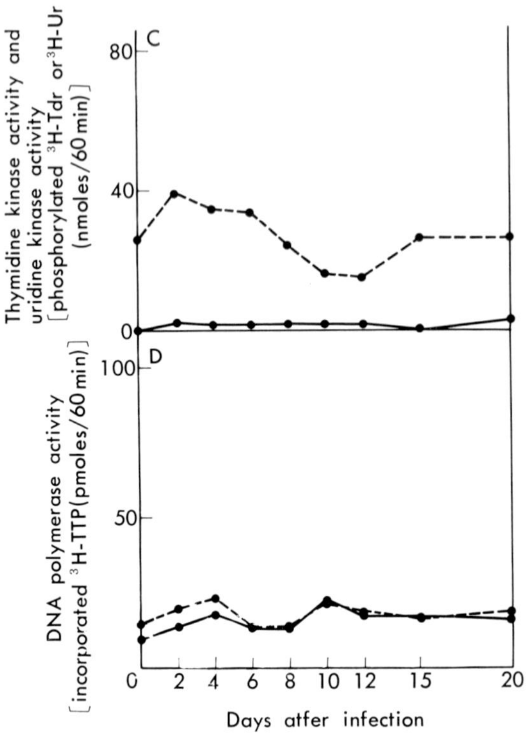

FIG. 2. Activity of thymidine kinase, uridine kinase, and DNA polymerase in mouse liver after infection with Friend virus

C. Activity of thymidine kinase (●——●) and uridine kinase (●- - -●).

D. Activity of DNA polymerase on templates of native DNA (●——●) and heat-denatured DNA (●- - -●). Enzyme activities were measured by the same methods as those described in the legend of Fig. 1.

crude extract of mouse spleen 8 days after infection with Friend virus was about 5 times more active than fractions from uninfected mouse spleen.

As shown in Figs. 3 A and B, on DEAE cellulose column chromatography of crude extracts of spleen from both mice infected with Friend virus and uninfected mice, thymidine kinase exhibited 1 peak and uridine kinase was separated into 3 peaks. The peak of thymidine kinase was eluted out with 0.01 M KCl solution, and Peak 1 of uridine kinase was eluted out with 0.01 M, Peak 2 with 0.1 M, and Peak 3 with 0.5 M KCl solution which contained 0.2 M Tris-HCl buffer, pH 8.0.

Summarizing the results of fractionation of thymidine kinase and uridine kinase, no enzyme form unique to virus-infected spleen was detected at all, although the specific activities of these enzymes were shown to increase remarkably after virus infection. However, the increases in the activities of thymidine kinase and uridine kinase after infection were not so remarkable when they were assayed by crude extract, as described above. This discrepancy may be due to interference by inhibitory, that is, dephosphorylating enzyme reactions, in crude extracts.

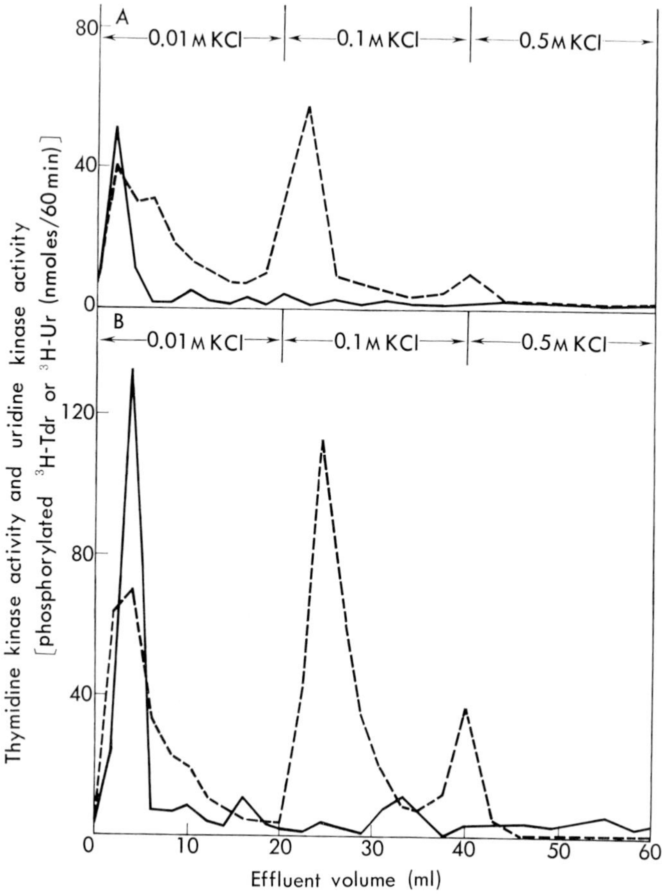

FIG. 3. DEAE-cellulose column chromatography of thymidine kinase and uridine kinase from spleens of control mice (A) and mice infected with Friend virus (B)

Enzyme extract (2.5 ml) was applied to a DEAE-cellulose column (1 × 5 cm) which was equilibrated with 0.2 M Tris-HCl buffer, pH 8.0, containing 0.01 M KCl and 0.01 M 2-mercaptoethanol. Tris-HCl buffers containing KCl were employed as stepwise eluents: 20 ml of 0.01 M, 20 ml of 0.1 M, and 20 ml of 0.5 M. The eluate was fractionated in about 2.5 ml each. The assays of thymidine kinase activity (——) and uridine kinase activity (----) were carried out by the same methods as those described in the legend to Fig. 1.

2. *DNA-dependent DNA polymerase*

Aposhian and Kornberg (*2*) have extracted phage-specific DNA polymerase from *Escherichia coli* infected with T_2 phage by phosphocellulose column chromatography, and Ono and Umehara (*17*) have found 3 molecular species of DNA polymerase in rat liver and some hepatomas. Thus, we examined the change of molecular species of DNA polymerase extracted from mouse spleen infected with Friend virus by the same procedure. As shown in Fig. 4 A, a crude extract of DNA polymerase from uninfected mouse spleen was separated by phosphocellulose column chromatography into 3 active peaks. These peaks exhibited ac-

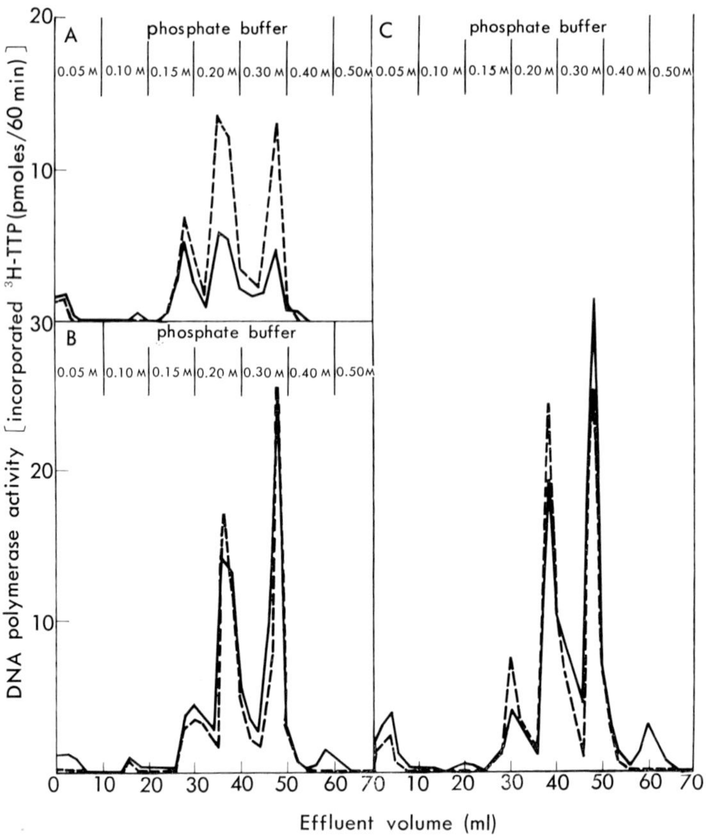

FIG. 4. Phosphocellulose column chromatography of DNA polymerase from spleens of control mice (A), 4 days after infection with Friend virus (B), and 8 days after infection (C)

Five ml of enzyme extract was applied to a phosphocellulose column (1 ×8 cm) which was equilibrated with 0.05 M phosphate buffer, pH 6.5, containing 0.01 M 2-mercaptoethanol. Phosphate buffers, pH 6.5, of the following concentrations containing 0.01 M 2-mercaptoethanol were used as stepwise eluents: 10 ml of 0.05 M, 10 ml of 0.1 M, 10 ml of 0.15 M, 10 ml of 0.2 M, 10 ml of 0.3 M, 10 ml of 0.4 M, and 10 ml of 0.5 M. Eluates from the column were fractionated in 2 ml each. The methods for assays of DNA polymerase activity using native DNA (——) and heat-denatured DNA (----) as the template were the same as those described in the legend to Fig. 1.

tivities on either native or heat-denatured calf thymus DNA as templates, and these 3 peaks were eluted out with 0.15 M, 0.20 M, and 0.30 M phosphate buffer, pH 6.5, respectively. A crude extract of DNA polymerase from mouse spleen infected with Friend virus was separated into 4 active peaks. The first 3 peaks corresponded to those separated from a crude extract of uninfected mouse spleen in regard to the position of the elution pattern, although the activity of each peak from infected mouse spleen increased remarkably over the corresponding peak in uninfected mouse spleen. However, the fourth peak of DNA polymerase, which was eluted out with 0.4 M phosphate buffer, pH 6.5, from a column charged with extract from infected spleen took only native DNA as a template. This peak was observed in a crude extract from mouse spleen 4 days after infection, and the activity of this peak obtained from mouse spleen 8 days after infection was higher than that of 4 days after infection (Figs. 4 B and C) and was even more remarkable in the spleen 30 days after infection (Fig. 5).

To determine whether the appearance of this DNA polymerase peak was really specific for Friend virus or resulted from the change of cellular population in the spleen induced by infection with the virus, we made the following test. Mice were given injections of 1 mg of acetylphenylhydrazine (per mouse for 4 days) to induce hemolytic anemia. As a result, the spleen enlarged, with the appearance of hematopoietic cells as in virus-infected spleens. On phosphocellulose column chromatography of a crude extract from the spleens of mice treated with acetylphenylhydrazine, the fourth active peak of DNA polymerase primed only by a native DNA was observed as that from mouse spleen infected with Friend virus (Fig. 6).

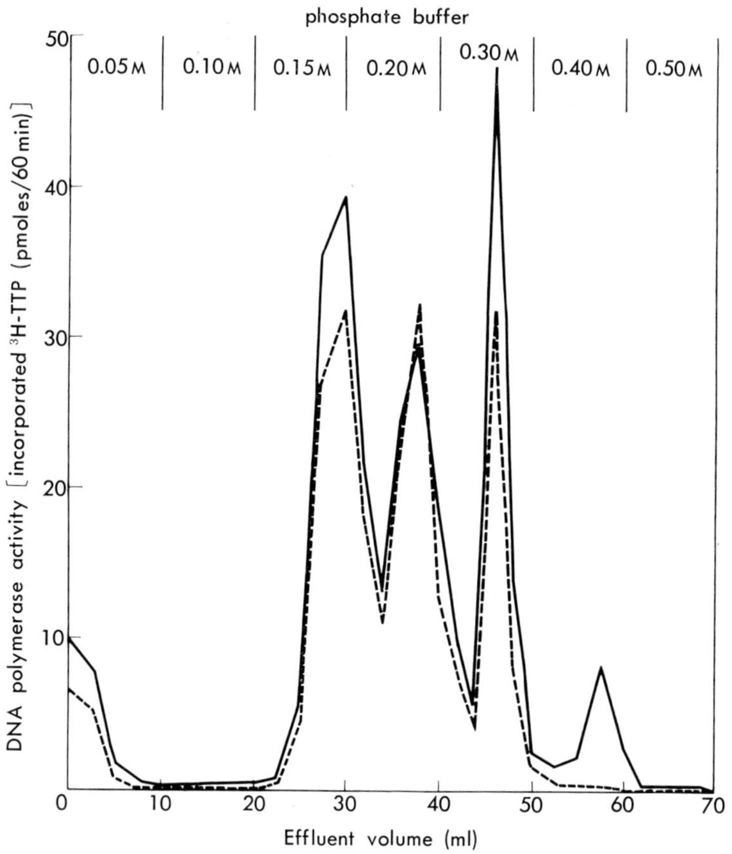

FIG. 5. Phosphocellulose column chromatography of DNA polymerase from mouse spleen 30 days after infection with Friend virus

The experimental procedures were the same as those of the experiment presented in Fig. 4. The activity on templates of native DNA (——) and heat-denatured DNA (- - - -) is shown.

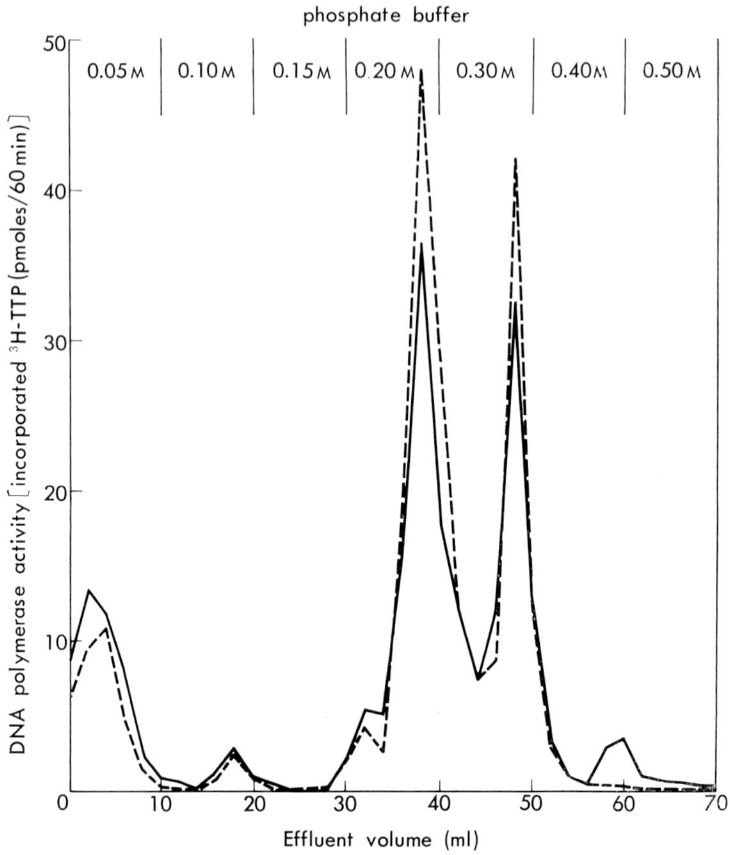

FIG. 6. Phosphocellulose column chromatography of DNA polymerase from spleens of mice treated with acetylphenylhydrazine

Acetylphenylhydrazine (1 mg / mouse) was injected once a day for 4 days and the mice were killed 2 days after final injection, as reported by Ito and Tatibana (*13*). The other experimental procedures were the same as those described in Fig. 4. The DNA polymerase activity on native DNA (——) and heat-denatured DNA (– – – –) templates is shown.

3. *RNA-dependent DNA polymerase*

The presence of RNA-dependent DNA polymerase in the particles of Friend virus was also expected, based on the report of Schlom *et al.* (*18*). Although this polymerase might be contained in the virus particle, the synthesis of the enzyme should be viewed as being carried out by the enzyme-forming machinery of the host cells, and it seemed reasonable to expect the presence of this polymerase also in the spleen producing viruses. Therefore, DNA synthesis depending on RNA extracted from mouse spleen infected with Friend virus, rA-rU, or r(AU), was tested using each peak of DNA polymerase activity separated as described above from spleen infected with Friend virus, and the results are presented in Table I. As shown in the table, so far, no stimulation of DNA synthesis by those templates has been found in any peak of DNA polymerase.

TABLE I. Comparison of DNA Polymerase Activity on Different Templates

Enzyme fraction	Templates						
	—	RNA	rA-rU	r(AU)	N-DNA[a]	D-DNA[b]	d(AT)
Peak 2	<1.0	<1.0	<1.0	<1.0	14.8	17.5	210.5
Peak 3	1.6	<1.0	<1.0	<1.0	11.1	18.0	106.3
Peak 4	1.6	<1.0	<1.0	<1.0	<1.0	<1.0	26.8

Each peak of DNA polymerase was fractionated from the extract of spleens of mice infected with Friend virus. The assays of DNA polymerase activity were carried out by the same method as those described in other experiments except that 5 μg each of RNA prepared from the spleens of mice infected with Friend virus, poly (rA : rU), r(AU) copolymer, calf thymus native or heat-denatured DNA, or d(AT) copolymer was used as the template instead of 120 μg of DNA in the reaction mixture.

[a] Native DNA. [b] Heat-denatured DNA.

The fractionation of DNA polymerase used in this test was started from the crude extract of the supernatant of spleen homogenate following high-speed (105,000$\times g$) centrifugation. Therefore, it was likely that RNA-dependent DNA polymerase would not be contained in the cell in a soluble form, even if it were present.

Next, we tested the presence of this enzyme activity in the high-speed (105,000$\times g$) centrifugation pellet after removing the precipitate formed by centrifugation at 10,000$\times g$. However, no significant activity was detected in this fraction either. This pellet fraction should contain the virus particles, if they were present. The negative result might be due to the fact that the amount of virus particles we collected in this fraction was not sufficient to exhibit a significant activity in our assay system.

Therefore, we searched for this enzyme activity in the low-speed (1,000$\times g$) centrifugation precipitate of spleen homogenate. This fraction is thought to contain the nuclei and plasma membrane. It was sonicated in the presence of 0.2% Triton X-100, then centrifuged at 30,000$\times g$ as described by Ackermann *et al.* (*1*), and the supernatant fraction was saved for enzyme assay. Some significant but low RNA-dependent DNA polymerase activity was found in this fraction.

DISCUSSION

Uridine kinase activity in the spleen of mice infected with Friend virus fluctuated considerably in the course of infection. However, the activity of enzyme fractions which were separated by starch zone electrophoresis and DEAE-cellulose column chromatography was increased remarkably by infection with Friend virus. These facts seemed to suggest that crude extract of enzyme from mouse spleen may involve inhibitor or phosphatase, which interferes with the kinase reactions. Gelbard *et al.* (*8*) have reported that the activity of partially purified uridine kinase from chorioallantoic membrane was increased by infection with Rous sarcoma virus. Therefore, these experiments seemed to suggest that the synthesis of uridine kinase may be induced to allow the multiplication of RNA virus and target cells in the spleen after virus infection.

The existence of altered uridine kinase which might be induced by Friend virus infection was assessed by experiments using electrophoresis and DEAE-cellulose column chromatography. Three peaks of uridine kinase activity were revealed in crude extract of enzyme from mouse spleen infected with Friend virus and also in the extract from normal mouse spleen. Gilliland and Symons (*9*) have reported that the induction of virus-specific uridine kinase was not observed after infection with cucumber mosaic virus, which is an RNA virus. These results suggest that the synthesis of uridine monophosphate after RNA virus infection depends on the uridine kinase in the host cells, and not on the virus-specific enzyme.

Although the DEAE-cellulose column chromatographic pattern suggested the existence of 3 molecular forms of uridine kinase, there remained the possibility that they showed different behavior in column chromatography depending on the degree of aggregation of subunits or by association with other proteins. Hashimoto *et al.* (*11*) fractionated thymidine kinase by electrophoresis using Pevikon and DEAE-cellulose column chromatography and found 1 molecular form in the enzyme extract from rat spleen and 2 molecular forms in the enzyme extract from Yoshida sarcoma cells as well as all other malignant cells they tested. However, in our experiment, thymidine kinase in mouse spleen consisted of only 1 molecular form and another enzyme form, such as Friend virus-specific thymidine kinase, was not detected after infection with the virus.

Three molecular forms of DNA polymerase were found in normal mouse spleen by phosphocellulose column chromatography, but this may be insufficient to consider them different molecular forms, as in the case of uridine kinase. Concerning DNA-dependent DNA polymerase, 1 unique molecular form of DNA polymerase which has the characteristic of taking only a native DNA as template was found to be induced by Friend virus infection. However, since this DNA polymerase was induced in spleens also by acetylphenylhydrazine treatment, one cannot insist that this enzyme is specific to Friend virus infection.

It has been reported that proliferation of erythroblasts is induced in the spleen by Friend virus infection, and also by the hematopoiesis induced after acetylphenylhydrazine treatment. Histological examinations have revealed the increase of erythroblasts in the spleens of mice infected with Friend virus as well as in those treated with acetylphenylhydrazine. From these facts, we can say that the appearance of a new peak of DNA polymerase activity after infection with Friend virus is likely to be due to the change in the cellular constitution of mouse spleen induced by the infection.

In extracts from regenerating rat liver and Morris hepatomas, Ono and Umehara observed 3 molecular forms of DNA polymerase by phosphocellulose column chromatography (*17*). Therefore, DNA polymerase primed by native DNA is not extracted from erythroblasts only. It appears necessary to study the function of DNA polymerase primed only by native DNA, and also the relation of the appearance of this DNA polymerase to the proliferation of erythroblasts.

Search for RNA-dependent DNA polymerase activity revealed that in spleen infected with Friend virus no soluble form of this enzyme was present, but it was detected in small amounts in the precipitate of low-speed centrifugation, which contains nuclei and plasma membrane. Although it is most likely that it is bound to the plasma membrane, a firm conclusion should await further experimentation.

Acknowledgment

This work was supported in part by a Grant-in-Aid for Scientific Research from the Ministry of Education of Japan.

REFERENCES

1. Ackermann, W. W., Murphy, W. H., Miller, B. A., Kurtz, H., and Backer, S. T. RNA-dependent DNA synthesis in cell free preparations of human leukemia cells. *Biochem. Biophys. Res. Commun.*, **42**, 723–729 (1971).
2. Aposhian, H. V., and Kornberg, A. Enzymatic synthesis of deoxyribonucleic acid. IX. The polymerase formed after T_2 bacteriophage infection of *Escherichia coli*: A new enzyme. *J. Biol. Chem.*, **237**, 519–525 (1962).
3. August, J. T., Cooper, S., Shapiro, L., and Zinder, N.D. RNA phage induced RNA polymerase. *Cold Spring Harbor Symp. Quant. Biol.*, **28**, 95–97 (1963).
4. Berns, K. I., Silverman, C., and Weissbach, A. Separation of a new deoxyribonucleic acid polymerase from vaccinia-infected HeLa cells. *J. Virol.*, **4**, 15–23 (1969).
5. Bollum, F. J. Thermal conversion of nonpriming DNA to primer. *J. Biol. Chem.*, **234**, 2733–2734 (1959).
6. Bresnick, E., and Karjala, R. J. End-product inhibition of thymidine kinase activity in normal and leukemic human leukocytes. *Cancer Res.*, **24**, 841–846 (1964).
7. Friend, C. Cell-free transmission in adult Swiss mice of a desease having the character of a leukemia. *J. Exp. Med.*, **105**, 307–318 (1957).
8. Gelbard, A. S., Kim, S. H., and Eidinoff, M. L. Nucleotide kinase activities in tissues infected with Rous sarcoma virus. *Cancer Res.*, **26**, 748–751 (1966).
9. Gilliland, J. M., and Symons, R. H. Partial purification and properties of ribonucleotide kinase in virus-infected and healthy plants. *Virology*, **33**, 221–226 (1967).
10. Haruna, I., Nozu, K., Ohtaka, Y., and Spiegelman, S. An RNA replicase induced by and selective for a viral RNA: Isolation and properties. *Proc. Natl. Acad. Sci. U.S.*, **50**, 905–911 (1963).
11. Hashimoto, T., Shiosaka, T., Toide, H., Okuda, H., and Fujii, S. Thymidine kinase from normal and tumor tissues. *GANN*, **60**, 41–47 (1969).
12. Hatanaka, M., and Dulbecco, R. SV40-Specific thymidine kinase. *Proc. Natl. Acad. Sci. U.S.*, **58**, 1888–1894 (1967).
13. Ito, K., and Tatibana, M. Operation of orotic acid pathway as the major source of pyrimidines in the hematopoietic mouse spleen. *Biochem. Biophys. Res. Commun.*, **23**, 672–678 (1966).
14. Keir, H. M., Subak-Sharpe, H., Shedden, W. I. H., Watson, D. H., and Wildy, D. Immunological evidence foı a specific DNA polymerase produced after infection by Herpes Simplex virus. *Virology*, **30**, 154–157 (1966).
15. Klemperer, H. G., Haynes, G. R., Shedden, W. I. H., and Watson, D. H. A virus-specific thymidine kinase in BHK 21 cells infected with Herpes Simplex virus. *Virology*, **31**, 120–128 (1967).
16. Magee, W., and Miller, O. V. Immunological evidence for the appearance of a

new DNA-polymerase in cells infected with vaccinia virus. *Virology*, **31**, 64–69 (1967).

17. Ono, T., and Umehara, Y. Heterogeneity of DNA polymerases in rat liver and hepatomas. *GANN Monograph*, No. 6, 96–107 (1968).
18. Schlom, J., Harter, D. H., Burny, A., and Spiegelman, S. DNA polymerase activities in virions of Visna virus, a causative agent of " slow " neurological disease. *Proc. Natl. Acad. Sci. U.S.*, **68**, 182–186 (1971).
19. Weissman, C., Simon, L., and Ochoa, S. Induction by an RNA phage of an enzyme catalyzing incorporation of ribonucleotides into ribonucleic acid. *Proc. Natl. Acad. Sci. U.S.*, **49**, 407–414 (1963).

GANN Monograph on Cancer Research 12, 1972

RNA-DEPENDENT RNA POLYMERASE FROM LEUKEMIA AND ASCITES TUMOR CELLS*

Ichiro HARUNA, Tsuneya OHNO, Nobumichi HOZUMI, and Itaru WATANABE

*Department of Molecular Biology School of Medicine, Keio University***

Both RNA-dependent RNA polymerase and its template RNA were found in Friend murine leukemia cells, poliovirus-infected HeLa cells, echovirus-infected FL cells, Ehrlich ascites tumor cells, and human leukemia cells. All enzyme fractions were shown to have a specific requirement for RNA from leukemia cells or virus-infected cells. The fractionation and characterization of the template RNA from Ehrlich ascites tumor cells are described. These results indicate that template RNA might be separated from ribosomal and transfer RNAs in tumor cells and might possess a different secondary molecular structure.

The RNA replicase (RNA-dependent RNA polymerase) of Qβ phage was first isolated by Haruna and Spiegelman (*3*) in 1965. This replicase has a strict template specificity, that is, it requires a specific RNA as its template. Qβ RNA replicase replicates Qβ RNA with Qβ RNA as a template but cannot synthesize RNA when any RNA such as r-RNA or t-RNA is used as a template. Further, neither the RNAs of plant viruses such as TMV and TYMV, nor the RNA of MS2 phage, which belongs to a different group of RNA phages (*10*), possesses template activity for Qβ RNA replicase. On the other hand, MS2 RNA replicase requires MS2 RNA for its template but cannot synthesize RNA with other RNAs, including Qβ phage RNA, as a template (*3*). If the same can be said for animal and/or plant RNA viruses, then by measuring the template activity against the RNA replicase of a certain virus, it might be possible to detect the presence of certain viral RNAs in RNA mixtures and to distinguish that viral RNA from other viral or nonviral RNAs. Therefore, an investigation into the nature and functions of certain RNA replicases and their template RNAs in leukemia and ascites tumor cells would certainly be important and could open an entirely new field for the study of oncogenic viruses. We have attempted to isolate an RNA-dependent RNA polymerase from leukemia and ascites tumor cells and to examine its dependence on certain specific RNAs. The results of these studies are presented and discussed herein.

* This work was supported in part by grants from the Scientific Research Fund of the Ministry of Education of Japan, the Waksman Foundation of Japan, and the Jane Coffin Childs Memorial Fund for Medical Research, U.S.A.

** Shinanomachi, Shinjuku-ku, Tokyo 160 (春名一郎, 大野典也, 穂積信道, 渡辺　格).

RNA-dependent RNA Polymerase in Transplantable Subcutaneous Solid Tumors of Friend Virus Leukemia (4)

Transplantable subcutaneous solid tumors of Friend virus leukemia were used for the primary study. The animals used were DDD mice obtained from the Institute of Medical Science, University of Tokyo. An outline of the method used for preparation of the enzyme and RNA is given in Chart 1. The method for assay of enzyme activity is described in Table I. An enzyme showing ribonucleotide-incorporating activity was prepared from a Friend virus-induced solid tumor. The results of 5 typical experiments are shown in Table II. Table III shows some of the general characteristics of the enzyme thus obtained. This enzyme had a clear requirement for template RNA, and RNA synthesis was observed only when all 4 ribonucleoside triphosphates were present. The omission of any one of the 4 triphosphates clearly reduced the incorporation of ^{3}H-UMP into the product. There was also an absolute requirement for bivalent magnesium ions. Addition of 20 μg of DNase and actinomycin D to the reaction

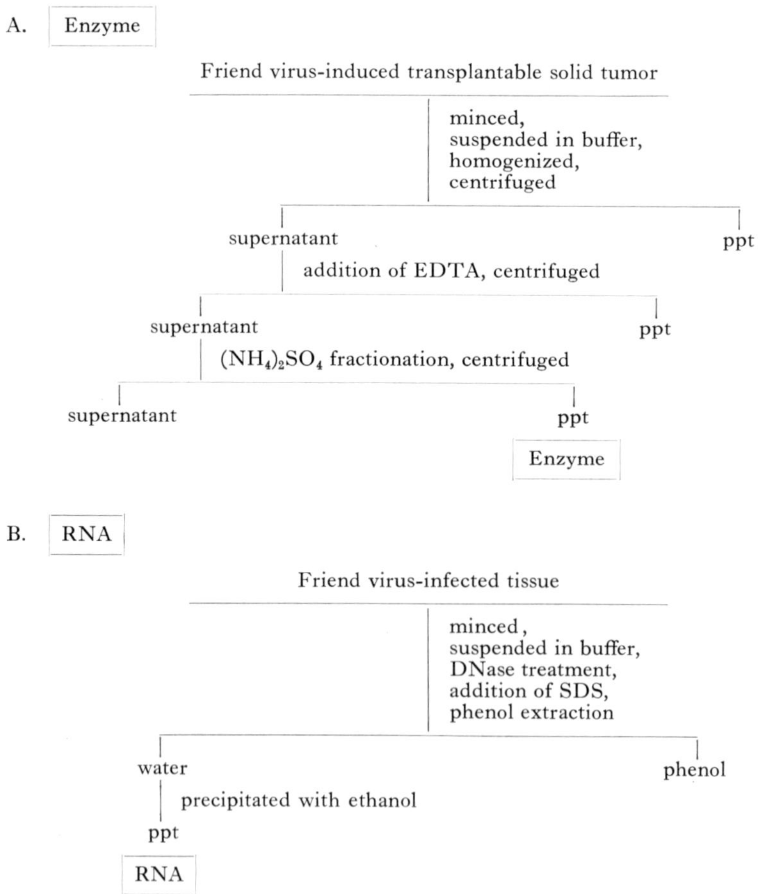

Chart 1. Preparation of the enzyme and RNA

TABLE I. Assay Condition for RNA-dependent RNA Polymerase

Tris-HCl, pH 7.4	21.0 μmoles
$MgCl_2$	3.2 μmoles
CTP, ATP, UTP, GTP	0.1 μmoles each
^{3}H-UTP	2×10^6 cpm/0.1 μmoles
Enzyme	20–30 μg
Template RNA	25–50 μg
Assay mixture	0.25 ml
Incubation	20 min at 36°

The reaction mixture was chilled in ice and 0.3 ml of 0.01 M Tris buffer, pH 7.4, and 0.1 ml of 80% trichloroacetic acid were added. The precipitate was collected on a membrane filter and washed 7 times with 5 ml of cold 5% trichloroacetic acid. The membrane was then dried and counted in a liquid scintillation counter.

TABLE II. Enzyme from Friend Virus-induced Transplantable Solid Tumor

Expt. No.	Template RNA	μg/0.25 ml	^{3}H-UMP incorporation (pmoles)
1	F.V. spleen RNA	0	9.6
	F.V. spleen RNA	25	49.2
2	F.V. spleen RNA	0	16.6
	F.V. spleen RNA	25	41.8
3	F.V. spleen RNA	0	36.2
	F.V. spleen RNA	25	61.2
	F.V. spleen RNA	50	74.0
	F.V. spleen RNA	75	99.8
4	F.V. spleen RNA	0	56.2
	F.V. spleen RNA	25	83.5
	F.V. spleen RNA	50	88.0
5	F.V. spleen RNA	0	30.0
	F.V. spleen RNA	25	45.2
	F.V. spleen RNA	50	54.0

F.V. spleen: Friend virus-infected DDD mouse spleen.

mixture had no significant effect, but the reaction was almost completely inhibited by 10 μg of RNase. As shown in Table IV, a stimulating effect was observed in the RNA from the transplantable solid tumor, but ribosomal and amino acid transfer-RNA of *Escherichia coli* and RNA from RNA phages (MS2, GA, Qβ) or from tobacco mosaic virus are not functional as templates. Based on these findings, this enzyme was considered to be an RNA-dependent RNA polymerase possessing template specificity. In each of the subcutaneous solid tumors, spleen and ascites tumor cells of Friend virus-infected mice, RNA-dependent RNA polymerase with template specificity and corresponding template RNA were detected.

TABLE III. Requirements of an Enzyme Isolated from Friend Virus-induced Transplantable Solid Tumor

Assay mixture in 0.25 ml	^{3}H-UMP incorporation (pmoles)
Complete	74.0
−GTP	46.6
−CTP	36.2
−ATP	32.6
$-Mg^{2+}$	0.0
DNase 10 μg	69.7
20 μg	68.1
RNase 10 μg	21.2
20 μg	20.8
Actinomycin D 40 μg	74.8
−RNA	36.2

Template RNA : RNA from Friend virus-infected mouse spleen.

TABLE IV. Template Specificity of Enzyme from Friend Virus-induced Transplantable Solid Tumor

Template	μg/0.25 ml	^{3}H-UMP incorporation (pmoles)
RNA from Friend virus-infected spleen	10	61.3
RNA from Friend virus-infected spleen	20	72.8
RNA from Friend virus-infected spleen	40	77.9
Qβ phage RNA	10	39.9
MS2 phage RNA	10	34.9
GA phage RNA	10	36.7
TMV RNA	10	37.3
t-RNA (*E. coli*)	10	35.8
r-RNA (*E. coli*)	10	41.9
DNA (calf thymus)	10	35.4
None		36.0

RNA-dependent RNA Polymerase in Animal RNA Virus-infected Cultured Cells (5, 6)

In order to establish the method for isolating RNA-dependent RNA polymerase and its corresponding template RNA, experiments were carried out using typical RNA viruses such as polio- and echoviruses. In the experiments with the poliovirus, an attenuated strain of poliovirus (Sabin 1) and HeLa cells were employed. The experiments with echovirus were done using echovirus 7 and FL cells. In each instance, we succeeded in isolating RNA-dependent RNA polymerase with template specificity and RNA with template activity. Part of the experimental data using poliovirus and HeLa cells is shown in Table V.

TABLE V. Enzyme from Poliovirus-infected HeLa Cells

Expt. No.	Template RNA	μg/0.25 ml	^{3}H-UMP incorporation (pmoles)
1	RNA from polio-infected HeLa cells	0	5.0
	RNA from polio-infected HeLa cells	19.4	15.2
2	RNA from polio-infected HeLa cells	0	19.3
	RNA from polio-infected HeLa cells	11.6	28.5
	Qβ phage RNA	4.0	20.9
3	RNA from polio-infected HeLa cells	0	11.3
	RNA from polio-infected HeLa cells	10.5	22.2

RNA-dependent RNA Polymerase in Ehrlich Ascites Tumor Cells (*7*)

After finding template RNA in Friend ascites tumor cells, studies were made on Ehrlich ascites tumor cells, which are not considered to be of viral origin. The presence of RNA-dependent RNA polymerase with template specificity and corresponding template RNA was also observed in these cells. This enzyme also required 4 different nucleoside triphosphates. The RNA synthetic reaction was stimulated by the addition of RNA from Ehrlich ascites tumor cells, but not phage RNA, TMV-RNA, ribosomal, and transfer RNA from rat liver or DNA as shown in Table VI. This observation suggested the presence of an RNA with template activity in Ehrlich ascites tumor cells. The presence of template RNA in Ehrlich ascites tumor cells, in which the virus was not thought to be present, brought up many problems and led us to investigate the possibility that RNA with template activity and RNA-dependent RNA polymerase might be present in human leukemic cells.

TABLE VI. Template Specificity of Enzyme from Ehrlich Ascites Tumor Cells

Template	μg/0.25 ml	^{3}H-UMP incorporation (pmoles)
RNA from Ehrlich ascites tumor cells	10	9.5
RNA from Ehrlich ascites tumor cells	40	17.0
Qβ phage RNA	10	4.5
MS2 phage RNA	10	5.5
GA phage RNA	10	5.4
TMV RNA	10	5.3
t-RNA (rat liver)	20	4.6
r-RNA (rat liver)	20	4.5
DNA (calf thymus)	10	4.0
None		5.0

RNA-dependent RNA Polymerase in Human Leukemia Cells (11)

We then attempted to detect the presence of template RNA and RNA-dependent RNA polymerase in the myeloblasts obtained from the peripheral blood of patients with acute myeloid leukemia. Although only 5 cases have been examined so far, RNA-dependent RNA polymerase with template specificity and the corresponding template RNA were found to be present in each case. Part of the results obtained are shown in Table VII.

TABLE VII. Enzyme from Acute Myeloid Leukemia Cells

Expt. No.	Template RNA	μg/0.25 ml	^{3}H-UMP incorporation (pmoles)
I–1	AML-RNA	0	9.7
	AML-RNA	8	27.6
I–2	AML-RNA	0	11.5
	AML-RNA	20	19.4
II	AML-RNA	0	11.7
	AML-RNA	20	16.9
III	AML-RNA	0	3.6
	AML-RNA	20	9.0
IV–1	AML-RNA	0	1.9
	AML-RNA	20	11.1
IV–2	AML-RNA	0	0.2
	AML-RNA	20	5.4
IV–3	AML-RNA	0	0.1
	AML-RNA	20	12.1
V	AML-RNA	0	2.2
	AML-RNA	20	16.7

Characterization of the Template RNA

When the template nucleic acid from Ehrlich ascites tumor cells was preincubated with 0.3 N KOH at 36° for 17 hr and neutralized, 90% of RNA synthesis was inhibited. This result indicated that the template for RNA polymerase is probably RNA. To provide further evidence of its RNA nature, the density of the template was examined by equilibrium density centrifugation in Cs_2SO_4. Most of the activity was found in the RNA region of the density gradient. These experiments substantiate the hypothesis that RNA was the template for the reaction. To examine the size of template RNA, RNAs from Ehrlich ascites tumor cells were analyzed by sucrose density gradient centrifugation. Template RNAs sediment at

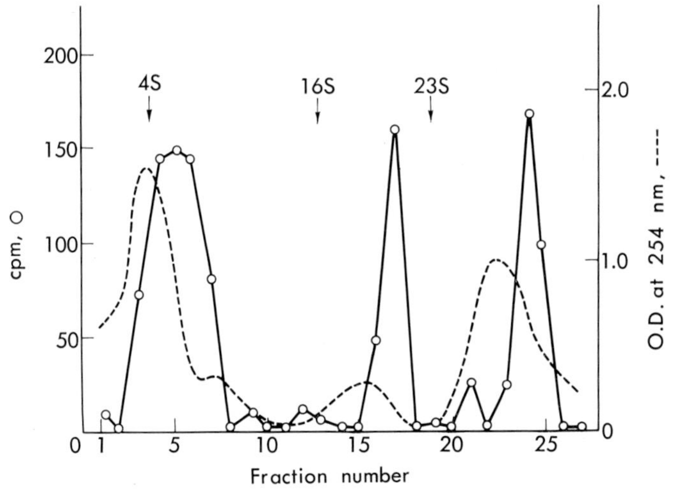

FIG. 1. Zonal centrifugation of template RNA in sucrose gradient
Ehrlich ascites tumor cell RNA (3.3 mg / ml) in 0.01 M Tris (pH 7.4) and 0.005 M $MgCl_2$ was layered over a 2.5–15% sucrose gradient containing 0.03 M Tris (pH 7.4) and 0.001 M $MgCl_2$, and centrifuged in a Spinco SW25–1 rotor for 18 hr at 21,000 rpm.

TABLE VIII. The Effect of Heat Treatment on the Nuclease Sensitivity of Template Activity of Ehrlich Ascites Tumor Cell RNA

Condition	^{3}H-UMP incorporation (pmoles)
1. Treated with 50 μg/ml deoxyribonuclease	3.80
2. Treated with 50 μg/ml ribonuclease	4.58
3. Treated with buffer only	4.76
4. Preincubated at 100° for 10 min, and treated with 50 μg/ml deoxyribonuclease	3.84
5. Preincubated at 100° for 10 min, and treated with 50 μg/ml ribonuclease	0.94
6. Preincubated at 100° for 10 min, and treated with buffer only	5.20

the 7S, 20S, and 34S positions (Fig. 1). RNAs having template activity were separated from ribosomal and transfer RNAs by zone centrifugation.

The nature of the template RNAs was investigated by determining their sensitivity to various treatments (Table VIII). When template RNAs in 0.1 xSSC (0.015 M sodium chrolide, 0.0015 M sodium citrate) were heated at 100° for 10 min and cooled quickly, the activity was not inhibited. Preincubation with 50 μg/ml of DNase or RNase at 36° for 30 min caused only a slight decrease in RNA polymerase activity. When template RNA was pretreated at 100° for 10 min, treatment with 50 μg/ml of RNase inhibited activity by more than 80%. These results suggest that template RNAs are in a double-strand state.

Nature of the Product

The product of the RNA-dependent RNA polymerase from Ehrlich ascites tumor cells was made acid soluble by treatment with 50 μg/ml of ribonuclease and 0.3 N KOH, and was resistant to 50 μg/ml of deoxyribonuclease.

Localization of Template RNA

To investigate the localization of template RNA in Ehrlich ascites tumor cells, cell homogenates were prepared in a homogenizer of the Emanuel-Chaikoff type and separated into nuclear and cytoplasmic fractions by centrifugation. Most of the activity was found in the nuclear fraction. Template RNA therefore seems to be located in the nuclei of the cells.

DISCUSSION

RNA-Dependent RNA polymerase with template specificity and its template RNA were found in Friend murine leukemia cells, poliovirus-infected HeLa cells, echovirus-infected FL cells, Ehrlich ascites tumor cells, and human leukemia cells.

Since poliovirus and Friend virus are RNA viruses, it was not surprising that viral RNAs were found in both the poliovirus-infected cells and the tissues from mice with Friend disease. However, the discovery of RNA with the same characteristics as viral RNA in Ehrlich ascites tumor cells was an unexpected finding. In 1961, Burdon and Smellie (*2*) extracted RNA-dependent RNA polymerase from Ehrlich ascites tumor cells, but they did not find any template specificity. Therefore, it may be said that self-replicating or viral RNA-like RNA was first detected in Ehrlich ascites tumor cells. However, the question remains whether or not RNA virus was present in the Ehrlich ascites tumor cells.

RNA having the same characteristics as self-replicating RNA or viral RNA was also found in myeloblasts in each of 5 cases of human acute myeloid leukemia examined. The next steps in pursuing this research are: (1) to confirm these findings by examining more cases of human leukemia, (2) to ascertain the presence or absence of self-replicating RNA in the leukocytes of healthy men (possibly in normal myeloblasts), and (3) to try to obtain more stable enzyme preparations from the small amount of the specimen by improving the method for purification of the enzyme.

From the results of studies on the nature of template RNA from Ehrlich ascites tumor cells (Table VIII), RNA having template activity might possess a special secondary molecular structure. At present, experiments are in progress to characterize the template RNA from other leukemia cells and to examine template activity of RNAs from Friend virus and echovirus.

The presence of an RNA-dependent RNA polymerase enzyme in leukemia and ascites tumor cells raises many questions concerning the mechanism of enzyme action, the nature of the template and the product, and the relationship between this enzyme and the RNA-dependent DNA polymerase in RNA tumor virus reported recently (*1*, *8*, *9*) for virus replication and cell transformation.

REFERENCES

1. Baltimore, D. Viral RNA-dependent DNA polymerase. *Nature*, **226**, 1209–1211 (1970).
2. Burdon, R. H., and Smellie, R. M. S. The incorporation of uridine 5′-triphosphate into RNA by enzyme fraction from Ehrlich ascites carcinoma cells. *Biochim. Biophys. Acta*, **51**, 153–162 (1961).
3. Haruna, I., and Spiegelman, S. Specific template requirements of RNA replicase. *Proc. Natl. Acad. Sci. U.S.*, **54**, 579–587 (1965).
4. Haruna, I., Ohno, T., Watanabe, I., and Ikawa, Y. Isolation of an RNA-dependent RNA polymerase from Friend murine leukemia cells. *Proc. Japan Acad.*, **46**, 1016–1021 (1970).
5. Haruna, I., Watanabe, I., Ohtaki, K., and Yamazaki, Z. Unpublished observations.
6. Haruna, I., Fukada, T., and Watanabe, I. Unpublished observations.
7. Ohno, T., Haruna, I., and Watanabe, I. Unpublihed observations.
8. Spiegelman, S., Burhy, A., Das. M. R., Keydar, J., Schlom, J., Travnicek, M., and Watson, K. Characterization of the products of RNA-directed DNA polymerases in oncogenic RNA viruses. *Nature*, **227**, 563–567 (1970).
9. Temin, H. M., and Mizutani, S. RNA-dependent DNA polymerase in virions of Rous sarcoma virus. *Nature*, **226**, 1211–1213 (1970).
10. Watanabe, I., Miyake, T., Sakurai, T., Shiba, T., and Ohno, T. Isolation and grouping of RNA phages. *Proc. Japan Acad.*, **43**, 204–209 (1967).
11. Watanabe, I., Haruna, I., Nakao, K., and Takaku, F. Unpublished observations.

DIFFERENTIATION OF LEUKEMIC CELLS

GANN Monograph on Cancer Research 12, 1972

DIFFERENTIATION OF LEUKEMIC MYELOBLASTS

Yasuo ICHIKAWA
*Department of Tumor Virus, Institute for Virus Research, Kyoto University**

The Ml cell line was established *in vitro* from a myeloid leukemia of SL strain mice. The cells of this line were cytologically identified as myeloblasts, whose normal differentiation appeared to be completely blocked. When these cells were seeded in soft agar on a harder agar layer containing conditioned medium from normal cells, single cells grew into colonies and differentiated into either macrophages or neutrophil granulocytes. The cell differentiation brought with it a conversion in the colony morphology, from solid to dispersed types. The percent of dispersed type colonies always increased with an increase in the concentration of conditioned medium. If a high concentration of conditioned medium was used, contact for 48 hr was sufficient to induce cell differentiation followed by loss of the colony-forming and leukemogenic capacity. This cell differentiation was suppressed by BUdR but not by FUdR.

A variety of conditioned media from normal cells appeared to contain both growth-stimulating and differentiation-stimulating factors for the Ml-line cells. The Ml-line cells themselves did not appear to produce the differentiation-stimulating factor as normal cells did. This is probably why cells of this line are allowed to grow without any sign of differentiation.

The differentiation-stimulating factor present in conditioned medium was relatively thermolabile, while the growth-stimulating factor was highly thermostable.

In many cases of leukemia, it is well known that great number of mature cells corresponding to the particular type of leukemia concerned appear in the peripheral blood and the sites of leukemic infiltration. This finding appears to suggest that leukemia cells retain the ability to differentiate. On the other hand, it is also a fact that no differentiated cells are found in cultures of long-term established lines of leukemia. The question thus arises whether only the cell clones whose differentiation is completely blocked are selected during long cultivation, or whether the absence of an essential substance required for cell differentiation leads to an apparent block of differentiation *in vitro*. In general, the differentiation of a certain cell type is at the same time accompanied by a regulation of the reproductive rate. The failure of leukemic cells to differentiate may be a favorable, if not indispensable, condition for their establishment *in vitro*.

* Kawara-machi, Shogoin, Sakyo-ku, Kyoto 606 (市川康夫).

In order to answer these questions, experiments were carried out with a cell line of myeloid leukemia. This line was chosen for 2 reasons; first, differentiation in the myeloid series is easily discernible by simple morphological methods; second, normal myeloblasts grow to form colonies and differentiate in soft agar culture (*4*, *6*, *7*, *12*, *14–17*), which was also used in the present experiments.

Experimental Procedures

A cell line, designated Ml, was established *in vitro* from a spontaneous myeloid leukemia of SL strain mice and has been maintained in this laboratory for about 3 years. The nuclei of the cells of this line are round or oval, and the cytoplasm is narrow, strongly basophilic, and peroxidase positive. No cells showed phagocytosis (Photos 1, 2, and 11). When cells were transplanted into isologous mice, generalized myeloid leukemia developed within 3 weeks. For cell culture, Eagle's minimum essential medium with a 4-fold concentration of amino acids and vitamins (EM) was used with 10% inactivated horse serum (HS). Cultures were incubated at 37° in a humidified atmosphere in which 5% CO_2 in air was continuously circulated. The cells grew in a suspension state, without adhering to the plate.

The main technique employed in these experiments was the soft agar technique. The Ml-line cells were seeded, 500 cells per 6-cm petri plate, in soft agar (0.33%) on a harder agar base (0.5%), and colonies were counted under an inverted microscope. Conditioned medium prepared from embryo cells, spleen, and peritoneal macrophages by the methods already reported (*6*, *7*) was added to the lower agar layer. The feeder cells, when present, were under the lower agar layer.

To check the rate of DNA synthesis in colony-composing cells, 2 ml of EM containing tritiated thymidine (1 μCi/ml, specific activity 5 Ci/mmole) was poured onto 12-day-old colonies and incubated for 2 hr. After being washed with EM, the colonies were picked up and smeared on a glass slide. In order to test the DNA synthesis of the cells exposed to conditioned medium, the cells were washed twice and 10^6 cells were incubated in 2 ml of EM with 10% HS and 0.05 μCi/ml tritiated thymidine for 12 hr. The cell smears were fixed in methanol and dipped in cold 10% trichloracetic acid for 10 min. After thorough washing with distilled water, the slides were dipped in Sakura NR-M2 emulsion at 45° and diluted 1:1 with distilled water. After exposure for 1 week at 4°, the slide was developed in Fuji Rendol.

Phagocytosis tests were undertaken as follows: a petri dish was inoculated with 5×10^6 cells, and India ink was added at a final concentration of 0.5%. After 4 hr of incubation at 37°, the cells were washed by centrifugation, and a drop of sediment was placed under a cover slip to be observed without staining, or a cell smear was stained with May-Grünwald-Giemsa.

Colony in Soft Agar

The Ml-line cells were seeded in soft agar on a harder agar layer containing conditioned medium, and the colonies were observed under an inverted micro-

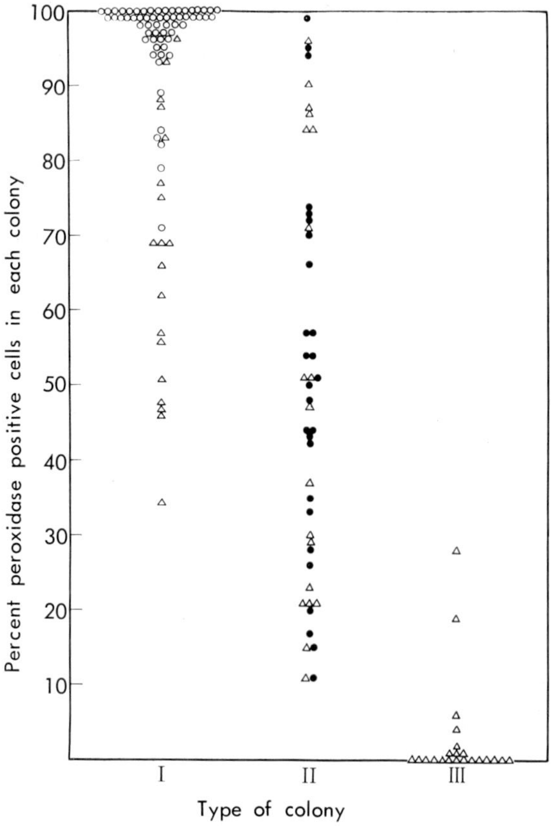

FIG. 1. Relationship between colony type and percent of peroxidase-positive cells found in the colony

Each dot represents one colony. Cell smears were made from 8-day-old (○), 10-day-old (●), and 12- to 14-day-old (△) colonies (*9*).

scope at various times after seeding. Colonies were classified as one of 3 types, I, II, and III, depending on the grade of dispersion of the colony-composing cells (Photos 3–6). Various types of colonies were picked up, smeared, and stained with May-Grünwald-Giemsa or tested for peroxidase reaction. The percents of peroxidase-positive cells in the three types of colonies are summarized in Fig. 1. The data indicate that the percent of peroxidase-negative cells in a given colony increased as the colony-composing cells dispersed in agar medium. The cytoplasm of these peroxidase-negative cells was wider and less basophilic than that of myeloblasts, and very often full of phagocytized substances (Photo 7). When Ml cells were seeded in soft agar containing 0.05% India ink, most of such cells present in type II and III colonies phagocytized carbon particles but the myeloblasts in type I colonies never did so (Photo 8). This cell type will be referred to as a macrophage. Type III colonies appeared to be composed almost purely of macrophages.

Autoradiography with tritiated thymidine was used to determine the rate of DNA synthesis in different colony types (Table I). The cells in type I colonies, as compared with those in type II, showed a higher incorporation rate of thymidine.

TABLE I. Cell Nuclei Labeled with ^{3}H-Thymidine

	Percent labeled	
Colony type	I	II
(average from 20 colonies)	47.0%	35.1%
Part of type II colony	Center	Periphery
(average from 8 colonies)	54.2%	35.2%

Two ml of EM containing tritiated thymidine (1 μCi/ml) was poured onto 12-day-old colonies and incubated for 2 hr. After being washed with EM, the colonies were picked up and smeared on a glass slide.

TABLE II. Cell Analysis of Type II Colonies (*9*)

Colony part	Myeloblast	Macrophage	Undetermined	Mitosis
Center	81	14	3	2
Periphery	39	56	5	0.4

Average from 8 colonies. Central and peripheral parts of 16-day-old colonies were separately picked up with a small spatula and smeared on a glass slide. Numbers indicate the percent of each cell type in a smear.

It is also evident that the cells located along the peripheral part of type II colonies were labeled about 20% less than the cells in the central part, suggesting, together with the cytological findings shown in Table II, that the DNA synthesis of macrophages was suppressed. This is also supported by the fact that cells from type II colonies always had a lower plating efficiency than did the cells from type I colonies (*9*).

Analyses of cell smears revealed that some of the type II colonies, less than 4% of the total colonies, contained neutrophil granulocytes instead of macrophages. Such colonies were always smaller than the other colony types and most of them had degenerated by 8 days after seeding. The cytoplasm of granulocytes was stained pink with PAS reaction, as reported by Ackerman (*2*) (see Photos 9 and 10).

These findings may be summarized as follows: the Ml-line cells differentiate to either macrophages or granulocytes when seeded in soft agar with conditioned medium. The appearance of differentiated cells in colonies brings with it a morphological change in the colonies, from the solid to the dispersed type. It is worth emphasizing that the same relationship between cell differentiation and colony morphology as described above has been reported also for normal hematopoietic cells (*6*, *7*, *15*).

Factors Affecting Cell Differentiation

1. Concentration of conditioned medium

Since contact with conditioned medium thus brought about cell differentiation accompanied by changes in the colony type, the effects of different concentrations of conditioned medium on colony type and number were tested. Although a

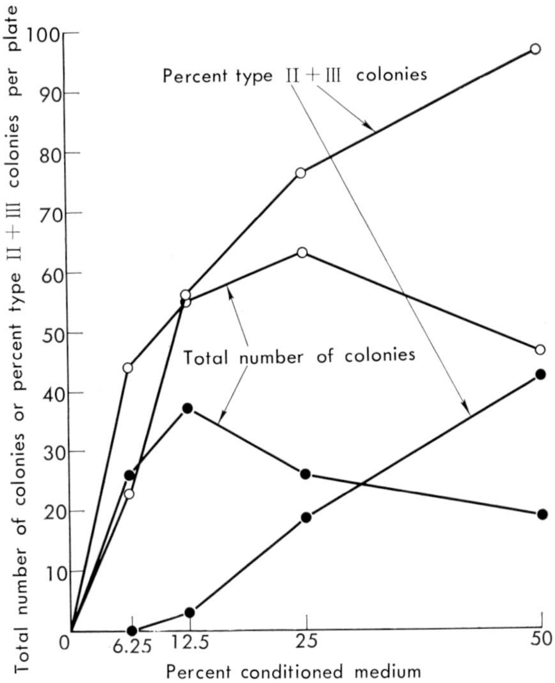

FIG. 2. Stimulation of cloning efficiency and induction of type II and III colonies by different concentrations of conditioned medium

Ml-line cells were seeded at 500 cells per plate, and colonies were counted 12 days after seeding. ○ results with conditioned medium from secondary embryo. ● results with conditioned medium from spleen macrophages (*9*).

higher concentration of conditioned medium was not always accompanied by a larger number of colonies, production of type II and III colonies was always stimulated by a high concentration of conditioned medium, suggesting the presence of an active substance in the conditioned medium (Fig. 2).

Another experiment was designed to test the colony-forming capacity of the cells that had been in contact with conditioned medium for 48 hr prior to the cloning in agar. The Ml cells that had been incubated for 48 hr with different concentrations of conditioned medium were divided into two groups: one group was seeded in soft agar to determine the number of colony formers, and the other was exposed to tritiated thymidine for 12 hr to test the rate of DNA synthesis. As shown in Fig. 3, incubation with increasing concentrations of conditioned medium led to a decrease in the number of colony formers. It should be noted that the decrease in colony-forming capacity was not always parallel to the decrease in the incorporation rate of tritiated thymidine.

2. *Length of contact with conditioned medium*

When type I colonies were observed after seeding, it was found that some of them changed into type II and III colonies, while some remained type I colonies. It appeared possible that there were 2 clones, one resistant to the effect of condi-

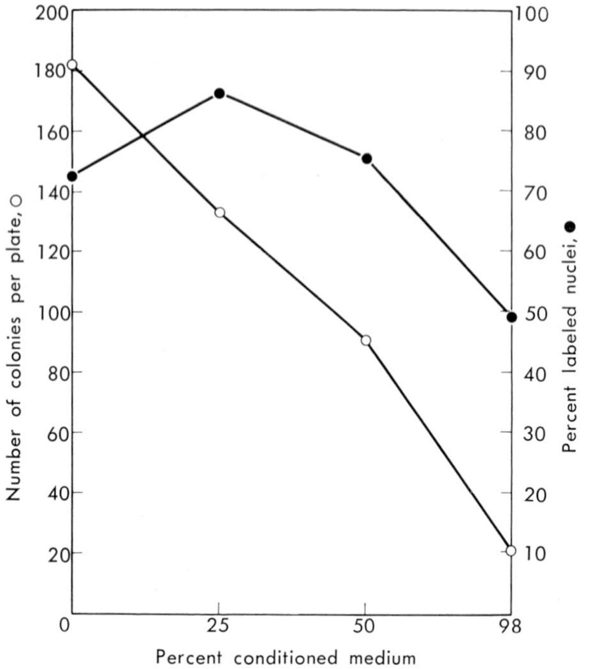

FIG. 3. Effect of 48-hr contact with different concentrations of conditioned medium

The incubated cells were washed twice and seeded at 500 cells per plate with 12.5% conditioned medium to determine the number of colony formers. Colonies were counted 12 days after seeding. The preincubated cells were also exposed to tritiated thymidine (0.1 μCi/10^6 cells/2 ml) for 12 hr (*10*).

tioned medium, and the other susceptible. Twice-recloned type I colonies were successively seeded for a third cloning with 25% conditioned medium, and the various types of colonies were counted at 8, 12, and 16 days after seeding. If colony type were determined by the cell clone, we would expect to find only type I colonies. When colonies were counted 8 days after seeding, a majority belonged to type I, but there was always an increase in the percent of dispersed-type colonies with increased incubation time (Fig. 4).

It was asked why a period of 10 days was necessary to bring about the conversion in colony types. Since it was technically difficult to apply a concentration of conditioned medium higher than 50% in the soft agar culture, the effect of higher concentrations of conditioned medium was tested by another system. Petri dishes were inoculated with 4×10^6 cells in 5 ml of 98% conditioned medium supplemented with 2% HS, and the cells were tested for phagocytosis after 48 hr. Although there were considerable variations in the results depending on the lot of conditioned medium, 40 to 90% of the cells showed active phagocytosis (Photo 12). The phagocytizing cells always showed extended cytoplasm, and their basophility was markedly decreased. It was also demonstrated that this treatment brought about a marked drop in the colony-forming capacity (*10*). The control cells which were incubated with EM did not show such a change (Photo 11). These results

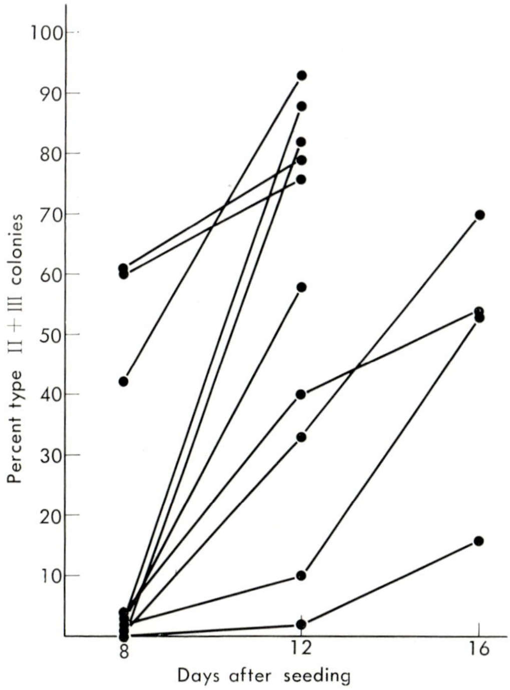

FIG. 4. Conversion of colony types with the time after seeding

Twice-recloned type I colonies were successively seeded at one colony per plate. Twenty-five percent conditioned medium from secondary embryo was used. Each line represents the percent of dispersed types of colonies in a plate at a given time after seeding.

are in good agreement with those of the next experiment, in which 80% conditioned medium was poured onto 10-day-old type I colonies. If poured with EM instead of conditioned medium, there occurred no changes in colony types. However, in the cultures poured with conditioned medium, a conversion of colony type from I to II was found after only 2 days (*10*).

The question arose as to whether this rapid differentiation might be due to a toxic effect of conditioned medium. If so, the effect would be nonspecific. Two lines of lymphoid leukemia, SCl (*13*) and CRLl (*11*), which were induced with SL and Rauscher viruses, respectively, were incubated with the conditioned medium and tested for phagocytosis. There were no signs of phagocytosis induced.

These results suggest that, if a high concentration of conditioned medium is used, contact for 48 hr is long enough to induce differentiation in Ml-line cells.

3. Source of conditioned medium

A variety of normal cells produced active conditioned medium which stimulated both colony formation and cell differentiation in cells of the Ml line. In contrast, conditioned medium from Ml cells stimulated colony formation more effectively than that from normal cells, but it had no effect on the induction of phagocytosis and morphological changes in colony type (*9*). This appears to be a mechanism that allows this line of cells to grow continuously without differentiation.

Inhibition by 5-Bromodeoxyuridine

For several cell types it has been reported that an appropriate concentration of 5-bromodeoxyuridine (BUdR) suppressed the manifestation of differentiated phenotype without interfering with cell replication (*1*, *3*,*5*, *18*, *19*). Therefore, I

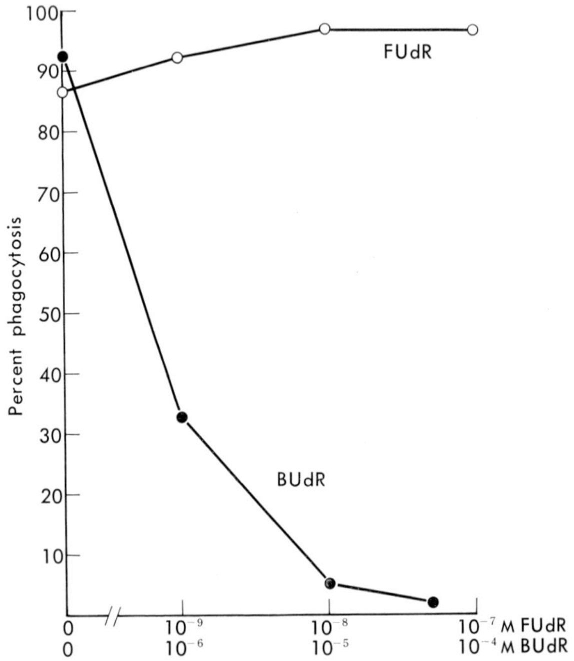

FIG. 5. Suppression by BUdR of the induction of phagocytosis

Ml-line cells were incubated with different concentrations of BUdR or FUdR for 72 hr. For the last 48 hr, conditioned medium was added at a final concentration of 44%. After being washed twice, the cells were tested for phagocytosis.

TABLE III. Inhibitory Effect of BUdR on the Induction of Phagocytosis

BUdR added	TdR added	No. of cells per plate after 3 days ($\times 10^6$)	Phagocytosis (%)
10^{-5} M	0	11	2.5
10^{-5} M	2×10^{-5} M	14	21.3
0	2×10^{-5} M	12	30.0
0	0	13	41.3

Ml-line cells were seeded at 5×10^6 cells per plate in EM with 2% HS. BUdR and TdR were added at the start of culture. Conditioned medium was added 24 hr later in a final concentration of 44%, adjusted so as not to change the concentration of BUdR and TdR. After another 48 hr, the cells were tested for phagocytosis.

was interested in testing whether this thymidine analogue inhibits the induction of phagocytosis in Ml-line cells.

First, Ml-line cells were cultured with different concentrations of BUdR (Sigma Chemical Co.) for 24 hr; then, conditioned medium was added at a final concentration of 44%, adjustment being made so as not to change the concentration of BUdR in the culture. After another 2 days, the cells were counted, washed twice, and tested for phagocytotic activity (Fig. 5). Increasing concentrations of BUdR suppressed the induction of phagocytosis by conditioned medium, with no readily discernible effect on cell growth up to 10^{-5} M. The suppression by BUdR was partially recovered by adding thymidine (TdR) at twice the molar concentration of the analogue (Table III). A similar analog, 5-fluoro-deoxyuridine (FudR) (F. Hoffman La Roche Co., gifted by Dr. Hamada of our institute), which could not be used at more than 10^{-7} M because of its toxic effect, always showed a slight enhancing effect on the induction of phagocytosis.

Some Properties of Differentiation-stimulating and Growth-stimulating Factors

The Ml-line cells produced colonies in soft agar and showed differentiation when exposed to a conditioned medium from normal cells. Without conditioned medium, the colony-forming efficiency was lower and the size of colonies was also smaller. It was also reported that the conditioned medium from Ml cells themselves stimulated colony formation but not differentiation.

The conditioned medium from normal cells thus had a mutually exclusive effect on Ml-line cells, stimulating cell division and inducing cell differentiation. If different substances were responsible for each of the activities of conditioned medium, the active substances might be separated from each other. Several experiments were undertaken to solve this problem, with the following results.

1. *Molecular size*

It was reported in a previous paper that a growth-stimulating factor for tumor cells was dialyzable (*8*). Experiments were designed to establish whether the differentiation-stimulating factor for Ml cells will pass through a dialysis membrane.

TABLE IV. Passage of Growth- and Differentiation-stimulating Factors through Dialysis Membrane (*10*)

Feeder layer	Dialysis membrane	No. of colonies per plate I	II	III	Total	Colony types II+III (%)
None	−	140	0	0	140	0
	+	127	0	0	127	0
Secondary embryo	−	139	89	2	230	39.6
	+	166	70	1	237	29.9

Ml-line cells were seeded at 500 cells per plate, and colonies were counted 12 days after seeding. Dialysis membranes were placed on top of a thin layer (1.5 ml) of 0.5% agar medium that had been poured onto the feeder layer. This table represents an average of the results from 4 experiments.

A dialysis membrane was placed on top of feeder cells and overlaid with a hard agar layer. The Ml cells were seeded in soft agar on the hard agar layer, as before. As shown in Table IV, the embryo feeder cells not only enhanced colony formation but induced conversion in colony types regardless of the presence of the dialysis membrane. In the next experiment, a dialysis bag containing 20 ml of conditioned medium was dipped in an equal volume of EM at 37° for 5 days. Phagocytosis-inducing activity for Ml-cells was detected in the dialysate, which enhanced colony formation as well. These findings suggest that both growth-stimulating and differentiation-stimulating factors can pass through a dialysis membrane.

There are some preliminary data suggesting a difference in the molecular size of the two factors. A conditioned medium was diluted 5-fold with fresh EM and then concentrated to the original volume by filtering it through a Diaflo membrane, UM10 (Amicon Co.), with a nitrogen pressure of 3.5 kg/cm². Phagocytosis-inducing activity was detected, with no detectable loss in activity, in the retention fluid but not at all in the filtrate. The filtrate, however, enhanced colony formation of Ml cells in soft agar culture, suggesting the smaller size of the growth-stimulating factor.

2. *Thermostability*

A conditioned medium was heated at 56, 70, and 100° for various lengths of time and was used for colony formation at a concentration of 50% (Table V). The growth-stimulating factor withstood heating at 70° for 30 min and even boiling for 10 min. In contrast, the differentiation-stimulating facor was relatively thermolabile. The increase in the number of colonies was accompanied by a decrease in the number of type II and III colonies, suggesting that increase in colony number might be due to deactivation of the differentiation-stimulating factor by heating.

This finding is supported by the following experiment, in which the effects of conditioned medium on cell growth, phagocytosis, and leukemogenicity were compared with each other (Table VI). Nonheated conditioned medium evoked phagocytosis in this line of cells and suppressed leukemogenic capacity. These activities of the conditioned medium were weakened by heating it at 70° for 30 min,

TABLE V. Thermostability of Conditioned Medium (*10*)

Treatment of conditioned medium	No. of colonies per plate	Colony types II+III (%)	No. of cells per colony
Untreated	187	48.2	33500
56° for 30 min	212	19.8	29600
70° for 10 min	209	1.9	23900
20 min	254	3.5	29200
30 min	228	0.0	17500
100° for 5 min	126	0.0	1800
10 min	97	0.0	1100
Without conditioned medium	6	0.0	200

The concentration of conditioned media was 50%. Ml-line cells were seeded at 500 cells per plate, and colonies were counted 12 days after seeding. Each calculation of the number of cells per colony was based on a count of 50 pooled colonies.

TABLE VI. Leukemogenicity of the Ml-line Cells Incubated with Conditioned Medium (*10*)

Incubated with	No. of cells per plate at the end of incubation ($\times 10^5$)	Cells with phagocytosis (%)	No of cells inoculated	Leukemia cases/ No. of recipients
EM	78	0.4	10^6	4/4
			10^5	3/3
			10^4	1/3
			10^3	1/5
Untreated conditioned medium	52	73.6	10^6	0/4
			10^5	0/4
			10^4	0/4
Conditioned medium heated at 70° for 30 min	120	30.8	10^6	5/5
			10^5	1/4
			10^4	0/4
			10^3	0/3

4×10^6 cells were incubated for 48 hr with EM (for control) or 98% conditioned medium, untreated or heated at 70° for 30 min. The incubated cells were counted, tested for phagocytotic activity, and intravenously inoculated into isologous adult mice. All surviving recipients were sacrificed 1 month after the transplantation and checked for enlargement of the spleen and lymph nodes.

while its growth-stimulating activity was unaffected. Since it was demonstrated that 2 factors, *i.e.*, growth-stimulating and differentiation-stimulating factors, were contained in conditioned medium, further purification studies are under way.

Note: As regards the dialyzable nature of the differentiation-stimulating factor, we have recently gotten some results that suggest its nondialyzability. Thus, no conclusions can yet be made regarding this problem.

REFERENCES

1. Abott, J., and Holtzer, H. The loss of phenotypic traits by differentiated cells. V. The effect of 5-bromodeoxyuridine on cloned chondrocytes. *Proc. Natl. Acad. Sci. U.S.*, **59**, 1144 (1968).
2. Ackerman, G. A. Histochemical differentiation during neutrophil development and maturation. *Ann. N.Y. Acad. Sci.*, **113**, 537 (1964).
3. Bischoff, R. and Holtzer, H. Inhibition of myeloblast fusion after one round DNA synthesis in 5-bromodeoxyuridine. *J. Cell Biol.*, **44**, 134 (1970).
4. Bradley, T. R. and Metcalf, D. The growth of mouse bone marrow cells *in vitro*. *Aust. J. Exp. Biol. Med. Sci.*, **44**, 287 (1966).
5. Coleman, A. W., Coleman, J. R., Kankel, D., and Werner, I. The reversible control of animal cell differentiation by thymidine analog, 5-bromodeoxy-uridine. *Exp. Cell Res.*, **59**, 319 (1970).
6. Ichikawa, Y., Pluznik, D. H., and Sachs, L. *In vitro* control of the development of macrophage and granulocyte colonies. *Proc. Natl. Acad. Sci. U.S.*, **58**, 488 (1966).
7. Ichikawa, Y., Pluznick, D. H., and Sachs, L. Feedback inhibition of the development of macrophage and granulocyte colonies. I. Inhibition by macrophages. *Proc. Natl. Acad. Sci. U.S.*, **58**, 1480 (1967).

8. Ichikawa, Y., Paran, M., and Sachs, L. The stimulation of tumor cell growth by a substance produced by normal and tumor cells. *J. Cell. Physiol.*, **73**, 43 (1968).
9. Ichikawa, Y. Differentiation of a cell line of myeloid leukemia. *J. Cell. Physiol.*, **74**, 223 (1969).
10. Ichikawa, Y. Further studies on the differentiation of a cell line of myeloid leukemia. *J. Cell. Physiol.*, **76**, 175 (1970).
11. Maeda, M., Notake, K., and Ishimoto, A. To be published.
12. Metcalf, D. Potentiation of bone marrow colony growth *in vitro* by the addition of lymphoid or bone marrow cells. *J. Cell. Physiol.*, **72**, 9 (1968).
13. Notake, K., Ichikawa, Y., Hanaoka, M., and Amano, S. A new long-term *in vitro* culture of normal and leukemic lymphocytes with special reference to a favourable simultaneous proliferation of leukemic virus and host cell. *Acta Haematol. Japon.*, **24**, 591 (1961).
14. Paran, M., and Sachs, L. The continued requirement for inducer for the development of macrophage and granulocyte colonies. *J. Cell. Physiol.*, **72**, 247 (1968).
15. Paran, M., Ichikawa, Y., and Sachs, L. Feedback inhibition of the development of macrophage and granulocyte colonies. II. Inhibition by granulocytes. *Proc. Natl. Acad. Sci. U.S.*, **62**, 81 (1968).
16. Pluznik, D. H., and Sachs, L. The cloning of normal " mast " cells in tissue culture. *J. Cell. Comp. Physiol.*, **66**, 319 (1965).
17. Pluznik, D. H., and Sachs, L. The induction of clones of normal " mast " cells by a substance in conditioned medium. *Exp. Cell Res.*, **43**, 553 (1966).
18. Silagi, S., and Bruce, S. A. Suppression of malignancy and differentiation in melanoic melanoma cells. *Proc. Natl. Acad. Sci. U.S.*, **66**, 72 (1970).
19. Stockdale, F., Okazaki, K., Nameroff, M., and Holtzer, H. 5-Bromodeoxyuridine: effect on myelogenesis *in vitro*. *Science*, **146**, 533 (1964).

EXPLANATION OF PHOTOS

PHOTO 1. Ml-line cells stained with May-Grünwald-Giemsa. ×1400

PHOTO 2. Ml-line cells showing positive peroxidase reaction. ×1400

PHOTO 3. Colonies in agar, 14 days after seeding. ×1.2, unstained.

PHOTO 4. Type I colony. ×55, unstained.

PHOTO 5. Type II colony. ×55, unstained.

PHOTO 6. Type III colony. ×55, unstained.

PHOTO 7. Macrophage found in a type II colony. Note the cytoplasm full of phagocytized substance. ×1400, stained with May-Grünwald Giemsa.

PHOTO 8. Macrophage that phagocytized carbon particles. ×1400, stained with May-Grünwald-Giemsa.

PHOTO 9. Some stages in the differentiation of granulocytes in a type II colony. ×500, stained with May-Grünwald-Giemsa.

PHOTO 10. Smear of a type II colony in which mature granulocytes showed positive PAS reaction. ×500

PHOTO 11. Ml-line cells incubated for 48 hr with EM and tested for phagocytosis. ×500, unstained.

PHOTO 12. Ml-line cells incubated for 48 hr with 98% conditioned medium and tested for phagocytosis. ×500, unstained.

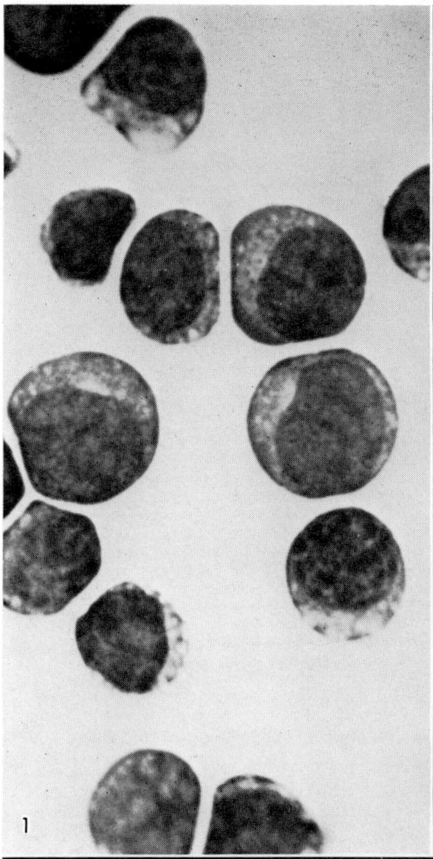
1

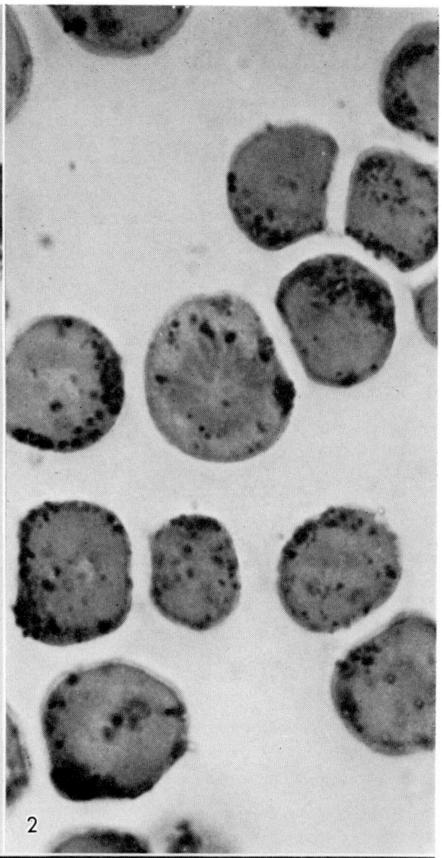
2

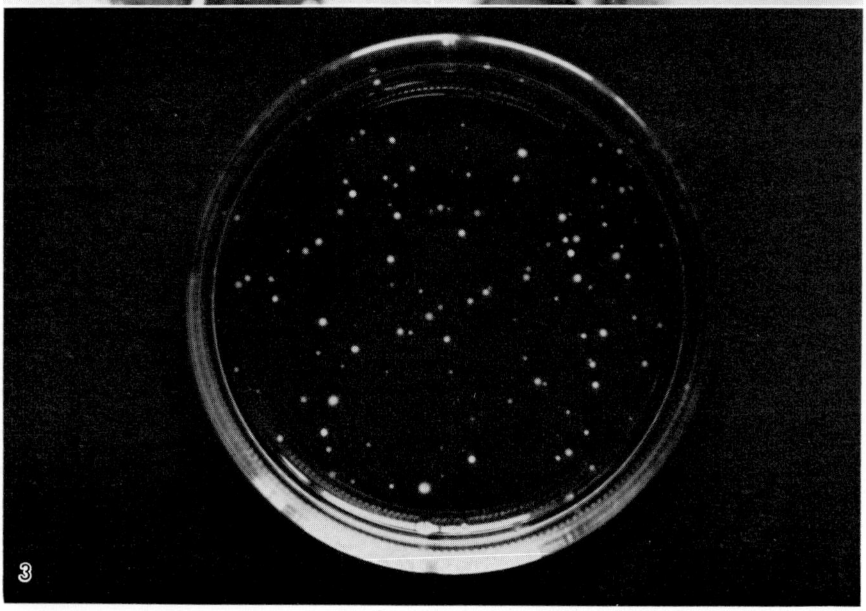
3

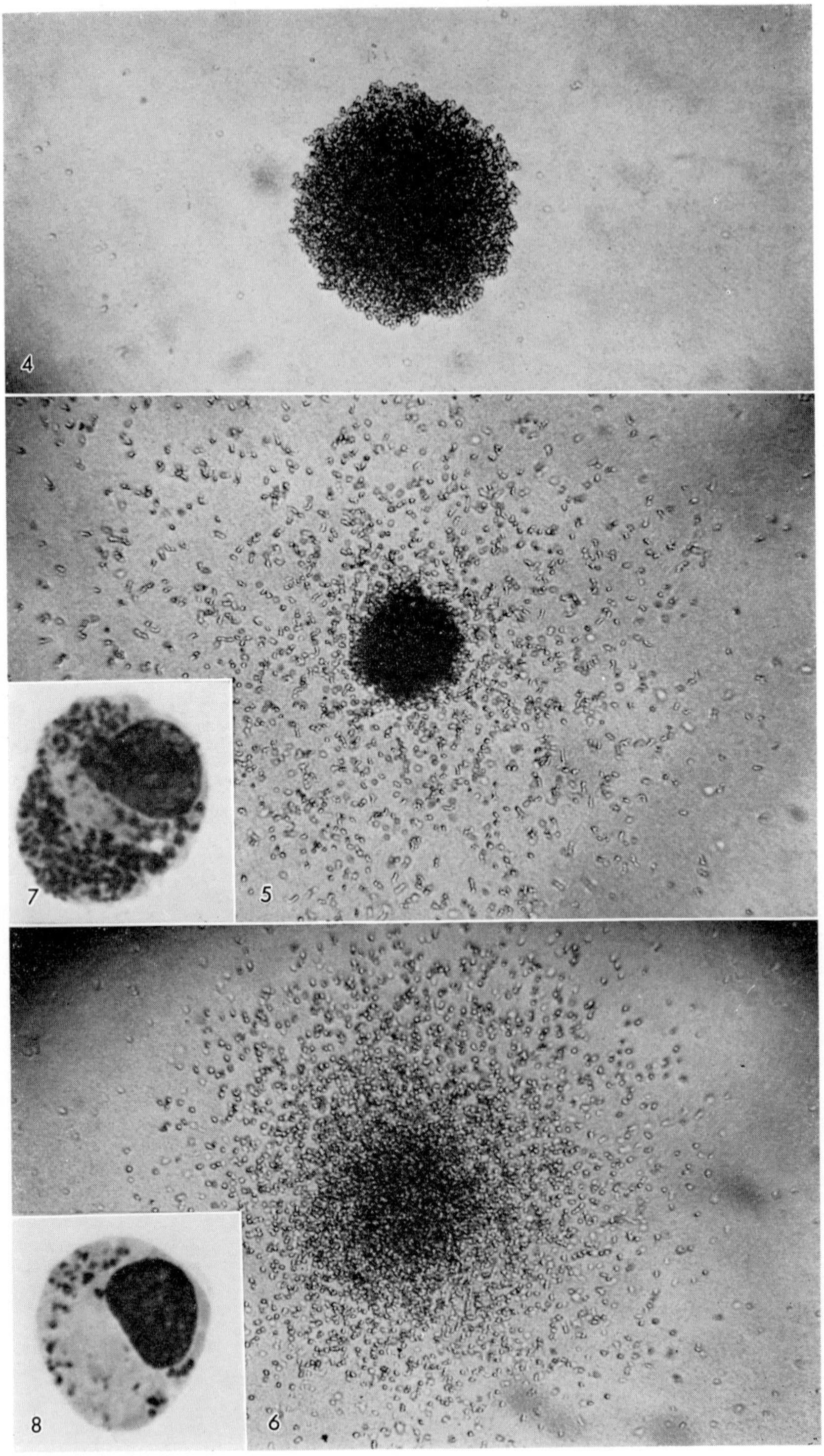
4
7
5
8
6

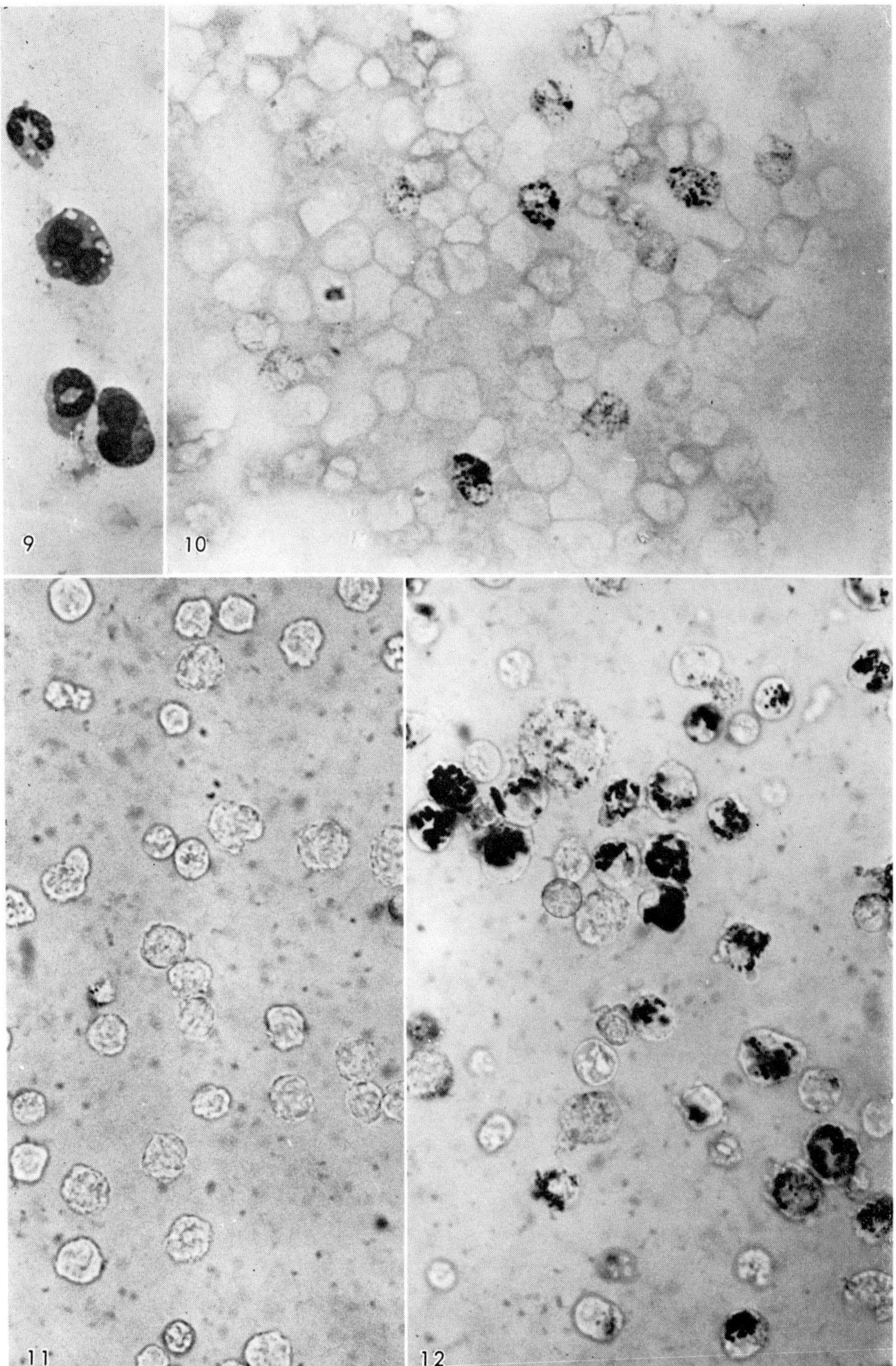
9
10
11
12

GANN Monograph on Cancer Research 12, 1972

PHENOTYPIC CHANGES IN FRIEND TUMOR CELLS

Mitsuru FURUSAWA,* Yoji IKAWA,** and Haruo SUGANO**
Laboratory of Embryology, Faculty of Science, Osaka City University and Department of Pathology, Cancer Institute***

Friend virus-induced mouse tumor cells that have been cultured *in vitro* for about 3 years have no " erythrocyte membrane-specific " antigen. When transplanted and cultured *in vivo* in a diffusion chamber, however, they synthesized the antigen(s) and in some case develop into anucleated erythrocytes. Some of them showed a strong erythrophagocytosis in the chamber.

There are several indications that tumor cells in higher animals reverse and transform themselves spontaneously to the " normally differentiated " state (*2*). The phenomenon, unusual but not wholly inconceivable, naturally arouses speculation from the medical viewpoint, and at the same time it would provide a useful means for the study of cell differentiation, since we can easily culture tumor cells *in vitro* and handle them in a clone level.

The present essay presents a summary of our investigations conducted over the last 3 years. Friend virus-induced tumor cells of a clonal culture *in vitro* manifest an ability to " differentiate " themselves into certain erythroid cells, characteristically capable of synthesizing antigenic molecules specific to the erythrocyte membrane (*5*), and the identification of these tumor cells has been established by the use of a specific antiserum, " anti-A," prepared by Furusawa and Adachi (*3*), which is reactive to the protein molecules of mouse erythrocyte (RBC) membrane. It has customarily been taken for granted that the criteria for cell differentiation are such things as morphological characteristics and the specific functions or the specific products of a given cell; all the same, if we look at ontogenic development from the viewpoint of cell sociology, it becomes important to stress the phenotypic specialization in the plasma membrane of the differentiated cell, *e.g.*, the " sorting-out " in embryonic cells and the metastasis of cancer would be counted as evidence of the important role played by the plasma membrane in cellular differentiation.

Adachi and Furusawa (*1*) indicated that their 3 structural molecules solubilized from the RBC membrane could be recognized as RBC-specific antigens, using Ouchterlony's agar plate. If a further generalization of this concept be allowed, it may lead one to assume that the proteins of the plasma membrane of

* Sugimoto-cho, Sumiyoshi-ku, Osaka 558 (古沢 満).
** Kami-Ikebukuro 1-37-1, Toshima-ku, Tokyo 170 (井川洋二, 菅野晴夫).

any differentiated cell are endowed with characteristics proper to each cell type and that they might afford one a fair criterion for the evaluation of differentiation.

Immunological Analysis of the Structural Molecules of RBC Membrane

1. Preparation of antiserum to RBC membrane protein

The method for preparation of the antiserum has been described in detail previously (*1*). The RBCs of 50 dd mice were hemolyzed in cold hypotonic phosphate buffered saline (0.005 M, pH 6.0). The ghost was collected from the hemolysate by centrifugation at $18{,}000 \times g$ for 15 min, and washed repeatedly with this buffer until the supernatant was completely free of hemoglobin color. Subsequently, the ghost was washed with 0.005 M phosphate buffered saline (pH 8.0) to remove the remaining hemoglobin. The washing was repeated until the ghost pad became pale pink in color. The resulting packed ghost was frozen overnight at $-20°$; then it was washed 3 times with cold distilled water. The resulting ghost suspension was 4 ml in volume. Four milliliters of the ghost suspension in a test tube was cooled at 0° in iced water, then 3 ml of butanol cooled at this temperature was added. The content of this tube was mixed thoroughly by pipetting vigorously for 15 min at 0°. The preparation was subsequently centrifuged for 4 min at $27{,}000 \times g$. Three phases were separated; a butanol phase, the lower aqueous phase, and an interfacial thin film. The lower phase was dialyzed overnight in isotonic buffered saline (pH 7.2) at 4°. The aqueous phase molecules were designated " antigen-A."

Adult female guinea pigs were given intramuscular injections of 1.0 ml of antigen-A with the Freund's complete adjuvant, 4 times, at intervals of 10 days. Three weeks after the last injection, the antisera were collected from each animal separately. These antisera were designated as " anti-A."

2. Agar diffusion test

The method was based on the Ouchterlony's procedure. The wells in agar plate were 9 mm in diameter, and the distance from edge to edge was 7 mm. The anti-A was absorbed with equal volume of packed RBCs at 37° for 60 min, and this treatment was repeated 3 times. Anti-A was absorbed with intact Ehrlich ascites tumor cells in a similar way. The serum was absorbed with one-half volume of mouse kidney and liver " microsomes," stirring at 37° for 60 min. This procedure was repeated twice. The anti-A was also absorbed with the " crushed " RBC ghost which was obtained from the packed RBCs of 3 times the quantity of the antiserum. The " crushed " RBC ghost was obtained by pounding the ghost with powdered dry ice using a mortar and pestle, and washing with isotonic saline (*1, 4*). Antigen-A was used as the test antigen for the diffusion test, in a concentration of 3–4 mg/ml protein.

In a double diffusion test, 3 lines of precipitation were observed in combination of antigen-A with anti-A (see Photo 1). In the absorption experiment, 3 lines could not be eliminated by the absorption of the anti-A with " microsomes " or with the surface of Ehrlich ascites tumor cells. On the other hand, the absorption with intact RBCs resulted in the elimination of the intermediate line.

The remaining 2 lines, however, could not be eliminated in this procedure. The complete elimination of the 3 lines was made possible by absorption with the " crushed " RBC ghost (Photo 1). The result of these absorption experiments appears to support the following explanations: 1) the antigenic molecules represented as 3 precipitin lines are specific to the RBC membrane and 2) the antigenic molecule represented as the intermediate line exists on the surface of the RBC, while antigenic molecules represented as the remaining 2 lines do not exist on its surface. This result indicates that the structural molecules of the RBC membrane may serve as a good criterion for erythroid differentiation.

3. Labeled-antibody staining

It has been demonstrated by Adachi and Furusawa (*1*) that the protein portion of the RBC membrane, the part remaining in the aqueous phase in butanol extraction, can be divided using Ouchterlony's agar plate into three antigenic fractions, which are specific to the RBC membrane. Labeled antibody staining with the anti-A was employed to ascertain the possibility of discriminating the erythroid cells from other sets of cells in mice. The procedures used in preparation of fluorescein-labeled antibody were reported in a previous essay (*3*). The direct staining method was adopted. Fresh cells were smeared on a slide glass with a Japanese paintbrush, dried for 10 min at room temperature, fixed in −20° acetone for 30 min, washed with phosphate buffered saline (pH 7.2), and finally stained with the FITC-conjugated antibody for 1 hr at 37°. The conjugated anti-A was adequately absorbed with the sediment (centrifuged at 16,000 $\times g$) obtained from a homogenate made up of mouse kidney and liver, which were completely deprived of RBCs by irrigation. The slide was then put into stirred buffered saline at room temperature for 10 min in order to wash out excess antibody.

The following observations were obtained in the case of the normal bone marrow. We found megakaryocytes giving negative, and also leucocytes revealing clear granules or leucocyte-like cells having annular nuclei giving negative. On the other hand, those thought to be in the erythroid cells were positive; the cytoplasm was fairly fluorescent, more so along the peripheral region, but it was negative in the nuclear domain. A comparison was made between normal, anemic, and transfused mice by cells to be classified in the erythroid. The results are shown in Table I. Several points can be deduced therefrom; the peculiar dis-

TABLE I. Fluorescence-positive Cells in Mouse Bone Marrow (*3*)

Condition of mouse	No. of animals tested	Cell count: positive/total nucleated	(%)
Normal	4	40/450	(8.9)
		39/707	(5.7)
		21/193	(10.9)
		16/279	(5.7)
Phenylhydrazine anemic	2	142/303	(47)
		208/404	(51)
Blood hypertransfused	2	8/4000	(0.2)
		0/4000	(0)

tribution of the ratios of positive cells to total nucleated, *viz.*, means of 7% in the normal animals, 49% in the anemic, 0.2% and none at all in the transfused. These ratios are what one might presume; the anemic state induced provoked a counteraction of intensive manufacturing of new RBCs, obviously increasing substantially nucleated erythroblasts, whereas the inhibited blood formation in the transfused naturally reduced the appearance of the nucleated within the time elapsed. As shown in Photo 2, this labeled anti-A stained exclusively in the cytoplasmic region or the cell membrane of the cells belonging to the RBC series in mouse bone marrow. It was concluded from the results of the present study that mouse erythroblasts at very early stages of their development already had the same specific antigens as those found in the membrane of the matured RBC, and that the labeled anti-A serves as a good reagent which can descriminate erythroid cells of even very early stages from other types of mouse cells.

Antigenicity of Friend Cells in the Spleen Foci

Ikawa *et al.* (*9*) histologically examined the spleen foci of Friend disease in early stages, which appeared in male DDD mice 3–12 days after inoculation with diluted Friend leukemic virus solution. The first appearance of Friend cells was observed in the periphery of the arterioles in the red pulp. They also examined the foci by electron microscopy and reported that the major part of the spleen foci in early stages was occupied by tumor cells, which resembled proerythroblasts or basophilic erythroblasts, and the most complex cells which might be interpreted as immature reticulum cells showed gradual transition into erythroblastic tumor cells (*8*). From the above results they concluded that the true nature of Friend cells in the foci was erythroblastic.

The Friend cells in the spleen foci reacted to the labeled anti-A and fluoresced, as shown in Photo 3, indicating that most of them are erythroblastic cells and have RBC-specific antigens; this supports Ikawa and Sugano's conclusion.

Antigenicity of Cultured Friend Cells

In October 1966, Ikawa and Sugano (*7*) established an ascites strain, SFAT-3, of Friend virus-induced leukemia by syngenic transplantation of early, focal, splenic lesions in male DDD mice. Since January 1968, they have maintained in clonal culture the above tumor *in vitro*, called TSFAT-3-Cl-1. The cytological characteristics and high heme synthesis of the ascitic and the *in vitro* cultured cells also support the view that the true nature of the cells is erythroblastic (*7*, *12*). Labeled-antibody staining, however, gave negative results, showing that the TSFAT-3-Cl-1 cells are lacking in RBC-specific antigens.

"*Differentiation*" *of TSFAT-3-Cl-1 Cells*

In marked contrast to the above findings, it was found that TSFAT-3-Cl-1 cells maintained in "intraperitoneal diffusion chamber culture" develop a tendency to "revert" to erythroid cells and to show erythrophagocytic activity.

Samples of the cultures (*ca.* 2×10^5 cells) were placed in a diffusion chamber, securely sealed with Millipore membrane pads of 0.45 μ pore diameter, and cultured in the peritoneal cavity of a 5-week-old male DDD mouse for 3 to 9 days.

1. Erythropoietic " differentiation "

Generally, the proportion of smaller cells was larger than had been found in the original culture, and in the most clear-cut cases, the predominant portion was occupied by polychromatophilic or normoblastic cells 10 to 15 μ in diameter. In some cases (5 out of 25 chambers) anucleated, hemoglobin-colored erythrocyte-like corpuscles were seen after Giemsa staining. These corpuscles were variable in size but mostly smaller than normal RBCs. It was also noted that there were cells very much like RBCs in size and shape, but stained light reddish blue.

Most striking was the fact, revealed by labeled-antibody staining, that in all the chamber cultures a great number of the tumor cells, which had previously shown negative fluorescence, now showed a positive cytoplasmic reaction (Photo 4). The proportion of converted cells ranged from 2 to 20% (only 1 case showed 90%). The nucleated erythrocyte-like cells are seen to fluoresce as strongly as normal RBCs, which can be easily recognized as such because of their small size, mostly smaller than normal RBCs. The erythrocyte-like elements staining light reddish blue with Giemsa solution gave a negative fluorescent reaction, which is a sure sign that they are not RBCs but are probably cell debris. As a control, a similar experiment with cultured lymphoblastic lymphoma cells (Lyb-1 and -2) gave completely negative results. The inference to be drawn from these results is that, rather than being contaminated from the outside of the chambers, the fluorescence-positive erythrocyte-like cells were newly formed, possibly by extrusion of the nuclei from the tumor cells during the culture. After treating the surface of the original TSFAT-3-Cl-1 cells with neuraminidase, they also showed a negative fluorescent reaction (5×10^5 cells were incubated at 37° for 1 hr in 1 ml mammalian Ringer's solution at pH 5.5 in the presence of 1 mg neuraminidase; 1 mg neuraminidase [Sigma] from *Cl. perfringens* releases 0.18 μmole of N-acetyl-neuramin-lactose at pH 5.0 at 37°), suggesting that the RBC-specific antigen expression may not include adaptive changes which result from the loss of sialomucin masking the cell surface during culture in a diffusion chamber, but instead may be due to a new synthesis of the specific antigenic molecules.

2. Erythrophagocytic " differentiation "

It was also confirmed that some of the TSFAT-3-Cl-1 cells that were kept in a diffusion chamber *in vivo* showed strong erythrophagocytosis. When the mixtures of TSFAT-3-Cl-1 (1×10^6 cells) and RBCs (1×10^7 cells) were cultured in the chamber *in vivo* for 3 days, there always appeared erythrophagocytic cells in proportions varying from 2 to 30%, but no phagocytic activity was found up to 24 hr. As shown in Photo 5, the cells engulfed with RBCs are mononuclear and 12 to 25 μ in diameter; in some specimens their cytoplasmic region is fully congested with the engulfed RBCs. Cytologically, they are quite different from the normal macrophage and very much like erythroblasts. So far as we tested, they did not eat Indian ink particles.

In short, we were able to demonstrate that the TSFAT-3-Cl-1 cells can retain their differentiating potency *in vitro* for a very long period, and that under experimental conditions they produce erythroid and erythrophagocytic cells.

Soule *et al.* (*13*) and Friend and her colleagues (*10*, *11*) have reported that virus-induced tumor cells demonstrated erythropoietic activity *in vitro*. The criteria they used, however, seem to be somewhat insufficient. Cytological observation alone does not provide concrete evidence for erythrocyte maturation, and Fe-uptake is not a unique characteristic limited to erythroid cells.

Morphological observations show that both the so-called Friend cells in the foci and the cultured TSFAT-3-Cl-1 resemble early erythroblasts, while the lack of RBC-specific antigens in the latter indicates that it is not erythroblastic. Thus, there are two possibilities. First, if we may assume that the origin of the TSFAT-3-Cl-1 is the Friend cell which had originally carried the RBC-specific antigens, the conclusion is inevitable that the Friend cell lost the antigens during *in vivo* culturing and became the TSFAT-3-Cl-1 having no specific antigens, and that later it resynthesized the antigens in the diffusion chamber. Second, one may instead take the view that the origin of TSFAT-3-Cl-1 is the forerunner of erythroblasts in the spleen foci, showing negative fluorescence and having no RBC-specific antigens, the implication being that presumptive erythroblastic tumor cells must have differentiated into erythroid cells under the present experimental conditions. In this case, of course, the TSFAT-3-Cl-1 shows a negative fluorescent reaction. These explanations are based on the fact revealed by Furusawa and Adachi (*3*) that the labeled anti-A stains specifically proerythroblasts to matured RBCs in the normal hematopoietic tissue. Further investigations are required to resolve this problem.

Apart from the above transformation, the present report contains an issue concerned with a peculiar phagocytic phenomenon, for which we offer the following possible explanations. One is that the cell that engulfed the RBCs is a macrophage, and that consequently the TSFAT-3-Cl-1 is, in all probability, the tumor cell originating from the so-called stem cell of mouse blood cells. With the malignant stem cell, Ichikawa (*6*) reported that the mouse myeloid leukemia cell can differentiate into granulocytes and macrophages *in vitro* by treatment with a conditioned medium. The other possibility is that the erythrophagocytic phenomenon need not be attributed to the phagocytic function of macrophages but is rather a newly developed function of the Friend tumor cell—a suggestion more easily acceptable, judging from the fact that the cell did not show any sign of preference for carbon particles, and from its morphological resemblance to erythroblasts rather than to macrophages. In this sense, the present use of the term erythrophagocytosis is not accurate and should be employed only with a somewhat restricted meaning; we incline by preference toward use of the term "quasi-phagocytosis" instead. Whatever the case may be, this two-way differentiation of the tumor cell into erythroid and phagocytic cells merits further investigation.

Before closing this discussion, it would be appropriate to comment on the present experimental procedure, *viz.*, the peculiar environment prevailing within the chamber. It is known that no differentiation has ever been observed when the TSFAT-3-Cl-1 was injected directly into the abdominal cavity. On the third day after the operation, the chamber was found to be covered with fibrous materials and filled with a gelatinous mass, both of which must hinder metabolic processes to no small extent. Could there be concealed any trigger capable of setting off a new phenotypic expression?

REFERENCES

1. Adachi, H. and Furusawa, M. Immunological analysis of the structural molecules of erythrocyte membrane in mice. I. Analysis of the aqueous phase molecules obtained by butanol fractionation of erythrocyte membrane. *Exp. Cell Res.*, **50**, 490–496 (1968).
2. Braun, A. C. Reversal of tumor growth. *In* "The Cancer Problem," Columbia University Press, New York and London, pp. 134–159 (1969).
3. Furusawa, M., and Adachi, H. Immunological analysis of the structural molecules of erythrocyte membrane in mice. II. Staining of erythroid cells with labelled antibody. *Exp. Cell Res.*, **50**, 497–504 (1968).
4. Furusawa, M., Kotani, M., Takeuchi, H., and Asayama, S. Some antigen similarities between mouse erythrocytes and Ehrlich ascites tumor cells. *Nature*, **207**, 1204 (1965).
5. Furusawa, M., Ikawa, Y., and Sugano, H. Development of erythrocyte membrane-specific antigen(s) in clonal cultured cells of Friend virus-induced tumor. *Proc. Japan Acad.*, **47**, 220–224 (1971).
6. Ichikawa, Y. Differentiation of a cell line of myeloid leukemia. *J. Cell Physiol.*, **74**, 223–234 (1969).
7. Ikawa, Y., and Sugano, H. An ascites tumor derived from early splenic lesion of Friend's disease: A preliminary report. *GANN*, **57**, 641–643 (1966).
8. Ikawa, Y., and Sugano, H. Spleen focus in Friend's disease: An electron-microscopic study. *GANN*, **58**, 155–160 (1967).
9. Ikawa, Y., Sugano, H., and Oota, K. Spleen focus in Friend's disease: Histological study. *GANN*, **58**, 61–67 (1967).
10. Patuleia, M. C., and Friend, C. Tissue culture studies on murine virus-induced leukemia cells: Isolation of single cells in agar-liquid medium. *Cancer Res.*, **27**, 726–730 (1967).
11. Rossi, G. B., and Friend, C. Erythrocytic maturation of (Friend) virus-induced leukemic cells in spleen clones. *Proc. Natl. Acad. Sci. U.S.*, **58**, 1373–1380 (1967).
12. Sassa, S., Takaku, F., Nakao, K., Ikawa, Y., and Sugano, H. Heme synthesis in Friend ascites tumor cells. *Proc. Exp. Biol. Med.*, **127**, 527–529 (1968).
13. Soule, H. D., Albert, S., Wolf, P. L., and Stansly, P. G. Erythropoietic differentiation of stable cell lines derived from hematopoietic organs of mice with virusinduced leukemia. *Exp. Cell Res.*, **42**, 380–383 (1966).

EXPLANATION OF PHOTOS

PHOTO 1. Precipitin patterns. Key: *A*, Aqueous-phase molecules obtained from mouse erythrocyte membrane; *Anti-A*, antiserum to aqueous-phase molecule; *Anti-A-R*, anti-A absorbed with intact mouse erythrocytes; *Anti-A-E*, anti-A absorbed with intact Ehrlich ascites tumor cells; *Anti-A-M*, anti-A absorbed with mouse kidney and liver "microsomes;" *anti-A-CR*, anti-A absorbed with "crushed" erythrocyte ghost (*1*).

PHOTO 2. Fluorescence photomicrograph of a smear of myeloid elements of mouse bone marrow showing reticulocyte (*R*) and erythroblast (*E*) with fluorescence, and negative myelocyte (*M*) (*3*).

PHOTO 3. Fluorescence photomicrograph of a smear of Friend cells in the spleen foci. Almost all the cells are fluorescent and contaminated erythrocytes show intense fluorescence. ×500

PHOTO 4. Fluorescence photomicrograph (a) and ordinary photomicrograph (b) of the same field. Two cells obtained from a diffusion chamber (TSFAT-3-Cl-1 cultured *in vivo* for 4 days) showing positive fluorescent reaction (a). ×500. Composite photograph showing fluorescence-positive anucleated cells obtained from the same chamber (c). ×600

PHOTO 5. "Erythrophagocytosis" by TSFAT-3-Cl-1 which was cultured in a diffusion chamber for 4 days with mouse erythrocytes. ×1,000

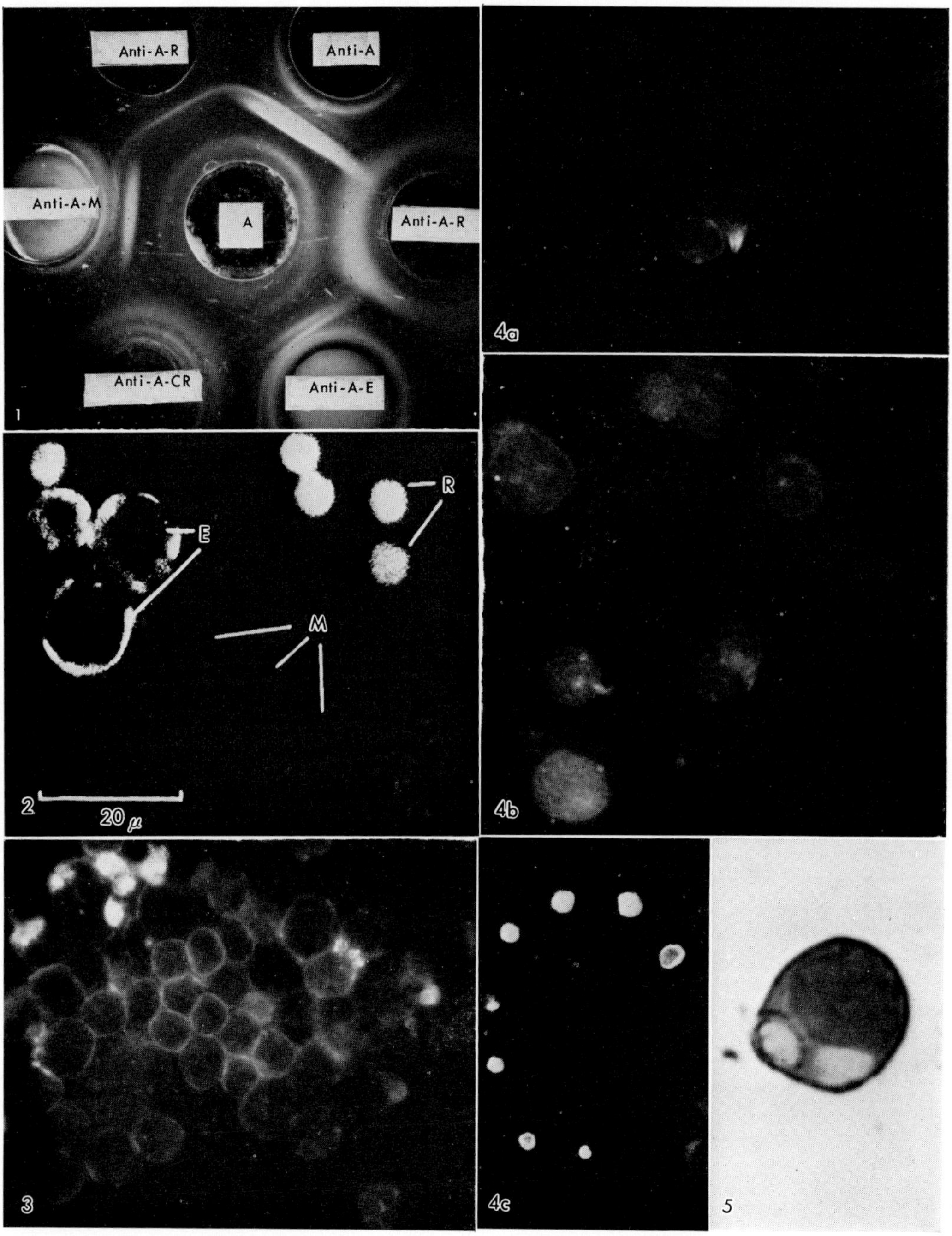
Anti-A-R
Anti-A
Anti-A-M
A
Anti-A-R
Anti-A-CR
Anti-A-E
1
R
E
M
2
20 μ
3
4a
4b
4c
5

RADIATION LEUKEMOGENESIS

FACTORS INVOLVED IN RADIATION LEUKEMOGENESIS

Kenjiro YOKORO, Takaaki ITO, and Nobutaka IMAMURA
*Department of Pathology, Research Institute for Nuclear Medicine and Biology, Hiroshima University**

The leukemogenicity of ^{90}Sr was compared with that of fractionated whole-body X-irradiation in a low-leukemia strain of mice.

Most of the leukemias induced by X-irradiation were thymic in origin and cytologically lymphoblastic, and their frequency was effectively lowered by thymectomy. In contrast, the leukemias induced by ^{90}Sr were not thymic in origin and, cytologically, were reticulum cell, stem cell, or lymphoblastic; their frequency was not modified by thymectomy. A unitary hypothesis is presented here on the basis of our observations of the histological changes in the lymphoid-myeloid systems of the mice treated in either of the above ways and of the tissue distribution of the residual radioactivity of ^{90}Sr-injected mice during the preleukemic period. Successful cell-free transmission of ^{90}Sr-induced leukemia strongly suggests that a virus may be involved in ^{90}Sr-induced leukemia and that the mechanisms of ^{90}Sr-induced and X-ray-induced leukemogenesis appear to be essentially the same.

The possible synergistic action of radiation and leukemogenic virus (passage A virus of Gross) in radiation leukemogenesis was analyzed in the rat. Both radiation and virus were necessary for induction of leukemia in young rats, while either one of them alone failed to induce the disease. Cell-free transmissibility of the induced leukemias indicated that the previously infected Gross virus multiplied in X-irradiated rats, transforming the target cells. Lymphomas developing at the site of " unirradiated thymus grafts " on thymectomized, X-rayed, and Gross-virus-infected rats carried the Gross tumor-specific cell-surface antigen. In radiation leukemogenesis in rats, and perhaps also in some other mammals, the primary inducer is viral. Radiation probably promotes interactions between the virus and its target cells. Immunosuppressive effects of radiation probably facilitate the proliferation of antigenically altered lymphoma cells.

In recent years, it has been shown that leukemia can be induced in mice almost at will by radiation, and considerable knowledge about the disease has been gained through systematic investigations (*41*, *42*). However, there are still some problems to be solved concerning the mechanism of radiation leukemogenesis. The

* Kasumi-cho 1-2-3, Hiroshima 734 (横路謙次郎, 伊藤隆明, 今村展隆).

present discussion is based mainly on the results of our recent experiments with mice and rats (*18–20, 46*). In experiments with mice, the relationship between the type of radiation used and the type of leukemia induced will be emphasized in connection with the role of the thymus. In experiments with rats, the possibility of synergism between radiation and the leukemogenic virus will be analyzed.

Experiments in Mice

1. A comparative study of the leukemogenicity of radiostrontium (^{90}Sr) and X-Irradiation in Mice

Radiostrontium (^{90}Sr), as a bone seeker, is selectively fixed in the bony tissue and induces osteogenic sarcomas (*2*). Finkel first reported that it also possesses a weak leukemogenic effect in mice (*7*). We observed a high incidence of leukemia in a low-leukemic strain of mice, and the leukemogenic effect of ^{90}Sr was compared with that of fractionated whole-body X-irradiation, which has been known to be one of the most effective means of inducing leukemia in mice (*25*).

Female ICR/JCL (CLEA) mice were used throughout the principal experiments. These mice derive from the ICR/Ha strain, in which the incidence of spontaneous leukemia is reported to be less than 1.0% (*3*).

Radiostrontium chloride, $^{90}SrCl$, purchased from the Radiochemical Centre, Amersham, Buckinghamshire, England, was diluted with physiological saline, and 1.0 μCi/g body weight was injected intraperitoneally into 5-week-old mice.

X-Irradiation was administered by a 180 kV X-ray unit at 25 mA with a HVL of 1.18 mm Cu, using 0.5 mm Cu and 0.5 mm Al filters, and delivered at a rate of 50 rad/min and a target-skin distance of 65 cm. A total of 680 R of whole-body X-irradiation was given in four doses of 170 R each at 5-day intervals beginning at 4 weeks of age, according to the schedule of Kaplan and Brown (*25*). Some mice received 1,000 R of partial-body X-irradiation over the right hind limb only, or combined with an injection of ^{90}Sr.

Thymectomy was performed at 3 weeks of age. Techniques used in preparation of leukemic cell suspensions and leukemic cell-free materials have been described elsewhere (*20*).

a) *Frequency and type of leukemia induced:* The experimental groups and data on the prevalence of leukemia developing up to 730 days after treatment are summarized in Table I. Unexpectedly, leukemia occurred at a high rate in mice injected with ^{90}Sr. ^{90}Sr alone was highly leukemogenic, showing an incidence of 61.8%. In contrast to X-irradiated mice, thymectomy never reduced the frequency of leukemia in ^{90}Sr-treated mice. In fact, it appeared to enhance the leukemogenicity, although this increase was not statistically significant. Fractionated whole-body X-irradiation was also highly leukemogenic, showing a prevalence of 77.3%, which was effectively lowered by thymectomy to 29.2% ($P<0.01$). Partial-body X-irradiation exhibited a weak additive effect to that of ^{90}Sr, and partial-body X-irradiation alone was also weakly leukemogenic. Among control mice, only 1 of 33 developed leukemia, after a long latent period.

A histogram of leukemia development is shown in Fig. 1. The peak of development in ^{90}Sr-treated mice was between 90 and 210 days after injection and

TABLE I. Incidence and Latency of Leukemia after Treatment with ^{90}Sr or X-Rays in Female ICR/JCL Mice†

Treatment	Incidence of leukemia (%)	Latency (days)
^{90}Sr Alone	21/34 (61.8)	95–713
Thymex+^{90}Sr	24/34 (70.6)	106–600
Whole-body X-ray	17/22 (77.3)	93–208
Thymex+whole-body X-ray	7/24 (29.2)	110–253
Local X-ray+^{90}Sr	13/16 (81.3)	86–678
Local X-ray alone	6/16 (37.5)	195–596
Untreated control	1/33 (3.0)	565

† Data up to 720 days after treatment.

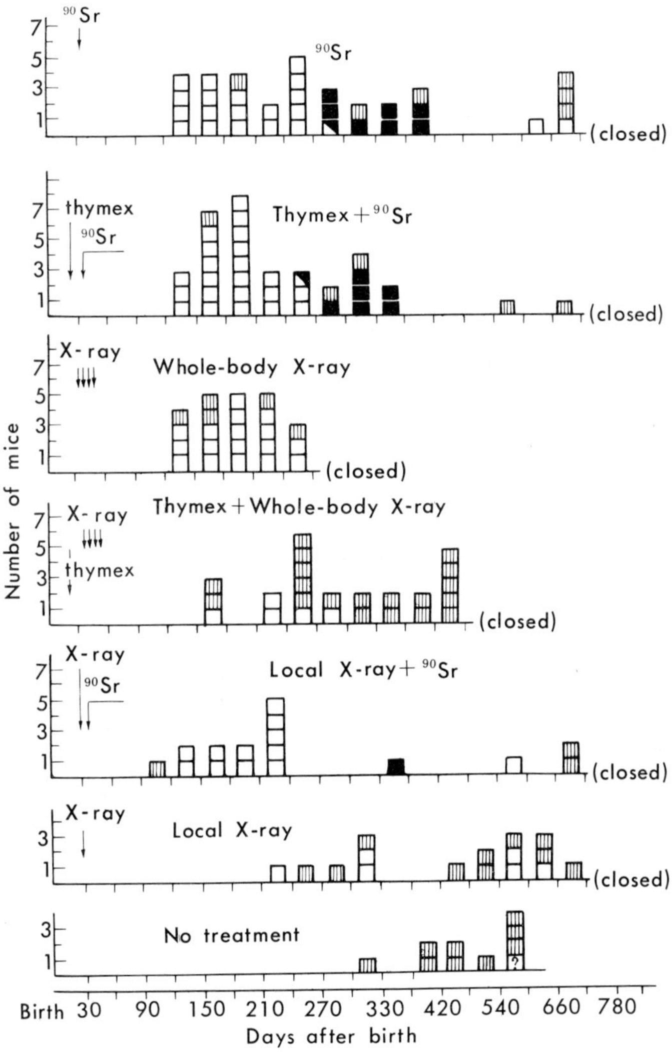

FIG. 1. Histogram of the latent periods of leukemia and osteogenic sarcoma induced by ^{90}Sr and X-rays

□ leukemia; ■ osteogenic sarcoma; ◣ leukemia+osteogenic sarcoma; ▥ others.

was not affected by thymectomy or additional partial-body X-irradiation. In whole-body X-irradiated mice, the peak was similar to that in ^{90}Sr-treated mice. In thymectomized whole-body X-irradiated mice and in nonthymectomized partially X-irradiated mice, leukemia developed but with a longer average latent period. In ^{90}Sr-treated mice, several cases of osteogenic sarcoma occurred after the peak of leukemia prevalence had passed. Some of these mice had both sarcoma and leukemia.

It is interesting to note that there was a rather distinct difference in cytological type between ^{90}Sr-induced and whole-body X-irradiation-induced leukemia. Leukemias induced by ^{90}Sr, including those occurring in thymectomized or partially X-irradiated mice, were not thymic in origin. These mice showed a systemic enlargement of lymph nodes with moderate to marked hepatosplenomegaly. The thymus was not involved. Some of these leukemias were lymphoblastic, but the majority of cases were either reticulum-cell or stem-cell type. In contrast to ^{90}Sr-induced cases, of 17 leukemias induced by fractionated whole-body X-irradiation, 16 were of thymic origin and cytologically lymphoblastic. The exceptional case, with no thymic tumor, was a stem-cell type. The leukemias induced by whole-body X-irradiation in thymectomized mice showed a systemic enlargement of lymph nodes with moderate hepatosplenomegaly and were lymphoblastic or stem-cell type. The leukemias induced by partial-body X-irradiation were macroscopically of nonthymic origin and cytologically were of the lymphoblastic or reticulum-cell type. No myeloid leukemia occurred in any group.

b) Transplantability and transmissibility of induced leukemia: The leukemias, whether induced by ^{90}Sr or by X-irradiation, were almost invariably transplantable into young adult ICR/JCL mice of both sexes, and the recipients died within about 4 weeks after inoculation. At autopsy, an invasion by leukemic cells in the peripheral blood, greatly enlarged lymph nodes, especially in the abdominal cavity, and hepatosplenomegaly were observed. Cytological studies revealed that the type of leukemia was the same as that of the cell donor, indicating acceptance of the grafted cells by the recipient.

In order to study the possible role of a virus in radiation leukemogenesis, leukemic cell-free extracts (filtrates or supernatants) of several leukemias induced by either ^{90}Sr or X-irradiation were inoculated into newborn ICR/JCL and ddN/JCL mice less than 24 hr after birth. In the original passage, of 8 cases of ^{90}Sr-induced leukemia, 5 were transmitted to recipient mice with a latency of 73 to 547 days, though the leukemogenic potency of extracts was rather low (9.1 to 33.3%). Of 4 cases of X-ray-induced leukemia, 3 were transmissible, with a latency of 240 to 465 days; the leukemogenic potency was also low (9.1 to 23.1%). Serial cell-free transmissions up to 4 consecutive animal passages were also achieved in 2 cases of leukemia originally induced by ^{90}Sr. Most of the leukemias induced by the extracts involved lymph nodes and spleen. In a few cases, thymic lymphomas were also observed. However, we have, thus far, been unable to demonstrate the presence of C-type virus particles in leukemic tissue of these mice.

2. *A comparative study of the response in the lymphopoietic and hematopoietic tissues to the administration of ^{90}Sr or whole-body X-irradiation*

In an attempt to elucidate the pathogenesis of ^{90}Sr-induced and X-ray-induced leukemias, hematological and patho-histological changes were studied in mice treated with either agent during the pre-leukemic period.

The strain, age, and sex of animals were similar to those of animals used in Sec. 1. Three groups of mice, the first group treated with ^{90}Sr, the second treated with fractionated whole-body X-irradiation, and the third untreated, were sacrificed regularly, 3 mice from each group being killed at a given interval up to 90 days after treatment. The doses and methods of treatment were also identical to those employed in Sec. 1. General hematological and histological examinations were performed on these mice. In another set of ^{90}Sr-treated mice, tissue distribution of residual radioactivity was estimated as a given interval up to 90 days after

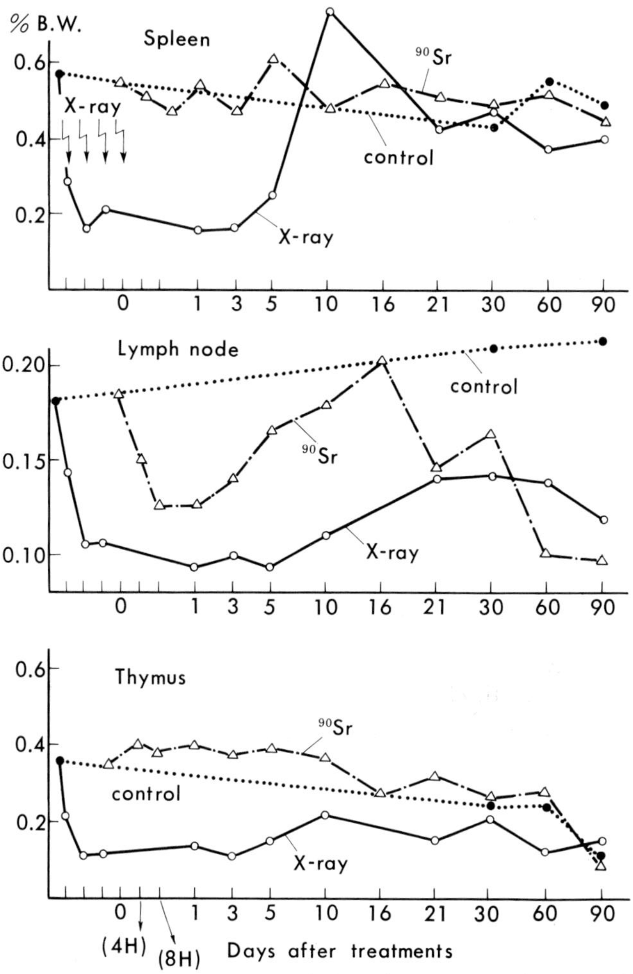

FIG. 2. Changes in spleen, mesenteric lymph node, and thymus weights following the treatment with X-rays (170R×4) or ^{90}Sr (1.0 μCi/g) in ICR/JCL mice

treatment, using the moist ashing method. Radioactivity was estimated with a Geiger-Müller counter.

a) Changes in the weight of the lymphoid tissue: Changes in the mean weight of the spleen, mesenteric node, and thymus of mice given either ^{90}Sr or whole-body X-irradiation are depicted in Fig. 2. A rapid and severe decrease of spleen weight in X-rayed mice was followed by swift recovery, showing a rebound on the tenth day. The weight settled down to the control level by the 21st day. A similar trend was observed in weight changes of the mesenteric node and thymus of X-rayed mice, though the recovery was slower and the weight never returned to the control level.

In contrast with such changes, there was little response in the lymphoid tissues

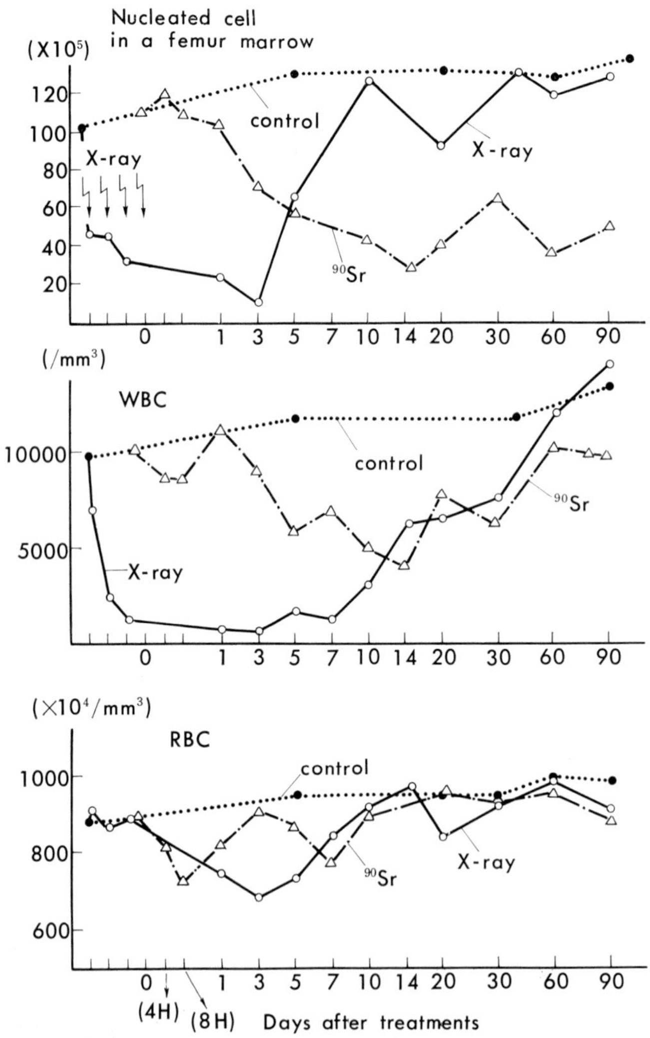

FIG. 3. Changes in nucleated cell in bone marrow, WBC, and RBC counts following the treatment with X-rays (170R×4) or ^{90}Sr (1.0 μCi/g) in ICR/JCL mice

of ^{90}Sr-treated mice except that of the mesenteric node, in which a moderate fluctuation, seen during the first 20 days, was followed by a distinct drop in weight on the 60th day.

b) Changes in the number of nucleated cells in femur marrow, WBC, and RBC (Fig. 3): A sharp fall in the number of nucleated cells in femur marrow of X-rayed mice was followed by vigorous regeneration, the number returning to the normal range by the tenth day, and no striking change was observed thereafter. This was well reflected in changes in the WBC. In ^{90}Sr-treated mice, on the contrary, there was a gradual and prolonged diminution in the number of nucleated marrow cells and the WBC, which had not returned to normal even after 90 days. With respect to RBC, there was no clear response to either treatment except a slight decrease in both groups during the early period. These changes observed in ^{90}Sr-treated mice could be attributed to the selective deposition of ^{90}Sr in the skeleton, from which the medullary hematopoietic tissue is continuously irradiated.

c) Residual radioactivity in various tissues of mice treated with 1.0 μCi/g of ^{90}Sr: From Fig. 4, it is clear that almost all radioactivity was traceable to the skeleton. The fixation of injected ^{90}Sr in the skeleton seemed to be very rapid and it reached a maximum as early as 4 hr after intraperitoneal administration. On

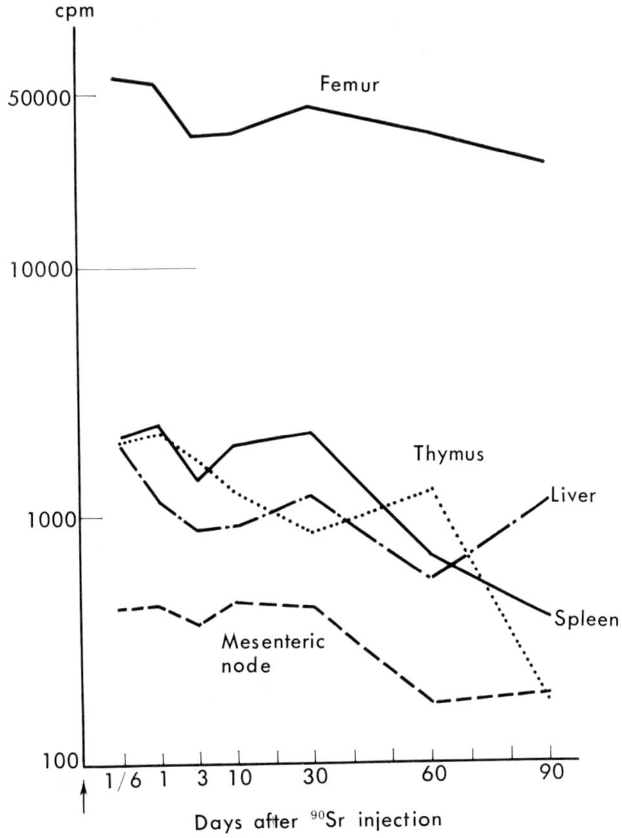

FIG. 4. Changes in residual radioactivity in various tissues following ^{90}Sr administration (1.0 μCi/g, i.p. injection)

the contrary, residual activity in various soft tissues was negligible, showing less than 1/50 of the activity of the skeleton throughout the observation period. These findings clearly explain why the pattern of radiation injury caused by ^{90}Sr is distinctly different from that due to whole-body X-irradiation.

d) *Histogenesis of leukemia induced by either ^{90}Sr or whole-body X-irradiation:* In whole-body X-irradiated mice, in which a high incidence of thymic lymphoma was observed, an initial leukemic lesion was found as early as 45 days after the termination of treatment in the deep cortex adjacent to the medulla of a lymphocyte-depleted lobe of the thymus as a small focus of accumulation of immature lymphoid cells with many mitotic figures (Photo 1). The other lobe appeared to be free from lymphomatous proliferation during this stage. The initial lesion increased in size over time, occupying the greater part of the lobe. Subsequently, it spread over the other lobe, and a macroscopic lymphoma was established by 90 days after the termination of treatment. This " unilateral development " of thymic lymphoma has been reported not only in radiation leukemogenesis (by whole-body X-irradiation) but also in spontaneous, viral, and chemical leukemogenesis (*38*).

In ^{90}Sr-treated mice, on the other hand, in which stem-cell or reticulum-cell type or nonthymic lymphoblastic leukemias predominate, a sustained hypoplastic state of the medullary hematopoiesis was characteristic. No conspicuous change was observed in the thymus throughout the experimental period. Instead, small foci of large polygonal cells with occasional mitotic figures were found in the deep cortex of lymph nodes of some mice sacrificed 90 days after treatment (Photo 2). These cell foci may represent the early appearance of nonthymic leukemia induced by ^{90}Sr.

3. *Discussion*

Through the aforementioned studies, our attention was focused on the role of the thymus in various aspects of radiation leukemogenesis and on the nature of induced leukemia. Many investigators have reported that removal of the thymus eliminates both the occurrence of spontaneous leukemia (*33*) and its induction by X-rays (*23*), chemicals (*28*), and viruses (*30*). We confirmed this in whole-body X-irradiated ICR/JCL mice. However, thymectomy did not lower the frequency of ^{90}Sr-induced leukemia but instead seemed to promote it. This may indicate that there is a difference in the leukemogenic mechanism between external irradiation with X-rays and internal irradiation with ^{90}Sr. The presence of the thymus appears to be a prerequisite for lymphoma induction by whole-body X-irradiation. In the induction of leukemia by ^{90}Sr, on the other hand, some extrathymic sites seem to play a role. From the pattern of injury caused by ^{90}Sr, ^{90}Sr-induced leukemia might be expected to be of bone marrow origin. However, most leukemias induced by ^{90}Sr were of the reticulum-cell, stem-cell, or lymphoblastic type. No myeloid leukemia was found in our studies. It has been suggested that the development of thymic lymphoma is not always the result of the direct effect of X-irradiation upon the thymus (*26*, *29*). Joneja and Stich (*22*) postulated on the basis of chromosomal changes in the hematopoietic tissue that whole-body X-irradiation produces leukemic progenitor cells in the bone marrow or spleen and that these cells migrate into the "injured thymus," where they proliferate. In the case of ^{90}Sr-induced leukemia, similar progenitor cells may be produced in the bone marrow by a direct effect of ^{90}Sr, after which they migrate into peripheral lymphoid tissues but not into the "intact thymus." Therefore we presume that leukemias develop unicentrically in the thymus after whole-body X-irradiation, whereas they develop multicentrically in the peripheral lymphoid tissues after ^{90}Sr injection. Furthermore, X-ray-induced leukemic progenitor cells, which have not as yet differentiated into any particular cell type, may be endowed with the capability of lymphoid differentiation in the thymus through an as yet unknown thymic factor. On the other hand, most of the ^{90}Sr-induced leukemic cells that settled in the peripheral lymphoid tissues without passing through the thymic environment might remain as primitive undifferentiated cell types (stem cells or reticulum cells). Our hypothesis is perhaps strengthened by the observation that the thymus does not seem to sustain any injuries due to ^{90}Sr injection, as it does after whole-body X-irradiation. This assumption may be further supported by the observation that ^{90}Sr-induced leukemias were not restricted to the lymphoid type, regardless of the presence or absence of the thymus.

In order to test our hypothesis, a small-scale experiment was performed in which local X-irradiation over the thymus region was performed on ^{90}Sr-injected mice. As anticipated, a significant increase in the frequency of lymphoblastic lymphoma originating in the thymus was observed among these mice as compared with mice given ^{90}Sr only (unpublished data). This may be interpreted by assuming that ^{90}Sr-injected mice were converted into a condition somewhat similar to that of whole-body X-irradiated mice by the additional X-irradiation of the thymus.

Several reports on the cell-free transmissibility of radiation-induced leukemia in mice indicate the participation of a leukemogenic virus as an inducing mechanism. The mechanism has been described as the activation by X-irradiation of a leukemogenic virus already present in the host (*11*). More recently, Huebner and Todaro (*16*) took the view that radiation, chemicals, and the normal aging process may favor the partial or complete activation (switching on) of viral information which is vertically transmitted from parent to offspring in switched-off form. This proposal is based on their hypothesis that the cells of all vertebrates contain information for producing C-type RNA viruses. Our success in cell-free transmission of ^{90}Sr-induced leukemia strongly suggests that a virus may take part in leukemia induction by ^{90}Sr and that the mechanisms of ^{90}Sr-induced and X-ray-induced leukemogenesis do not differ in their essential nature.

Experiments in Rats

1. Induction of leukemia in rats by a combination of radiation and virus

There is little doubt that some tumors in both mammals and birds are caused by oncogenic viruses, and, if there are any oncogenic viruses in human tumors, leukemia seems to be one of the most likely candidates. On the one hand, with respect to the mechanism of radiation leukemogenesis, it is reasonable to suppose that somatic mutation may play a dominant role, since ionizing radiation is known to be a powerful mutagen. But there is ample evidence indicating that the situation is more complex; the implication of leukemogenic virus in radiation leukemogenesis in mice has been well documented by several investigators including ourselves (*6*, *12*, *14*, *15*, *19*, *21*, *31*). However, in attempting to analyze the role of viruses in radiation leukemogenesis, the mouse does not seem to be wholly satisfactory, due to the fact that many mouse strains are naturally infected with leukemogenic virus and that whole-body X-irradiation alone produces leukemia at a high rate. On the other hand, it seems advisable to use rats because the frequency of radiation-induced leukemia in rats is generally low (*34*), and because, thus far, no rat leukemogenic viruses have ever been isolated. That is, the rat is a cleaner experimental medium than the mouse. Furthermore, certain strains of rats show a high susceptibility during the early postnatal period to leukemogenic viruses of mouse origin.

The present studies were undertaken to clarify the respective roles played by radiation and virus in the induction of leukemia in rats.

A highly inbred strain of Wistar/Furth (W/Fu) rats of both sexes were used throughout the present studies. The frequency of spontaneous leukemia in this strain has been reported to be low, and spontaneous leukemia occurs only in older rats (*27*).

A leukemic female W/Fu rat that had been injected at birth with the rat-adapted passage A virus of Gross (*36*) was obtained through the courtesy of Dr. H. Okano, Cancer Institute, Kyushu University School of Medicine, Fukuoka. A leukemic cell-free filtrate containing the virus was prepared from the rat by a procedure described by Levinthal *et al.* (*30*). The virus has since been maintained in our laboratory through successive cell-free passages in W/Fu rats by inoculating 0.1 ml of leukemic filtrate intraperitoneally within 48 hr after birth of the recipients. The virus preparation was stored in an electric deep freezer at $-100°$ until used.

The X-irradiation factors were identical to those employed in the mouse experiments described in the previous section of this paper.

In the principal experiment, 76 rats of both sexes were divided into 5 groups. In the first group, the rats received 600 R of whole-body X-irradiation delivered in 4 doses of 150 R each at 5-day intervals. The irradiation was started when rats were 4 to 5 weeks of age. They were then inoculated intraperitoneally with 0.4 ml of Gross virus a few hours after the last X-irradiation. In the second group, rats received fractionated whole-body X-irradiation alone, and the third group of rats were inoculated with the virus alone, with a dose and time schedule identical to that of the first group. In addition, 2 litters of newborn rats were inoculated intraperitoneally, within 48 hr after birth, with 0.05 ml of the same lot of the virus preparation in order to certify the leukemogenic activity of the virus. Two litters of untreated rats served as controls. The experiment was terminated on the 400th day after treatment.

a) *Frequency of leukemia* : The experimental groups and the occurrence of leukemia in various groups up to 400 days after treatment are summarized in Table II. Neonatal inoculation of Gross virus in this strain of rats showed a high leukemogenicity, as previously reported (*36*). All 15 rats developed thymic lym-

TABLE II. Leukemia Induction in Wistar/Furth Rats with X-Rays and Gross Virus

Treatment	No. of rats	Leukemia cases	Latency (days)
Gross virus alone (at 48 hr after birth)	15	15	80–90
Gross virus alone (at 8 weeks of age)	15	0	—
X-Ray alone[a]	12	0	—
X-Ray[a]+Gross virus[b]	20	11	77–213

[a] 600 R whole-body X-irradiation, divided into 4 equal doses at 5-day intervals, started at 4–5 weeks of age.

[b] Inoculated immediately after the last X-irradiation (at 7–8 weeks of age).

phomas within 90 days after viral inoculation. However, the susceptibility of the rat to the virus appeared to decrease rapidly as the age of the rats increased; no leukemia occurred when the virus was inoculated at 7 to 8 weeks of age. Fractionated whole-body X-irradiation, started at 4 to 5 weeks of age, was also ineffective in eliciting leukemia up to 400 days after the termination of X-irradiation. No leukemia development was observed in the control group. In contrast to the above groups, 11 out of 20 rats (55%) that received a combined treatment of X-irradiation and virus inoculation developed leukemia with a latent period of from 77 to 213 days. Seven of these cases of induced leukemia occurred with a shorter latent period, from 80 to 120 days, and originated in the thymus; these cases were similar to those observed in susceptible strains of mice (*10*) and W/Fu rats after neonatal virus inoculation. Three of the 4 remaining cases were nonthymic lymphoid leukemia, and one was myeloid leukemia of the chloroma type; the latent period of the myeloid leukemia was much longer than that of the thymic lymphoma. There was no clear difference in the prevalence of leukemia between sexes, perhaps because the number of the rats was small; there were 6 cases in females (50.0%) and 5 cases in males (62.5%).

b) *Leukemogenicity of the cell-free filtrates prepared from the leukemic tissue of the induced leukemias:* Two leukemic cell-free filtrates were prepared from 2 thymic lymphomas induced by a combination of X-irradiation and Gross virus injection. These preparations were inoculated into each of 2 litters of newborn W/Fu rats within 48 hr after birth to test their leukemogenic activity. All but 1 (*i.e.*, 13 out of 14) of the recipients developed thymic lymphomas with a latent period of from 65 to 110 days, thus indicating the persistence and multiplication of the Gross virus originally inoculated into the host.

2. *Further analysis of the role of radiation and virus in radiation leukemogenesis in rats*

In an attempt to strengthen our understanding of the mechanism involved in radiation leukemogenesis, the respective roles played by radiation and virus were analyzed in more detail. In this experiment, a special condition was established in order to rule out the direct leukemogenic effect of X-irradiation in induction of thymic lymphoma.

The strain and age of experimental animals and the dose and time schedules of virus inoculation and X-irradiation were practically identical to those of Sec. 1, with the exception of a slight increase in X-ray dose.

The cytotoxic effect of antiserum against the Gross tumor-specific cell-surface antigen upon induced lymphoma cells was tested *in vitro* according to a technique devised by Gorer and O'Gorman (*8*).

W/Fu rats were thymectomized at 4 weeks of age. They subsequently received 680 R of whole-body X-irradiation in 4 split doses at 5-day intervals started at 5 weeks of age, and a few hours after the last exposure Gross virus was inoculated intraperitoneally. Immediately after the virus inoculation, the rats were grafted subcutaneously on the back with syngeneic neonatal whole thymus tissue. Our anticipation was that lymphoma might develop in the grafted thymus which had not been irradiated. Two other groups, one without virus inoculation, the other without X-irradiation, served as controls.

a) *Frequency of leukemia:* Experimental groups and the frequency of leukemia are shown in Table III. As anticipated, 15 out of 25 rats that were thymectomized, X-rayed, virus-infected, and grafted with neonatal thymus developed lymphomas at the site of the thymus graft within 110 days after treatment. The lymphomas appeared in the subcutaneous tissue of the back as grayish spherical tumor masses (Photo 3). Histological examination revealed that they consisted of lymphoblastic cells identical to those of the thymic lymphoma *in situ* (Photo 4). The lymphomas were localized during the early stage but later became generalized lymphoid leukemia with the appearance of numerous tumor cells in the peripheral blood.

TABLE III. Incidence of Leukemia in Variously Treated W/Fu Rats

Treatment				Leukemia cases/ No. in group	Leukemia incidence (%)	Latency (days)
Thymex	X-Ray	Virus	Thymus graft			
+	−	+	+	0/23	0	—
+	+	−	+	0/18	0	—
+	+	+	+	15/25	60	50–110

No leukemia occurred in control groups up to 350 days after treatment, in which either X-irradiation or virus infection was omitted.

b) *Cytotoxic test of the induced lymphoma cells:* In brief, lymphoma cells showed a very high cytotoxic index when incubated *in vitro* with antiserum to the Gross-tumor-specific cell-surface antigen. This indicates that these lymphoma cells are carrying the Gross-virus-related antigen.

c) *Leukemogenicity of cell-free filtrates prepared from lymphomas that developed at the site of thymus graft:* As in Sec. 1, 2 leukemic cell-free filtrates were prepared from lymphomas that developed at the site of the neonatal thymus graft. These preparations were then inoculated into each of 2 litters of syngeneic newborn rats within 48 hr after birth in order to test their leukemogenicity. All of the recipients (10/10) developed thymic lymphomas with a latent period of from 41 to 70 days. From these findings, it is clear that Gross virus actively participates in induction of lymphomas at the site of the nonirradiated thymus graft.

Next, an important question arises as to whether the lymphomas developing in the thymic graft are derived from the cells of the donor, which had never been exposed to X-irradiation, or from cells that entered the graft secondarily from the previously X-irradiated tissue of the host. In order to clarify this, chromosomal analysis of the lymphoma cells using the sex chromosome as indicator and observation of the transplantation behavior of lymphoma cells in the parental and F_1 hybrid recipients are currently under way in our laboratory. Preliminary results suggest that most of the lymphomas developed at the site of the thymus graft are, in fact, derived from the grafted donor cells which had never been X-irradiated.

d) *Immunological status of variously treated rats:* In order to learn more about the concrete role of radiation in radiation leukemogenesis, experimental groups identical to those in Sec. 2 were subsequently tested for immunological competence at a given interval up to 50 days after treatment; the tests used were Jerne's spleen plaque-forming cell method (*17*) and measurement of serum hemolysin and hemagglutinin titers against sheep red blood cells.

In brief, the number of hemolytic plaque-forming cells in the spleen and serum antibody titers was much lower throughout the experimental period in X-rayed, thymectomized, virus-infected rats than in nonirradiated, thymectomized, virus-infected rats. A sustained lymphopenia in the peripheral blood and a hypoplastic state in the lymphoid tissues were also observed in the former group. These results indicate that whole-body X-irradiation is an effective means of prolonging and intensifying the immunosuppressive state of the thymectomized, virus-infected host.

3. *Discussion*

In Sec. 1, it was clearly demonstrated that both radiation and virus are necessary for the induction of leukemia in young rats; leukemia failed to develop after the application of either treatment alone. Furthermore, cell-free transmissibility of the induced lymphomas indicated that the originally infected Gross virus had been multiplying in X-irradiated rats, leading to malignant transformation of the target cells. The results of Sec. 2 strengthen our view that Gross virus acts as the prime inducer of the disease and that X-irradiation promotes interaction between Gross virus and its target cells and the proliferation of antigenically altered lymphoma cells through its immunosuppressive effect on the host. The sequence of events appears to be analogous to that demonstrated by Kaplan (*24*) in C57BL mice, in which a leukemogenic virus was vertically transmitted from the parents.

In our previous studies (*40*, *45*), it was shown, in adult RF mice, that whole-body X-irradiation followed by inoculation of either Gross or Moloney virus significantly increased the frequency of myeloid leukemia without affecting that of thymic lymphoma. We ascribed this phenomenon to the acceptance of viruses by the myeloid precursor cells during a period of heightened proliferating activity after X-irradiation. Graffi (*9*) showed that the frequency of myeloid leukemia was raised in the Graffi virus-infected mice by the additional treatment with either X-irradiation or polycyclic hydrocarbons. Similarly, Lieberman *et al.* (*32*) demonstrated that small doses of X-irradiation or urethane potentiated the leukemogenic activity of a cell-free agent prepared from radiation-induced lymphomas in C57BL mice. Jenkins and Upton (*21*) also reported an enhancement of leukemia frequency by pre-irradiation of the host inoculated with cell-free preparations of radiation-induced leukemia in RF mice. The aforementioned effect of radiation in viral leukemogenesis is still not wholly understood; it is not clear whether it is due to its immunosuppressive effect, to alteration of lympho-myeloid activity, or to viral gene activation. We are inclined to attribute the present experimental results to a sequence in which X-irradiation alters the hematopoietic and lymphopoietic systems of young adult rats, inducing the system to revert to the neonatal state during the recovery phase. This confers on an adult rat a susceptibility to Gross virus, which in turn leads to the eventual development of leukemia.

In Sec. 2, the prime importance of preconditioning of the host was unequivocally demonstrated by showing the origination of lymphomas from unirradiated cells.

The effect of radiation (*13*) and inoculation of leukemogenic viruses (*4*, *5*, *17*, *35*, *37*) in suppressing immunologic responses has been well documented. A dual effect by both agents might also contribute to making the host tolerant to the inoculated virus and to facilitating the proliferation of leukemic cells which have acquired a new antigenic property.

We usually use the term " radiation carcinogenesis " without much consideration and assume that the mechanism may be an almost universal one. However, the evidence obtained from our experiments indicates that the mechanism is complex. For instance, the induction of mammary tumors in rats by X-irradiation appears to be the result of the direct effect of radiation on the mammary epithelial cells, though the real mechanism has not been established (*1*). In this case, hormones act as either promotors or inhibitors of the growth rate of the induced tumor (*44*). Therefore, in the case of mammary tumorigenesis, radiation may play the primary role as a carcinogen, and the carcinogenic effect may be influenced by the hormonal environment of the host. On the contrary, in radiation leukemogenesis, as reported here, the situation is reversed; a virus appears to be the prime inducer, while conditions favoring interaction between the virus and the target cells are facilitated by radiation. These findings offer a good example of the etiological complexity of radiation carcinogenesis.

Finally, the usefulness of the rat in leukemia research should be emphasized. As mentioned before, there is little doubt that, in mice, leukemias either developing spontaneously or induced by radiation or chemicals are essentially viral in nature. Furthermore, it has been widely assumed that all vertebrate cells carry the C-type RNA viral genome which is vertically transmitted from parents to offspring in switched-off form (*16*). However, the evidence in the rat seems too meager to merit acceptance of this hypothesis at the present moment. To the best of our knowledge, no unequivocal data have been presented on the role of viruses in rat leukemogenesis, though there have been a few reports suggesting its involvement (*39*, *43*). Thus, the rat seems to be a suitable tool in analyzing the complex mechanisms involved in leukemogenesis.

REFERENCES

1. Bond, V. P., Schellabarger, V. P., Cronkite, E. P., and Fliedner, T. M. Studies on radiation-induced mammary gland neoplasia in the rat. V. Induction by localized irradiation. *Radiation Res.*, **13**, 318–328 (1960).
2. Brues, A. M., Lisco, H., and Finkel, M. P. Carcinogenic action of some substances which may be a problem in certain industries. *Cancer Res.*, **7**, 48 (1947).
3. Buffett, R. F., Grace, J. T. Jr., and Mirand, E. A. Properties of a lymphocytic leukemia agent isolated from Ha/ICR Swiss mice. *Proc. Soc. Exp. Biol. Med.*, **116**, 293–297 (1964).
4. Ceglowski, W. S., and Friedman, H. Immunosuppressive effect of Friend and Rauscher leukemia disease viruses on cellular and humoral antibody formation. *J. Natl. Cancer Inst.*, **40**, 983–995 (1968).
5. Dent, P. B., Peterson, R. D. A., and Good, R. A. A defect in cellular immunity during the incubation period of passage A leukemia in C3H mice. *Proc. Soc. Exp. Biol. Med.*, **119**, 869–871 (1965).
6. Duplan, J. F., and Latarjet, R. Studies on the mechanism of radiation-induced leukemogenesis in C57BL mice. *Cancer Res.*, **26**, 395–399 (1966).
7. Finkel, M. P. Relative biological effectiveness of internal emitters. *Radiology*, **67**, 665–672 (1956).
8. Gorer, P. A., and O'Gorman, P. The cytotoxic activity of isoantibodies in mice. *Transplant. Bull.*, **3**, 142–143 (1956).
9. Graffi, A. Chloroleukemia of mice. *Ann. N.Y. Acad. Sci.*, **68**, 540–558 (1957).
10. Gross, L. Development and serial cell-free passage of a highly potent strain of mouse leukemia virus. *Proc. Soc. Exp. Biol. Med.*, **94**, 767–771 (1957).
11. Gross, L. Attempt to recover filtrable agent from X-ray-induced leukemia. *Acta Haematol.*, **19**, 353–361 (1958).
12. Gross, L. Serial cell-free passage of a radiation-activated mouse leukemia agent. *Proc. Soc. Exp. Biol. Med.*, **100**, 102–105 (1959).
13. Hasek, M., and Lengerova, A. Immunology. *In* "Mechanisms in Radiobiology," ed. by M. Errera and A. Forssbery, Academic Press, New York, pp. 207–229 (1960).
14. Hiraki, K., Irino, S., Sota, S., and Ikejiri, K. Leukemogenic activity of cell-free filtrates from radiation-induced leukemia of RF mice. *Acta Haematol. Japon.*, **25**, 816–821 (1962).
15. Holmberg, E. A. D., Vasquez, C., de Pasqualini, C. D., Pavlovsky, A., and Rabasa, S. L. A cellular passage of ^{32}P-induced leukemia: An electron microscopic study. *Cancer Res.*, **27**, 198–204 (1967).
16. Huebner, R. J., and Todaro, G. J. Oncogenes of RNA tumor viruses as determinants of cancer. *Proc. Natl. Acad. Sci. U.S.*, **64**, 1087–1094 (1969).
17. Imamura, N., Takizawa, S., Nishihara, E., Yamasaki, T., and Yokoro, K. Immunosuppressive effect of leukemogenic viruses. *Proc. Hiroshima Univ. RINMB.*, **11**, 54–61 (1970).
18. Ito, T. Leukemogenic effect of radiostrontium (^{90}Sr) in mice: A comparative study of leukemogenicity of ^{90}Sr and X-rays. I. Incidence and characteristics of ^{90}Sr-induced and X-ray-induced leukemias. *Acta Haematol. Japon.*, **33**, 415–431 (1970).
19. Ito, T. Leukemogenic effect of radiostrontium (^{90}Sr) in mice: A comparative study of leukemogenicity of ^{90}Sr and X-rays. II. Transmissibility of the induced

leukemias, alkaline phosphatase activity and cytogenetic changes of leukemic cells. *Acta Haematol. Japon.*, **33**, 432–448 (1970).
20. Ito, T., Yokoro, K., Ito, A., and Nishihara, E. A comparative study of the leukemogenic effect of strontium-90 and X-rays in mice. *Proc. Soc. Exp. Biol. Med.*, **130**, 345–350 (1969).
21. Jenkins, V. K., and Upton, A. C. Cell-free transmission of radiogenic myeloid leukemia in the mouse. *Cancer Res.*, **23**, 1748–1755 (1963).
22. Joneja, M. G., and Stich, H. F. Chromosomes of tumor cells. IV. Cell population changes in thymus, spleen and bone marrow during X-ray-induced leukemogenesis in C57BL/6J mice. *J. Natl. Cancer Inst.*, **35**, 421–434 (1965).
23. Kaplan, H. S. Influence of thymectomy, splenectomy and gonadectomy on incidence of radiation-induced lymphoid tumors in strain C57 black mice. *J. Natl. Cancer Inst.*, **11**, 83–90 (1950).
24. Kaplan, H. S. On the natural history of the murine leukemias: Presidential address. *Cancer Res.*, **27**, 1325–1340 (1967).
25. Kaplan, H. S., and Brown, M. B. A quantitative dose-response study of lymphoid-tumor development in irradiated C57 black mice. *J. Natl. Cancer Inst.*, **13**, 185–208 (1952).
26. Kaplan, H. S., Hirsch, B. B., and Brown, M. B. Indirect induction of lymphomas in irradiated mice. IV. Genetic evidence of the origin of the tumor cells from the thymic grafts. *Cancer Res.*, **16**, 434–436 (1956).
27. Kim, U., Clifton, K. H., and Furth, J. A highly inbred line of Wistar rats yielding spontaneous mammo-somatotropic pituitary and other tumors. *J. Natl. Cancer Inst.*, **24**, 1031–1055 (1960).
28. Law, L. W., and Miller, J. H. The influence of thymectomy on the incidence of carcinogen-induced leukemia in strain DBA mice. *J. Natl. Cancer Inst.*, **11**, 425–437 (1950).
29. Law, L. W., and Potter, M. Further evidence of indirect induction by X-radiation of lymphocytic neoplasms in mice. *J. Natl. Cancer Inst.*, **20**, 489–493 (1958).
30. Levinthal, J. D., Buffett, R. F., and Furth, J. Prevention of viral lymphoid leukemia of mice by thymectomy. *Proc. Soc. Exp. Biol. Med.*, **100**, 610–614 (1959).
31. Lieberman, M., and Kaplan, H. S. Leukemogenic activity of filtrates from radiation-induced lymphoid tumors of mice. *Science*, **130**, 387–388 (1959).
32. Lieberman, M., Haran-Ghera, N., and Kaplan, H. S. Potentiation of virus leukemogenesis in C57BL mice by X-irradiation or urethane. *Nature*, **203**, 420–422 (1964).
33. McEndy, D. P., Boon, M. C., and Furth, J. On the role of thymus, spleen and gonads in the development of leukemia in a high-leukemia stock of mice. *Cancer Res.*, **4**, 377–383 (1944).
34. Moloney, W. C., Boschetti, A. E., and Dowd, G. Observations on leukemia in Wistar and Wistar Furth rats. *Blood*, **26**, 341–353 (1965).
35. Odaka, T., Ishii, H., Yamamura, K., and Yamamoto, T. Inhibitory effect of Friend leukemia virus infection on the antibody formation to sheep erythrocytes in mice. *Japan. J. Exp. Med.*, **36**, 277–290 (1966).
36. Okano, H., Kunii, A., and Furth, J. Electron microscopic study of leukemia induced in rats with Gross virus. *Cancer Res.*, **23**, 1169–1175 (1963).
37. Peterson, R. D. A., Hendrickson, R., and Good, R. A. Reduced antibody forming capacity during the induction period of passage A leukemia in C3H mice. *Proc. Soc. Exp. Biol. Med.*, **114**, 517–520 (1963).
38. Siegler, R. Pathology of murine leukemia. *In* "Experimental Leukemia," ed. by

M. A. Rich, North-Holland Publishing Co., Amsterdam, pp. 51–95 (1968).
39. Svec, F., and Hlavay, E. Transmission of a filtrable agent from rat leukemia induced by X-ray irradiation and treatment with methylcholanthrene. *Acta Haematol.*, **26**, 252–260 (1960).
40. Takizawa, S., Ito, A., and Yokoro, K. Role of the mouse lymphoma virus of Moloney in induction of myeloid leukemia by X-irradiation. *Acta Haematol. Japon.*, **29**, 42–48 (1966).
41. Upton, A. C. The role of radiation in the etiology of leukemia. *In* "Proceedings of the International Conference on Leukemia-Lymphoma," ed. by C. J. D. Zarafonetis, Lea & Febiger, Philadelphia, pp. 55–70 (1968).
42. Upton, A. C., and Cosgrove, G. E., Jr. Radiation-induced leukemia. *In* "Experimental Leukemia," ed. by M. A. Rich, North-Holland Publishing Co., Amsterdam, pp. 131–158 (1968).
43. Weinstein, R. S., and Moloney, W. C. Virus-like particles associated with chloroleukemia in the rat. *Proc. Soc. Exp. Biol. Med.*, **118**, 459–461 (1965).
44. Yokoro, K., and Furth, J. Relation of mammotropes to mammary tumors. V. Role of mammotropes in radiation carcinogenesis. *Proc. Soc. Exp. Biol. Med.*, **107**, 921–924 (1961).
45. Yokoro, K., Takemoto, H., and Kunii, A. Role of mouse lymphoma virus in induction of myeloid leukemia by X-ray. *Annu. N.Y. Acad. Sci.*, **114** (Art. I), 203–212 (1964).
46. Yokoro, K., Ito, T., Imamura, N., Kawase, A., and Yamasaki, T. Synergistic action of radiation and virus in induction of leukemia in rats. *Cancer Res.*, **29**, 1973–1976 (1969).

EXPLANATION OF PHOTOS

PHOTO 1. "Unilateral development" of thymic lymphoma found in a mouse sacrificed 45 days after the termination of fractionated whole-body X-irradiation. The atrophic lobe (on the right) has been replaced by neoplastic cells, while the other lobe maintains normal architecture without any lymphomatous lesion. ×40

PHOTO 2. A small area showing large polygonal cells with some mitotic figures, found in the deep cortex of the cervical lymph node of a mouse sacrificed 90 days after ^{90}Sr inoculation. This may represent the early appearance of nonthymic leukemia induced by ^{90}Sr. ×400

PHOTO 3. The macroscopic appearance of the lymphoma developed at the site of "unirradiated thymus graft" on a thymectomized, X-rayed, Gross virus-infected rat sacrificed 89 days after treatment.

PHOTO 4. The histological appearance of the lymphoma shown in Photo 3. ×400

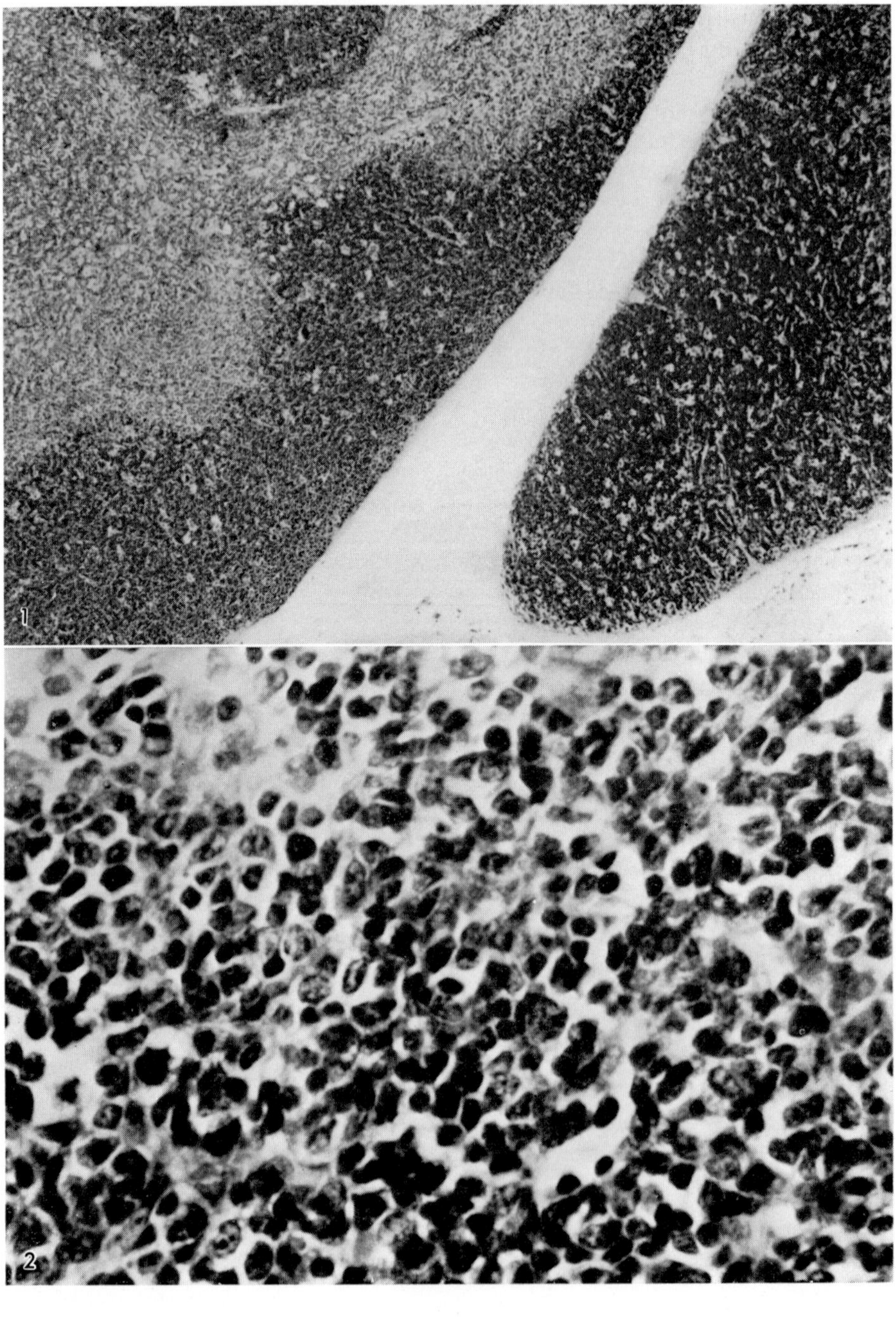

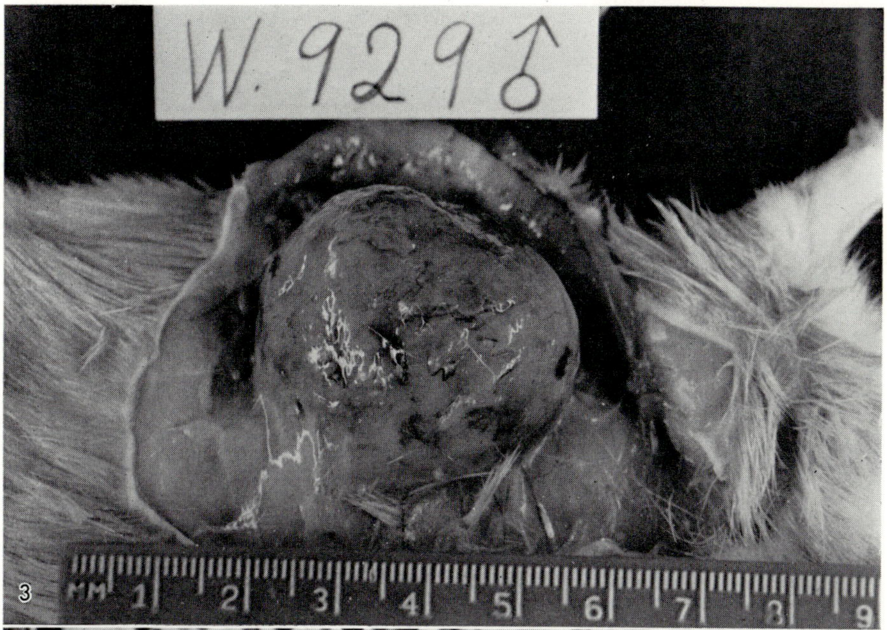
W. 929 ♂
MM 1 2 3 4 5 6 7 8 9
3

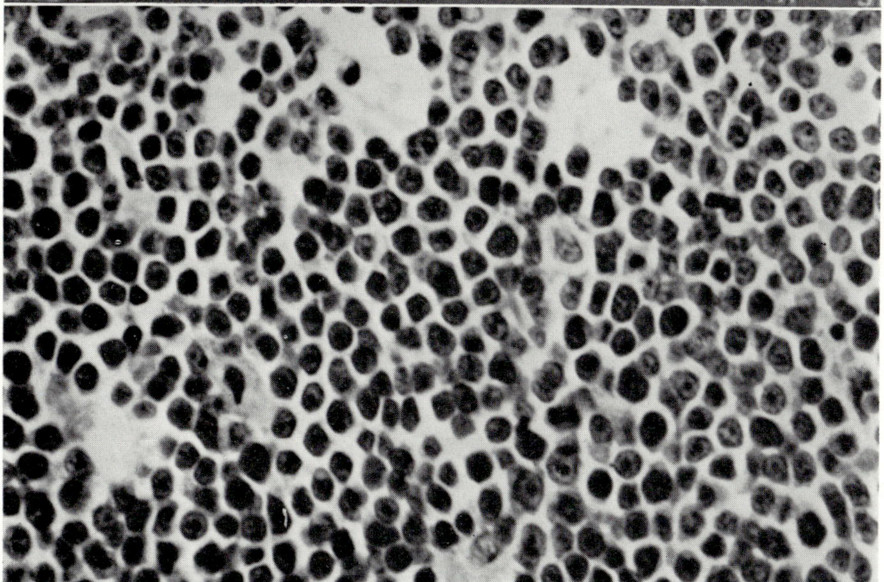
4

GANN Monograph on Cancer Research 12, 1972

RADIATION-INDUCED LEUKEMIA IN C57BL/6J MICE*

Tsutomu KASUGA, Jun-ichiro HAYAKAWA,† Takeshi FURUSE, and Yuhko IWAI

*Section of Pathology, Division of Physiology and Pathology, National Institute of Radiological Sciences***

It is well known that C57BL/6J mice are strongly resistant to the transmission of exogenous oncogenic virus and do not develop spontaneous tumor except for a few lymphoreticular neoplasms. The majority of tumors induced in this strain of mice by radiation were virus-dependent thymic lymphomas, while a few of them were reticulum cell sarcoma-type thymomas, which had no viral particles. The repopulation of thymic cells after the fourth irradiation was performed by large lymphocytes and/or reticular cells in the medulla, and regenerated renewed cortex was established between the medulla and the old exhausted cortex by 21 days after the fourth exposure. Siegler has stated that thymoma is created at the small contracted thymus consisting of only the reticulum cells. In our present experiment, microscopic atypical cell-foci in the medulla were found in the relatively small repopulated thymus 100 days after the first irradiation. The incidence of thymic lymphoma in mice induced by cell-free filtrate was 15.6%, and its latency was about 1 year. The virus particles and viral life cycles were easily identified by electron-microscopy in small thymomas in the early stage but were hard to locate in large thymomas in the present study. The relationship between the action of the virus and the kinetics of the infected target cells is also discussed. The results presented herein, in which thymic lymphoma with refractory anemia was positive to the direct Coomb's test, indicates that thymic lymphoma is a disease that produces an autoimmune disorder similar to the human refractory anemia/thymoma syndrome, as described by Eyster and Barnes. Since daily fractionated irradiation with 10 R/day at a high dose rate induced granulocytic leukemia (15.2% incidence) with a shorter latency but no lymphoma in the C57BL/6J mice, the following hypothesis is proposed. The pathology of radiation-induced leukemia is chiefly determined by certain target cells which include various endogenous factors on the host's side, such as differences in the radiosensitivity of the cells, immunogenetic factors, *etc.*
The tumorigenicity of high LET (linear energy transfer) radiation which is only partially understood was also discussed.

* This work was supported by a grant from the Science and Technology Agency and a grant from the Ministry of Education of Japan.

† Division of Radiation Hazards

*** Anagawa 4-9-1, Chiba 280 (春日　孟, 早川純一郎, 古瀬　健, 岩井攸子).

Since extensive work has been done by Kaplan, Furth, Upton, and others, all the problems involved in the mechanism of radiation leukemogenesis seem to have been clarified. In fact, however, radiation carcinogenesis is understood poorly and fragmentarily, except for leukemogenesis in mice (*63*). To date, it has been postulated that the carcinogenic potential of radiation is produced by the interrelationships among the mode of radiation, degree of tissue damage, immunogenetic background of the irradiated host, and kinetics of activated oncogenic viruses (*51*, *54*, *60*, *66*). The two-stage mechanism of carcinogenesis has been, in general, accepted (*2*). Radiation-induced leukemia, especially lymphocytic lymphoma, in mice is due to the interaction between a proper destruction and subsequent regeneration of tissues containing target cells, and the viral kinetics of latent endogenous virus which has become oncogenic by irradiation (*9*, *20*, *21*, *36*, *40*). There have been several reports on prevention and promotion of radiation-induced leukemia based on experiments with mice, which have a rather high incidence of spontaneous leukemia (*22*, *35*, *38*, *41*, *59*). Therefore, for the analytical study of radiation leukemogenesis, C57BL/6J strain mice are the best material, because they have a very low incidence of spontaneous tumors, such as lymphomas and reticulum cell sarcomas, and no incidence of spontaneous myeloid leukemia (*8*). They respond less to exogenous oncogenic viruses (*45*) and have immunobiological feature (*49*), such as the $H\text{-}2^b$ locus (*57*). Moreover, no instances of induction of leukemia in offspring by transmission of viruses from a leukemic mother mouse of the C57BL strain have been observed (*33*). In the present experiments, X-irradiation was performed under the following conditions: 200 kV, 20 mA, a half-value layer of 0.5 mm copper and 0.5 mm aluminum, FSD=50 cm, and a dose rate of 77 R/min.

Incidence of Spontaneous Tumor in C57BL/6J Strain Mice

The incidence of spontaneous tumors, such as thymic and non-thymic lymphomas and reticulum cell sarcomas, is very low in C57BL/6J mice, and the tumors appear late in life (*8*, *63*). The C57BL/6J strain mice used for all the present experiments were bred by sister-brother mating in the farm of the Oomura Institute of Experimental Animals, beginning in 1967. The original colony at the institute was obtained from the National Cancer Institute, N.I.H., Bethesda, U.S.A.

TABLE I. Frequency of Spontaneous Tumor in C57BL/6J Strain Mice

	No. of mice	No. of tumors	Incidence (%)	Latency (days)
NIRS (1970)	182	3[a]	1.6	>365
Duplan (1965)[b]	42	?	2.5	?
Lieberman and Kaplan (1959)	74	1	1.3	565

[a] Lymphoma consisting of splenomegaly and hepatomegaly without enlarged thymus.

[b] Duplan's data were presented at the NIRS (National Institute of Radiological Science) Seminar in 1965.

The incidence of spontaneous tumors in C57BL/6J mice used was 1.6%, as low as the incidence reported by others (Table I; refs. *7*, *36*). Spontaneous and experimental myeloid leukemia have never been reported in mice of this strain.

Pathology of the Radiation-induced Thymomas

For the induction of thymic lymphoma, C57BL/6J mice 6 weeks of age and 9 weeks of age were exposed to whole-body irradiation, four fractionated exposures at 4-day intervals (170 R×4 times). In the case of mice irradiated at 6 weeks of age, thymomas developed predominantly in early adult life (Table II), and its incidence was high. The tumors induced in the mice irradiated after 9 weeks of age appeared during adult life, and their incidence was relatively low. Their histology revealed not only thymoma and lymphocytic lymphoma but also myeloid leukemia, though only a few (Tables II and III).

TABLE II. Incidence of Tumors in C57BL/6J Mice Irradiated at Age 6 and 9 Weeks

Type of tumor	No. of mice with tumors	Number of tumor-bearing animals dying each month after X-irradiation[a]														
		1	2	3	4	5	6	7	8	9	10	11	12	13	14	15
Irradiated at age 6 weeks:[b]																
Thymoma	13	—	—	1	4	8	—	—	—	—	—	—	—	—	—	—
Lymphoma	2	—	—	—	—	3	—	—	—	—	—	—	—	—	—	—
Total	16	—	—	1	4	11	—	—	—	—	—	—	—	—	—	—
Irradiated at age 9 weeks:[c]																
Thymoma	37	—	—	—	7	13	4	6	3	2	—	1	1	—	—	—
Lymphoma	15	—	—	—	2	4	2	1	4	—	—	1	1	—	—	—
Myeloid	2	—	—	—	—	—	1	—	—	—	—	—	1	—	—	—
Total	54	—	—	—	9	17	7	7	7	2	—	2	3	—	—	—

[a] C57BL/6 strain mice used were irradiated in 4 equal fractions at 4-day intervals.
[b] Sixteen out of 19 female mice were positive.
[c] Two hundred mice were examined, including 66 males and 134 females.

TABLE III. Incidence and Histology of Leukemia in C57BL/6 Mice, in Four Equally Fractionated Exposures of Irradiation at 4-Day Intervals (Total: 680 R)

	No. of mice	Thymoma	Lymphoma	Myeloid	Total
Irradiated at age 6 weeks:					
Female	19	13 (68.4)	3 (15.8)	—	16 (84.2)
Irradiated at age 9 weeks:					
Male	66	9 (13.6)	3 (4.5)	—	12 (18.2)
Female	134	28 (20.9)	12 (8.9)	2 (1.5)	42 (31.3)

Figures in parentheses are percentages.

1. General histology of thymomas

The majority of radiation-induced thymomas showed a usual lymphocytic lymphoma pattern, *i.e.*, a starry-sky pattern (Photo 1A, arrow), and a few of them showed a pattern of reticulum cell sarcoma or histiocytic sarcoma with prominent phagocytic activity and without the starry-sky pattern (Photo 2A).

2. Electron microscopy of thymomas

Thymoma tissues in the early and late stages, benign thymus tissues, and benign lymph nodes were fixed with 2.5% glutaraldehyde fixative buffered with 0.1 M sodium cacodylate with 1% $CaCl_2$ solution at 15° for 1 hr and were also post-fixed with 1% cacodylate-buffered osmium tetroxide solution at 0° for 30 min. The specimens were dehydrated by graded ethanol and then embedded in Epon-Araldite mixture. Thick sections were provided for light microscopy and for trimming the block. The blocks were cut with glass knives in a Porter-Blum MT-2-type microtome. A Hitachi 11-Ds-type electron microscope was used. The lead hydroxide and uranyl acetate double-staining method proved satisfactory for the examination. The lymphocytic thymoma cells were closely analogous to benign thymic lymphocytes with sparse organelles, such as mitochondria, endoplasmic reticulum, and so on. The intercellular spaces of small thymomas were broadened but those of large thymomas were very considerably narrowed (Photo 1). A small number of thymomas were reticulum cell sarcoma-type thymomas with ergastoplasms of rough and smooth surfaces, lysosomes, mitochondria, and so on, and also with prominent ectoplasmic zones. Certain desmosomes were not found (Photo 2). The presence of reticulum cell sarcoma-type thymomas induced by radiation in C57BL/6J mice has not been reported previously. Thymomas induced by 7, 12-dimethylbenz[*a*]anthracene, consisting mainly of functional reticulum cell sarcoma-type thymomas, were reported by Stutman (*56*), and 75% of human thymomas are epithelial reticular thymomas (*65*).

3. Histogenesis of the radiation-induced thymomas

It has been said that lymphocytes in the thymic cortex are 4 times as radiosensitive as thymic lymphocytes in the medulla of rats, determined by using the method of local X-irradiation (*58*), and lymphocytes in the medulla of mice are highly resistant to the action of corticosteroid (*16*). Although the repopulation of intracortical lymphocytes starts from the intracortex itself and not from the medulla, and the repopulation of lymphocytes occurs 5 days after a single X-irradiation, recovery of the thymus after a four-fractionated irradiation is much different from that of the thymus after a single irradiation, and the weight of asymmetric recovered thymus never returns to the control level, even 20 days after irradiation (*54*). In our present experiments, the four-fractionated irradiation group mice were sacrified, after 24 hr, 3, 7, 14, and 21 days, and at different intervals up to 3 months. The histology of the thymus taken from the sacrified mice was examined. The medulla consisted of large hyperplastic lymphocytes and reticular cells, and the cortex was occupied by an almost equal number of large and small lymphocytes in the regenerating thymus after the third exposure to irradiation (Photo 3A). Small lymphocytes in the thymus, 24 hr after the fourth exposure to irradiation, were markedly reduced not only in the cortex but also in the medulla (Photo 3B). By 7 days after irradiation, small lymphocytes had completely disappeared from the cortex, and only necrobiotic reticular tissues remained in the cortex. However, small lymphocytes reappeared in the medulla composed of hypertrophic Hassal corpuscles and activated reticulum cells (Photo 3C). After 21 days, regenerated renewed cortex was established between the medulla and the old exhausted cortex (Photo 3D). The bilateral thymic lobes were slightly asymmetric. Multicentered foci of large atypical lymphocytes were also investigated in the contracted regenerated thymic medulla 100 days after the first irradiation (Photo 3E, F). On the other hand, the contracted thymus of nonirradiated mice treated with cell-free filtrate was composed of atypical uniform reticulum cells (Photo 4). The role of Hassal corpuscles is to clear away degenerated lymphocytes (*3*, *54*, *55*). The irradiated thymus of mice is repopulated by surviving reticular cells (*5*), which probably act by partial regulation of lymphocytic growth activity under normal conditions (*16*). The development of thymoma is related to dedifferentiated reticulum cells of the medulla in the small contracted thymus (*30*, *54*). Sato has indicated, by means of the cell-counting method, that the population of atypical large cells begins to appear at the 35th day after final irradiation and that the number of such cells increases exponentially (*52*). It has been reported by Metcalf that the mean time of the cell cycle of large lymphoma cells is 7.6 hr and that of medium sized cells is 20.2 hr (*44*). The microscopic foci of lymphomas are found in the regenerating thymus after irradiation, and their incidence is 84% at 50 days and 97% at 100 days after irradiation (*29*).

Relationship between the Development of Thymomas and Oncogenic Virus

Fresh thymoma tissues, 100 to 200 mg in weight, taken from the irradiated C57BL/6J mice were made into 10% tumor homogenate in physiological saline solution. This tumor homogenate was centrifuged 3 times at 4,000 rpm at 0° for 20 min per time and was passed through a Gelman #GA-9 membrane filter (0.1 μ hole). The resulting 10% cell-free filtrate was injected into the peritoneal cavity of C57BL/6J 21-day-old mice (0.25 ml/mouse). The injected mice were examined until the termination of their lives. All of the mice injected were examined histologically. The incidence of lymphoma induced by cell-free filtrate was 15.6%, and its latency was about 1 year (Table IV). One out of 5 cases of lymphoma induced by cell-free filtrate was a thymic lymphoma (Photo 5), the incidence of which was less than in the results reported by others (*32*, *36*, *37*). Administration of cell-free filtrate into newborn mice induces thymic lymphoma in the range of 17 to 100% (*36*, *37*). Serial passage of radiation-induced lymphoma virus (RLV) through young adult mice leads to increased incidence of lymphoma (*9*, *32*, *36*). Inoculation of RLV into an irradiated host and/or an irradiated host treated with bone marrow cells promotes the induction of thymoma and its latent period becomes shorter (*9*, *13*, *14*, *32*). The incidence of lymphoma which develops from nonirradiated thymus grafted into the irradiated host after thymectomy becomes higher (*25–27*, *34*). Haran-Ghera and Peled, and Duplan

TABLE IV. Lymphoma Incidence in C57BL/6 Mice Treated with Filtrates of Radiation-induced Thymoma

	Age at injection (days)	No. of mice	Mice with lymphoma		Average latent period (days)
			No.	%	
NIRS (1970)	21	32	5	15.6	357
Lieberman and Kaplan (1959)	1	59	10	17	582
Lieberman *et al.* (1964)	20	9	6	66	212
	20	16	1	6.2	366
	1	10	10	100	117
	1	15	0	0	>388
Duplan (1965)†	30	45	19	42	—
	1	43	16	37	—

† Duplan's data were presented at the NIRS Seminar in 1965.

and Latarjet have stated that thymoma induction is produced by a close relation between the amount of target cells and that of viruses (*9*, *14*). It has been reported that passaged A virus and/or Molony virus inoculated into thymectomized mice induces myeloid leukemia (*11*, *66*), and that a high incidence of thymoma occurs in nonirradiated newborn mice treated with cell-free filtrate of spontaneous myeloid leukemia from RF mice (*18*, *50*, *60*, *63*). Recently, a valuable report appeared which clarified the role of leukemogenic virus in the induction of leukemia by radiation. Mouse Gross lymphoma virus induces thymic lymphoma with a high incidence in irradiated W/Fu rats which have no endogenous oncogenic virus (*67*). On the basis of these facts, it is postulated that the histology of leukemia induced by murine leukemogenic virus might be determined by the interrelation between a certain host factor and the situation of the target cells, because murine leukemogenic virus easily adapts to environmental conditions (*24*, *28*, *30*, *66*) but does not adapt to immunogenetic factors in the host, as was shown by experiments using Friend virus (*49*). It appears that the induction of lymphoma by RLV is not constant but varies by case (*9*, *36*). In the present experiments, ultrastructural viral budding was rare in the thymic lymphocytes of normal thymus. In general, the viral kinetics were most active in small thymomas weighing less than 100 mg in an early stage and were not so active in large thymomas (Photos 6, 7, and 8, and Table V). Although it has been reported that virus particles were pooled in reticulum cells in an experiment involving inoculation of murine leukemia virus (*42*), no virus budding was observed in reticulum cell sarcoma-type thymomas (Photo 3 and Table V). Virus particles in the thymoma of C3H mice are sparsely distributed in the intracellular spaces of tumor cells and are abundant in the spleen of the host (*12*). The ultrastructural category of RLV, which is found in the irradiated host, belongs to the " C " type described by Bernhard (*6*, *12*, *15*, *50*). Lieberman and Kaplan have reported that the highest incidence of thymic lymphomas was induced by inoculation of the cell-free filtrate taken from the precancerous small thymus after irradiation (*36*). On the other hand, according to our electron-microscopic observations, the life cycle of viruses was identified constantly in the small thymoma and was hard to find in large ones. These findings might imply

TABLE V. Frequency of Virus Particles and Budding Formation found in Various Tissue Cells by Electron Microscopy

	Virus sER	Particles rER	Budding on cell membrane	Intracellular space
Normal thymus	±	±	±	±
Thymoma				
Early	++++	++	+++	++++
Late				
Lymphocytic	+++	+++	+	++
Reticular cell	±	−	−	−
Benign lymph node†	+	−	−	+

† The lymph node material examined was not taken from enlarged retroperitoneal nodes in mice suffering from thymoma.

that leukemogenic viruses are marked during a turnover stage of the tumor cells when they are proliferating exponentially. Moreover, these findings indicate that, although the action of virus on leukemogenesis is needed for the malignant transformation of target cells, the later autonomous proliferation of the malignant transformed target cells can progress without the aid of continuous stimulation by the virus.

Direct Coomb's Test in C57BL/6J Mice with Refractory Anemia/Thymoma Syndrome

The thymus produces and supplies immune competent cells under the control of immune competent precursor cells in the bone marrow (*46*). One of the mechanisms that dramatically inhibit radiation-induced thymoma (*9*, *20*, *53*) is the action of deoxycholate-resistant cells in the bone marrow (*4*). The irradiated and/or thymectomized mice suffer from a notable immune suppression, which is cured by bone marrow cell transplantation (*7*, *13*, *43*, *45*, *53*). Barnes' report on whether or not thymoma in mouse causes an autoimmune disease is of great interest (*1*). In our experiment, after a single irradiation with 600 R, blood from the 20 irradiated mice was sampled at intervals of 4 weeks for examination of antiglobulin test results, A/G ratio, disc electrophoresis, peripheral blood cell count, and hematocrit. The antiglobulin test (Coomb's test) was carried out by the direct method. The A/G ratio in serum-protein was calculated from the density distribution of protein on cellulose-acetate membrane electrophoresis. The sera were also analyzed by disc electrophoresis. Only 1 case suffering from localized thymoma with continuous anemia (Ht=35 to 46) was positive to direct Coomb's test. The immune reaction had appeared during a limited period between 12 and 16 weeks after whole-body irradiation. A relative increase of α-postalbumin and β-transferrin (Fig. 1), and a temporary decrease of A/G ratio (1.1) were seen in this case only (Fig. 2). Human refractory anemia/thymoma syndrome is positive to direct Coomb's test (*1*, *10*, *46*). On the other hand, Haran-Ghera and his co-workers have reported that the degree of immune depression in mice is related to the amount of leukemogenic agent released during a

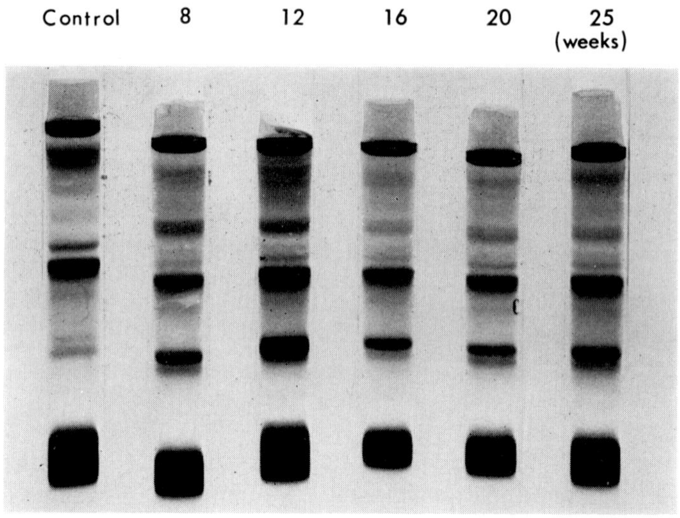

FIG. 1. Disc electrophoresis pattern of serum of C57BL/6J mice bearing radiation-induced thymoma

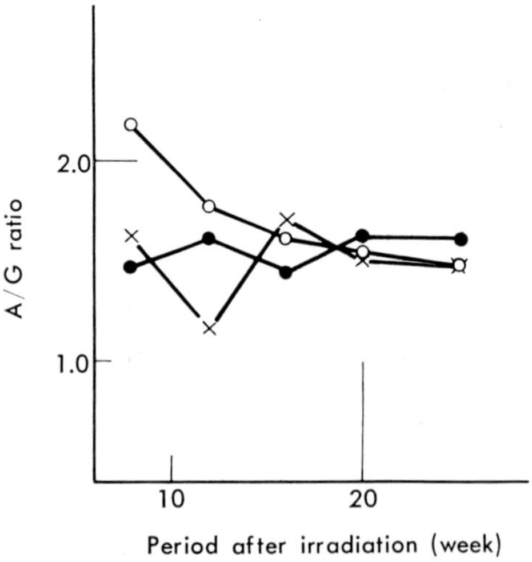

FIG. 2. A/G ratio in serum-protein of C57BL/6J mice bearing thymoma and no thymoma

○ nonirradiated group; ● X–600R without thymoma; × X–600R bearing thymoma.

limited period of 5 to 10 days after irradiation (*13*, *14*). It has also been reported that recovery from immune depression in thigh-shielded irradiated mice begins immediately and proceeds until the control level is reached, but that of non-thigh-shielded irradiated mice does not return to the control level even 20 days after irradiation (*53*). Therefore, it is possible that the refractory anemia/thymoma syndrome in mice positive to direct Coomb's test is also an autoimmune disease similar to that of human beings.

Relationship between the Method of Irradiation and Myeloid Leukemia in Mice

Radiation-induced lymphoma is more frequent in female mice than in male mice when they are irradiated as young adults (*19*), while radiation-induced myeloid leukemia is much more frequent in male mice than in female mice when irradiation occurs in adulthood (*62, 63*). Although it has been reported that protracted X-irradiation produces less myeloid leukemia than a single irradiation (*60, 63*), the opposite has also been reported (*41*). The mice used in these experiments were LAF_1 and mice of other strains with a higher incidence of spontaneous myeloid leukemia. No attempt has been made to date to induce granulocytic leukemia in C57BL/6J mice.

1. Multifractionated low-LET irradiation and myeloid leukemia

For multifractionated irradiation, C57BL/6J mice were exposed to daily fractionated whole-body irradiation with 10 R/day and fractionated whole-body irradiation with 25 R twice a week (50 R/week) and 100 R/2 weeks (200 R/month), beginning at 10 weeks of age. All the irradiated mice were examined histologically. The total dose given to each group was 1000 R. The incidence of leukemia in C57BL/6J mice induced by multifractionated irradiation in the present experiment is given in Table VI as compared with the above-mentioned four-fractionated irradiation group. As shown in this table, a slightly higher incidence (15.2%) of granulocytic leukemia (Photos 9 and 10) and no lymphoma were observed in the 10 R-daily irradiated group. The latency of granulocytic leukemia was less than 7 months after the first irradiation. A histological diagnosis of granulocytic leukemia was determined in compliance with the definition of Dunn (*8*). Continuous irradiation promotes not only an increase of tumor incidence (*41*) but also a shortening of the latent period (*35, 41*). Different responsiveness of the hematopoietic cell series to continuous γ-irradiation has been reported, showing that lymphocytes decrease severely with continuous exposures up to 2.2 R daily, erythrocytes and platelets were reduced with 4.4 R daily, and the granulocytic cell series decreased with 8.8 R per day (*17, 41*). It has been shown that γ-rays are more effective on hematopoietic cells than X-rays (*17*). The radiosensitivity of normoblasts and myelocytes is similar in rats (50 R/day) (*31, 39*).

TABLE VI. Influence of Various Fractionated Irradiation on Histology and Latency of Leukemias in C57BL/6J Strain Mice

Irradiation (fraction times)	No. of mice	Thymoma	Lymphoma	Myeloid	Latency (days)
10R × 100	13	—	—	2	<70
50R × 20	29	—	—	1	90
100R × 10	17	1	—	—	<25
170R × 4	19	13	3	—	90–150

Duration of irradiation: 10R × 100 = 5 months, 50R × 20 and 100R × 10 = 5 months, and 170R × 4 = 2 weeks.

Continuous hyperplasia of the granulocytic cell series has been shown, by the use of tritiated thymidine, to begin just after the first irradiation (*39*). In thymectomized mice, the incidence of lymphocytic leukemia decreases markedly, while that of myeloid leukemia increases notably (*43*). Not only radiation-induced lymphoma but also radiation-induced myeloid leukemia is virus-dependent (*18*). On the basis of the above facts, it is induced that the mechanism of production of myeloid leukemia by means of 10 R/day-irradiation is related to a certain balance of interaction between the activated release of viruses (*13*) and the least radiosensitive myelogenous cells in the bone marrow.

2. *High-LET irradiation and myeloid leukemia*

A single intermediate dose of not only low-LET but also high-LET radiation is highly leukemogenic, and the incidence of both myeloid and lymphoid leukemia becomes higher when irradiated with an increasing dose rate and/or when the dose given is increased by using low-LET radiation (*23, 38, 47, 48, 60, 61, 63, 64*). The leukemogenicity of high-LET radiation (1 to 5 MeV fast neutrons) is, in general, less dependent on not only the accumulated dose given but also the different dose rates. For the induction of myeloid leukemia, although the relative biological effectiveness (RBE) of high-LET radiation in comparison with low-LET radiation in a single irradiation is 0.7, the RBE of daily continuous irradiation is 16.0. Also, for the induction of thymic lymphoma, the RBE of a single irradiation is 1.0; however, the RBE of continuous irradiation is 3.3 (*64*). By means of continuous fast-neutron irradiation, lymphoid leukemia with an incidence higher than 50% has been induced even in mice that were thigh-shielded during irradiation (*48*). Continuous irradiation using high-LET radiation prevents the induction of solid tumors, such as pulmonary tumor, except hormone-dependent tumors (*35, 41, 64*).

Acknowledgments

We gratefuly acknowledge the opportunity for and assistance in this work given us by Drs. T. Yamamoto and H. Sugano, the electron-microscopic aid of Mr. H. Miyamoto of Tokyo Medical and Dental University, and the encouragement of Drs. T. Terasima and T. Tsuchiya.

REFERENCES

1. Barnes, R. D. Refractory anaemia with thymoma. *Lancet.*, **31**, 1464 (1966).
2. Berenblum, I., and Trainin, N. Application on the two-stage mechanism of carcinogenesis to leukemogenesis with low doses of X-rays as initiating factor. *In* "Radiobiology," ed. by P. L. T. Ilbery, Butterworths, London, pp. 98–101 (1961).
3. Blau, J. N. A phagocytic function of Hassall's corpuscles. *Nature*, **208**, 564–567 (1965).
4. Blomgren, H. The influence of the bone marrow on the repopulation of the thymus in X-irradiated mice. *Exp. Cell Res.*, **58**, 353–364 (1969).
5. Carnes, W. H., Kaplan, H. S., Brown, M. B., and Hirsch, B. B. Indirect induction of lymphomas in irradiated mice. III. Role of the thymic grafts. *Cancer Res.*, **16**, 429–433 (1956).

6. de Harven, E. Morphology of murine leukemia viruses. *In* " Experimental Leukemia," ed. by M. A. Rich, North-Holland Publishing Co., Amsterdam, pp. 97–129, (1968).
7. Doell, R. G., de Vaux St. Cyr, C., an Grabar, P. Immune Reactivity prior to development of thymic lymphoma in C57BL mice. *Int. J. Cancer*, **2**, 103–108 (1967).
8. Dunn, T. B. Normal and pathologic anatomy of the reticular tissue in laboratory mice, with a classification and discussion of neoplasms. *J. Natl. Cancer Inst.*, **14**, 1281–1433 (1954).
9. Duplan, J. F., and Latarjet, R. Studies on the mechanism of radiation-induced leukemogenesis in C57BL mice. *Cancer Res.*, **26**, 395–399 (1966).
10. Eyster, M. E., and Jenklins, D. E., Jr. Erythrocyte coating substances in patients with positive direct antiglobulin reactions: Correlation of γG globulin and complement coating with underlying diseases, overt hemolysis and response to therapy. *Am. J. Med.*, **46**, 360–371 (1969).
11. Gross, L. Transmission of myelogenous leukemia by filtrates. *In* " Oncogenic Virus," Pergamon Press, London and New York, pp. 214–215 (1961).
12. Gross, L., and Feldman, G. G. Electron microscopic studies of radiation-induced leukemia in mice. Virus release following total-body X-irradiation. *Cancer Res.*, **28**, 1677–1685 (1968).
13. Haran-Ghera, N., Lieberman, M., and Kaplan, H. S. Direct action of a leukemogenic virus in the thymus. *Cancer Res.*, **26**, 438–442 (1966).
14. Haran-Ghera, N., and Peled, A. The mechanism of radiation action in leukemogenesis: Isolation of a leukemogenic filtrable agent from tissues of irradiated and normal C57BL mice. *Brit. J. Cancer*, **21**, 730–738 (1967).
15. Hoffman, H., and Darveniza, N. Electron microscopic studies of a transplantable, radiation-induced mouse leukemia. *In* " Radiobiology," ed. by P. L. T. Ilbery, Butterworths, London, pp. 161–169 (1961).
16. Ishidate, M., Jr., and Metcalf, D. The pattern of lymphopoiesis in the mouse thymus after cortisone administration or adrenalectomy. *Aust. J. Exp. Biol. Med. Sci.*, **41**, 637–649 (1963).
17. Jacobson, L. O. The hematologic effects of ionizing radiation. *In* " Radiation Biology," ed. by A. Hollaender, McGraw-Hill Book Co., New York, Vol. I, pp. 1029–1090 (1954).
18. Jenkins, V. K., and Upton, A. C. Cell-free transmission of radiogenic myeloid leukemia in the mouse. *Cancer Res.*, **23**, 1748–1755 (1963).
19. Kaplan, H. S. Influence of age on susceptibility of mice to the development of lymphoid tumors after irradiation. *J. Natl. Cancer Inst.*, **9**, 55–56 (1948).
20. Kaplan, H. S. Influence of thymectomy, splenectomy, and gonadectomy on incidence of radiation-induced lymphoid tumors in strain C57 Black mice. *J. Natl. Cancer Inst.*, **11**, 83–90 (1950).
21. Kaplan, H. S., and Brown, M. B. Further observations on inhibition of lymphoid tumor development by shielding and partial-body irradiation of mice. *J. Natl. Cancer Inst.*, **12**, 427–436 (1951).
22. Kaplan, H. S., Marder, S. N., and Brown, M. B. Adrenal cortical function and radiation-induced lymphoid tumors of mice. *Cancer Res.*, **11**, 629–633 (1951).
23. Kaplan, H. S., and Brown, M. B. A quantitative dose-response study of lymphoid tumor development in irradiated C57 Black mice. *J. Natl. Cancer Inst.*, **13**, 185–208 (1952).

24. Kaplan, H. S. On the etiology and pathogenesis of the leukemias: A review. *Cancer Res.*, **14**, 535–548 (1954).
25. Kaplan, H. S., and Brown, M. B. Development of lymphoid tumors in non-irradiated thymic grafts in thymectomized irradiated mice. *Science*, **119**, 439–440 (1954).
26. Kaplan, H. S., Brown, M. B., Hirsch, B. B., and Carnes, W. H. Indirect induction of lymphomas in irradiated mice. II. Factor of irradiation of the host. *Cancer Res.*, **16**, 426–428 (1956).
27. Kaplan, H. S., Carnes, W. H., Brown, M. B., and Hirsch, B. B. Indirect induction of lymphomas in irradiated mice. I. Tumor incidence and morphology in mice bearing nonirradiated thymic grafts. *Cancer Res.*, **16**, 422–425 (1956).
28. Kaplan, H. S. Radiation-induced leukemia in mice. A progress report. *In* " Radiation Biology and Cancer," University of Texas Press, Austin, pp. 289–302 (1958).
29. Kaplan, H. S. Early microscopic diagnosis of lymphosarcoma *in situ* in thymus of irradiated mice. *Federation Proc.*, **19**, 399 (1960).
30. Kaplan, H. S. The role of radiation in experimental leukemogenesis. *Natl. Cancer Inst. Monograph*, **14**, 207–220 (1964).
31. Lamerton, L. F. Cell proliferation under continuous irradiation. *Radiat. Res.*, **27**, 119–138 (1966).
32. Latarjet, R., and Duplan, J. F. Experimentals and discussion on leukemogenesis by cell free extracts of radiation-induced leukemia in mice. *Int. J. Radiat. Biol.*, **5**, 339–344 (1962).
33. Law, L. W. Transmission studies of a leukemogenic virus, MLV, in mice. *Natl. Cancer Inst. Monograph.*, **22**, 267–285 (1966).
34. Law, L. W., Bradley, T. R., and Rose, S. Reversal of the thymus-dependent influence in radiation leukemogenesis of C57BL mice. *J. Natl. Cancer Inst.*, **31**, 1462–1477 (1963).
35. Lesher, S., Sacher, G. A., Grahn, D., Hamilton, K., and Sallese, A. Survival of mice under duration-of-life exposure to gamma rays. II. Pathologic effects. *Radiat. Res.*, **24**, 239–277 (1965).
36. Lieberman, M., and Kaplan, H. S. Leukemogenic activity of filtrates from radiation-induced lymphoid tumors of mice. *Science*, **130**, 387–388 (1959).
37. Lieberman, M., Haran-Ghera, N., and Kaplan, H. S. Potentiation of virus leukemogenesis in C57BL mice by X-irradiation of urethane. *Nature*, **203** (4943), 420–422 (1964).
38. Lindop, P. J., and Rotblat, J. Long-term effects of a single whole-body exposure of mice to ionizing radiation. II. Causes of death. *Proc. Royal Soc.* (*London*), *Ser. B*, **154**, 350–368 (1961).
39. Lord, B. I. The effects of continuous irradiation on cell proliferation in rat bone marrow. *Brit. J. Haematol.*, **10**, 496–506 (1964).
40. Lorenz, E., Congdon, C. C., and Uphoff, D. Prevention of irradiation-induced lymphoid tumors in C57BL mice by spleen protection. *J. Natl. Cancer Inst.*, **14**, 291–299 (1953).
41. Lorenz, E., Hollcrofi, J. W., Miller, E., Congdon, C. C., and Schweisthal, R. Longterm effects of acute and chronic irradiation in mice. I. Survival and tumor incidence following chronic irradiation of 0.11 R per day. *J. Natl. Cancer Inst.*, **15**, 1049–1058 (1955).
42. Masurovsky, E. B., and Rich, M. A. Early development of murine leukemia virus in thymus. *Federation Proc.*, **25**, 375 (1966).

43. Metcalf, D., Wiadrowski, M., and Bradley, R. Analysis of the role of the thymus in leukemia development with the use of thymectomy and thymys grafts. *Natl. Cancer Inst. Monograph*, **22**, 571–583 (1966).
44. Metcalf, D., and Wiadrowski, M. Autoradiographic analysis of lymphocyte proliferation in the thymus and in thymic lymphoma tissue. *Cancer Res.*, **26**, 483–491 (1966).
45. Miller, J. F. A. P. The thymus and the development of immunologic responsiveness: The thymus directs the maturation of immunologic capabilities by means of a humoral mechanism. *Science*, **144**, 1544–1551 (1964).
46. Miller, D. G. The immunologic capability of patients with lymphoma. *Cancer Res.*, **28**, 1441–1448 (1968).
47. Mole, R. H. Patterns of response to whole-body irradiation: The effect of dose intensity and exposure time on duration of life and tumors. *Brit. J. Radiol.*, **32**, 497–501 (1959).
48. Nowell, P. C., and Cole, L. J. Late effects of fast neutrons *versus* X-rays in mice: Nephrosclerosis, tumors, longevity. *Radiat. Res.*, **11**, 545–556 (1959).
49. Odaka, T., and Matsukura, M. Inheritance of susceptibility to Friend mouse leukemia virus. VI. Reciprocal alteration of innate resistance or susceptibility by bone marrow transplantation between congenic strains. *J. Virol.*, **4**, 837–843 (1969).
50. Parsons, R. F., Upton, A. C., Benders, M. A., Jenkins, V. K., Nelson, E. S., and Johnson, R. E. Electron microscopic observations on primary and serially passaged radiation-induced myeloid leukemias of the RF mouse. *Cancer Res.*, **22**, 728–736 (1962).
51. Reif, A. E. Radiation carcinogenesis at high dose-response level: A hypothesis. *Nature*, **190**, 415–417 (1961).
52. Sato, C. Cell population analysis of radiation leukemogenesis in mice. *Tohoku J. Exp. Med.*, **96**, 97–109 (1968).
53. Sato, C. Earlier recovery of lymphopoiesis and immunological response by bone marrow shielding after leukemogenic irradiation in mice. *GANN*, **60**, 393–400 (1969).
54. Siegler, R., Harrell, W., and Rich, M. A. Pathogenesis of radiation-induced thymic lymphoma in mice. *J. Natl. Cancer Inst.*, **37**, 105–121 (1966).
55. Siegler, R., and Rich, M. A. Pathogenesis of murine leukemia. *Natl. Cancer Inst. Monograph*, **22**, 525–541 (1966).
56. Stutman, O., Yunis, E. J., and Good, R. A. Carcinogen-induced tumors of the thymus. I. Restoration of neonatally thymectomized mice with a functional thymoma. *J. Natl. Cancer Inst.*, **41**, 1431–1452 (1968).
57. Tennant, J. R., and Snell, G. D. Some experimental evidence for the influence of genetic factors on viral leukemogenesis. *Natl. Cancer Inst. Monograph*, **22**, 61–72 (1966).
58. Trowell, O. A. Radiosensitivity of the cortical and medullary lymphocytes in the thymus. *Int. J. Radiat. Biol.*, **4**, 163–173 (1962).
59. Upton, A. C. Leukemogenesis: Role of viruses and cytological aspects. *In* "Symposium on cellular and aetiology of late somatic effects of ionizing radiation," Academic Press, London and New York, pp. 67–82, (1962).
60. Upton, A. C., Furth, W. J., and Kimball, A. W. A comparison of the induction of myeloid and lymphoid leukemias in X-radiated RF mice. *Cancer Res.*, **18**, 842–848 (1958).
61. Upton, A. C. Comparative aspects of carcinogenesis by ionizing radiation. *Natl. Cancer Inst. Monograph*, **14**, 221–242 (1964).

62. Upton, A. C., Jenkins, V. K., Walburg, H. E., Jr., Tyndall, R. L., Conklin, J. W., and Wald, N. Observations on viral, chemical, and radiation-induced myeloid and lymphoid leukemias in RF mice. *Natl. Cancer Inst. Monograph*, **22**, 329–347 (1966).
63. Upton, A. C., and Cosgrove, G. E., Jr. Radiation-induced leukemia. *In* "Experimental Leukemia," ed. by M. A. Rich, North-Holland Publishing Co., Amsterdam, pp. 131–158 (1968).
64. Upton, A. C., Randolph, M. L., and Conklin, J. W. Late effects of fast neutrons and gamma-rays in mice as influenced by the dose rate of irradiation: Induction of neoplasia. *Radiat. Res.*, **41**, 467–491 (1970).
65. Watanabe, H. A pathological study of thymoma. *Acta Pathol. Japon.*, **16**, 323–358 (1966).
66. Yokoro, K., and Ito, T. Role of host factors in induction of leukemia by radiation and virus. *Acta Pathol. Japon.*, **18**, 362–371 (1968).
67. Yokoro, K., Ito, T., Imamura, N., Kawase, A., and Yamasaki, T. Synergistic action of radiation and virus in induction of leukemia in rats. *Cancer Res.*, **29**, 1973–1976 (1969).

EXPLANATION OF PHOTOS

PHOTO 1. Radiation-induced thymoma in late stage, lymphocytic lymphoma type. Cells are poor in organelles. ×12,500. Photograph 1A is low-power view of the same case and shows the presence of large reticular cells, starry-sky pattern (arrow). ×1,200

PHOTO 2. Radiation-induced thymoma in late stage, reticulum cell sarcoma-type. Cells with abundant organelles and prominent ectoplasmic zone are closely associated with each other. ×10,320. Photograph 2A is a low-magnification view of the same case. ×1,200

PHOTO 3. Regeneration and atypical cell development in the thymus after fractionated irradiation. A: thymus just before the fourth irradiation; ×600. B: thymus 24 hr after the fourth irradiation; ×600. C: seven days after irradiation, the cortex is completely necrobiotic, and hypertrophic Hassal corpuscles are seen in the medulla; ×600. D: twenty-one days after irradiation, regenerated renewed cortex is established between the regenerated medulla and the old exhausted cortex; ×300. E: atypical cell focus occurs in the medulla; ×600. F: high magnification of Photo 3E; ×1,200. The long arrows indicate the cortex-medulla boundary.

PHOTO 4. Small contracted thymus, consisting of only atypical and immature reticular cells, 32 days after injection of cell-free filtrate (RLV). ×1,200

PHOTO 5. Thymoma of C57BL/6J mouse induced by cell-free filtrates. Slightly tumorous enlarged lymph nodes of neck and retroperitoneum, and nonremarkable spleen are seen.

PHOTOS 6 and 7. Viruses in the tumor cells of radiation-induced thymoma, lymphocytic lymphoma type. Arrows show mature virus particles (" C " type of Bernhard), and *ev* indicates the immature viral genomes. The arrow in Photo 5 indicates viral budding. ×25,000

PHOTO 8. Viral life cycle in tumor cells. 8a to 8d show that on the plasma membranes, and 8A to 8D show those on the smooth-surfaced membranes. ×48,000

PHOTOS 9 and 10. Myelogenous leukemia in C57BL/6J mice induced by multifractionated daily irradiation with 10 R/day. 9: periostal invasion of granulocytic leukemia cells (×600), and these tumor cells were metastatic to liver, kidneys, spleen, *etc.* 10: higher magnification of leukemia cells in the bone marrow of Photo 9 (×1,200), and differentiated pattern of granulocytic cell series with abundant mitotic figures can be seen.

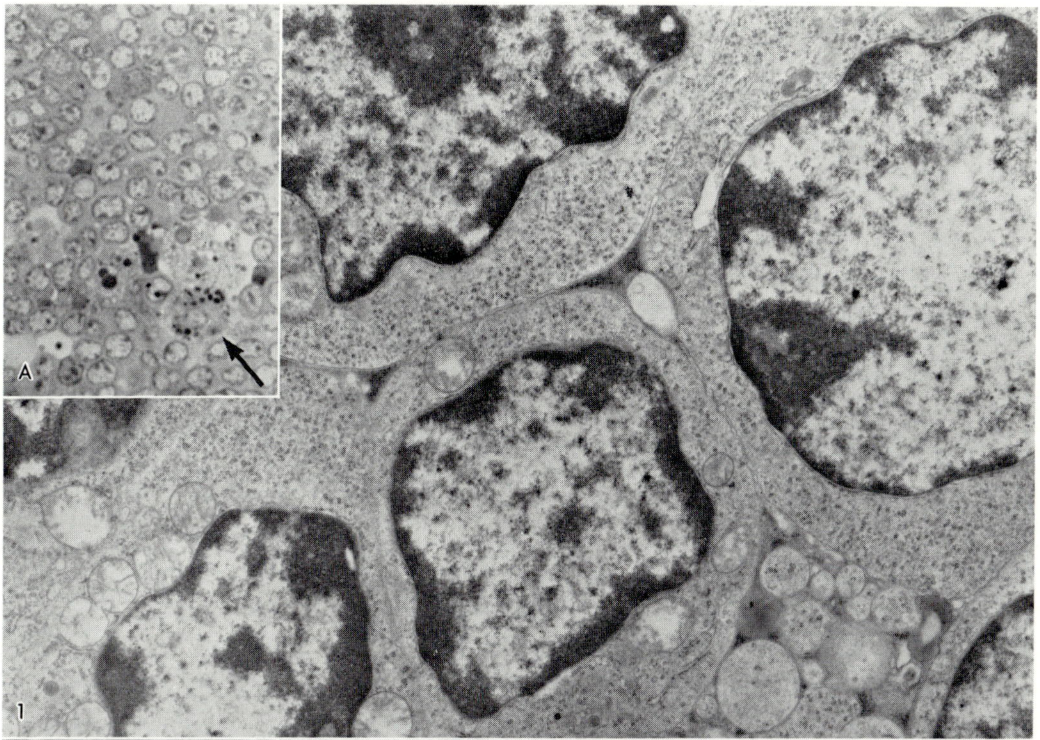
A
1

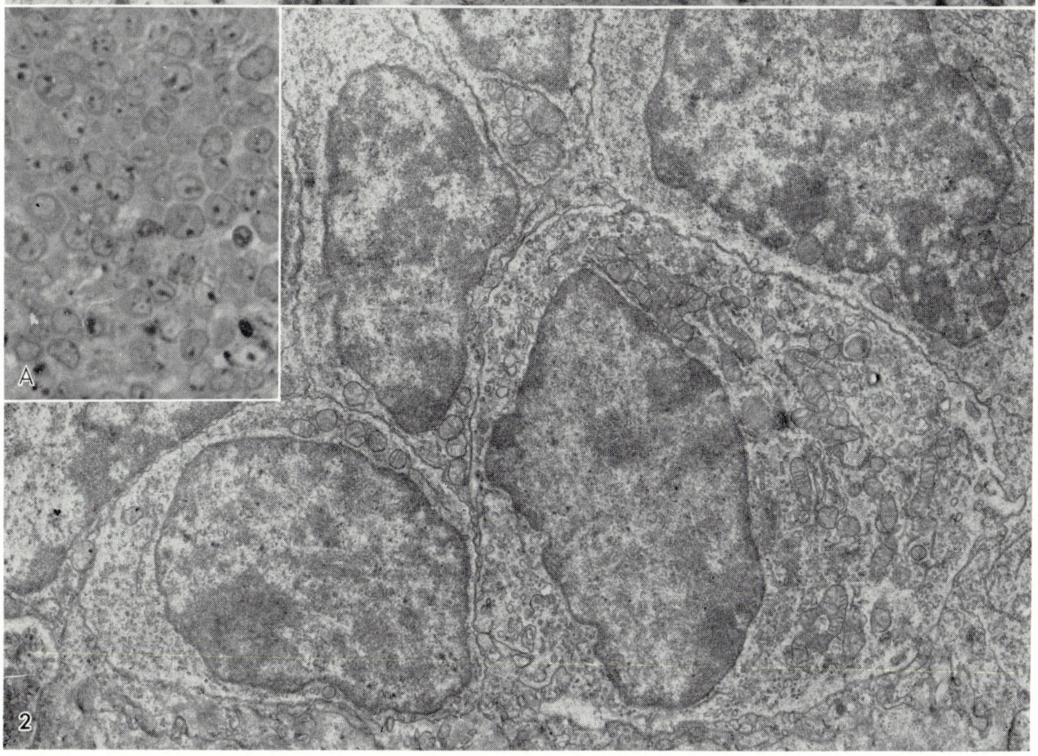
A
2

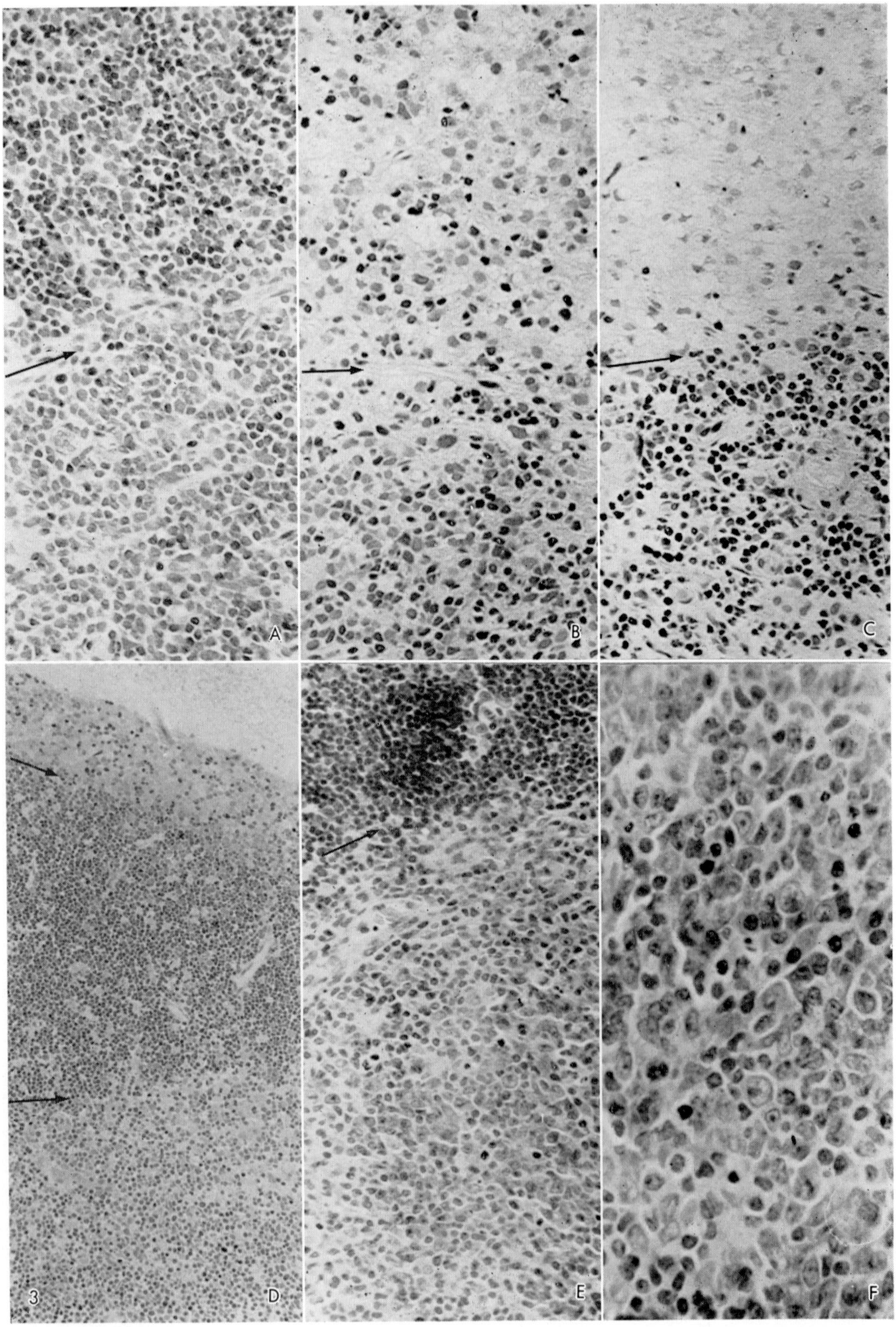
A
B
C
3
D
E
F

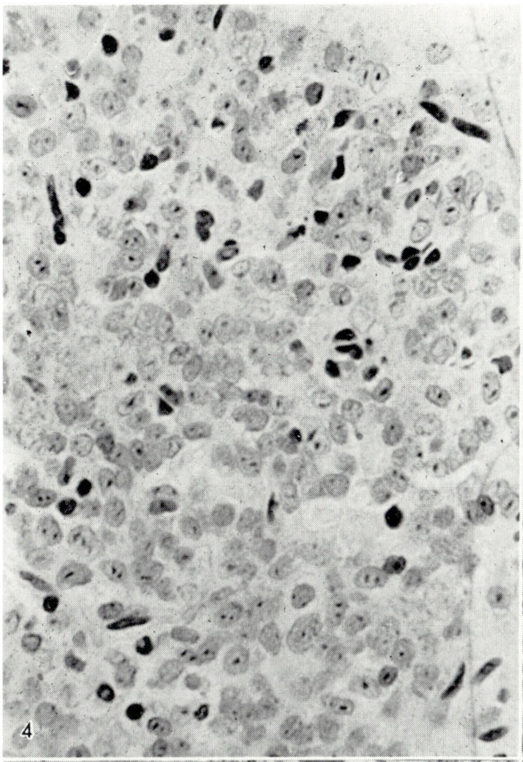
4

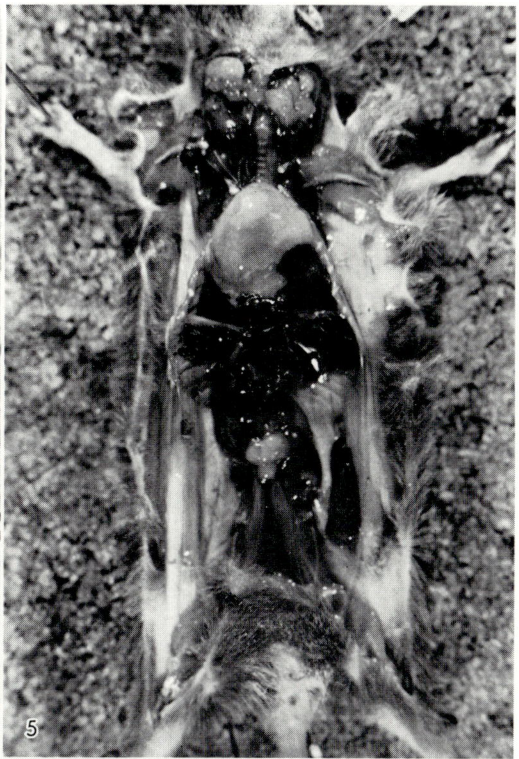
5

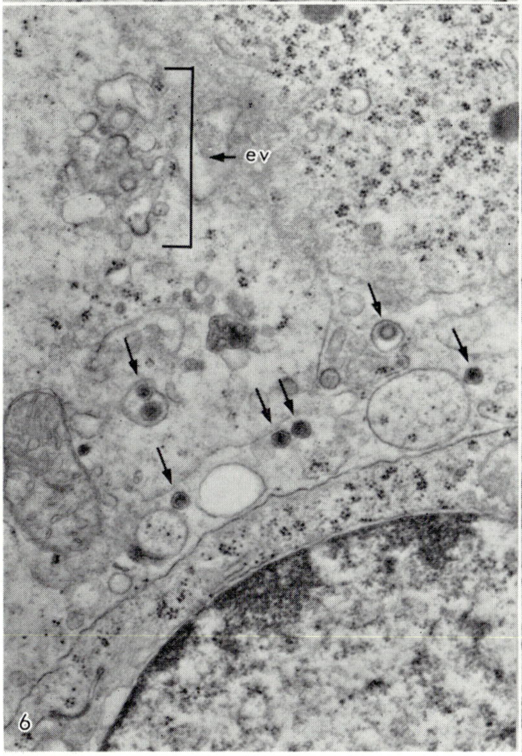
ev
6

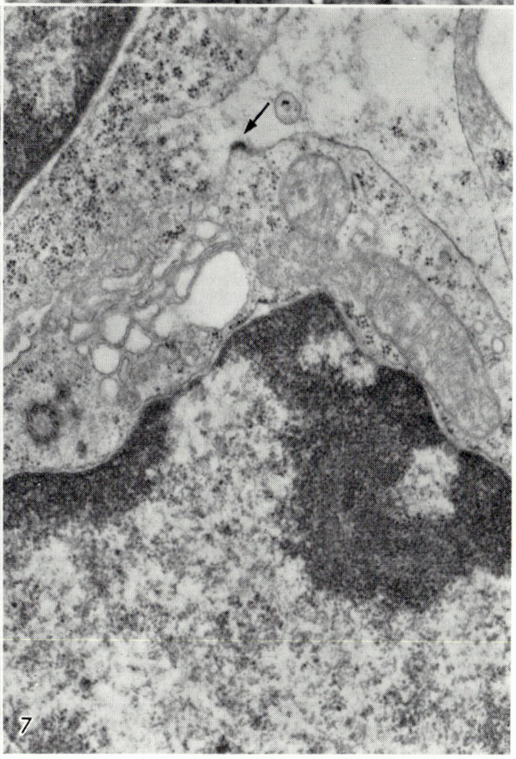
7

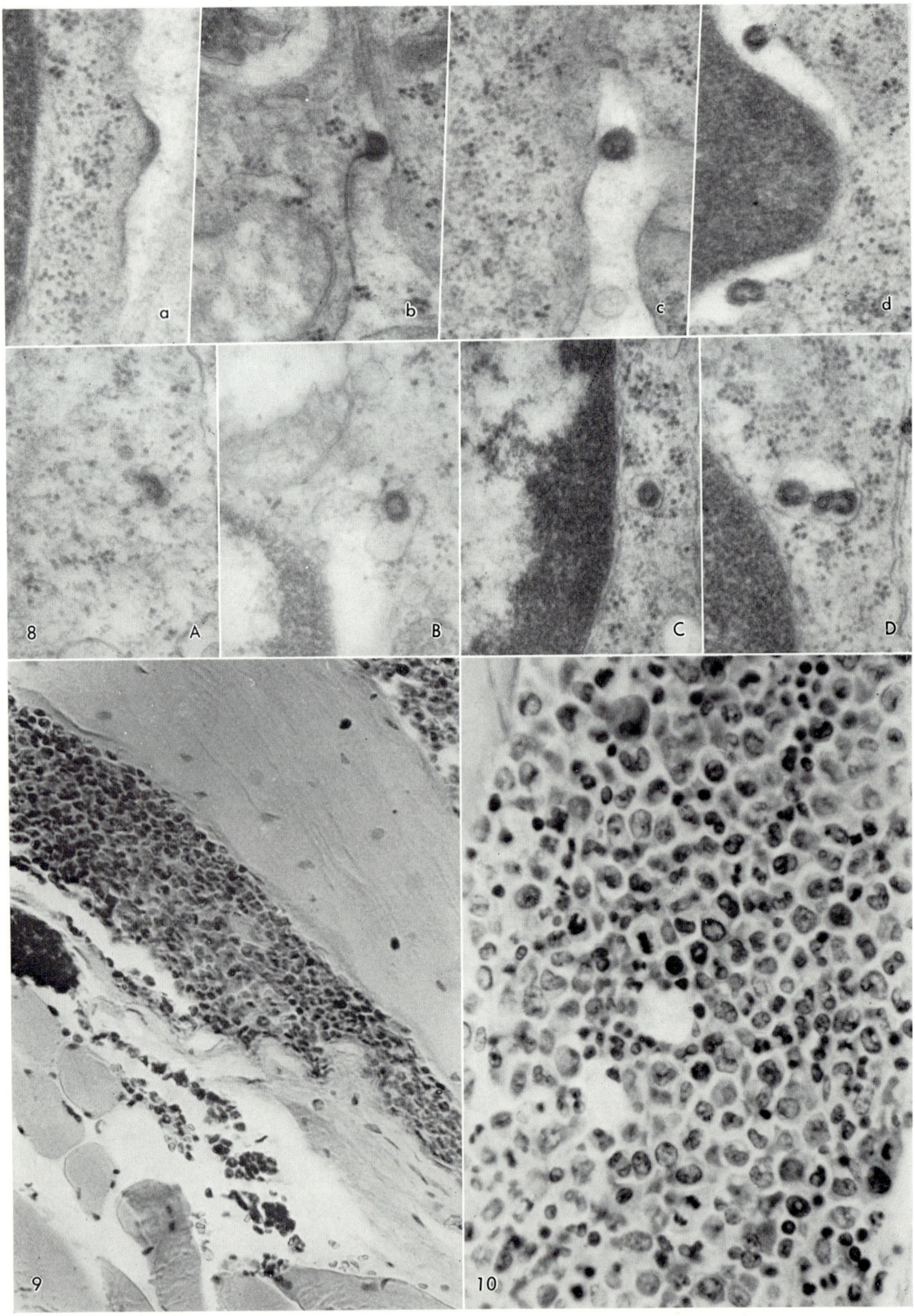
a
b
c
d
8
A
B
C
D
9
10

CHEMICAL LEUKEMOGENESIS

GANN Monograph on Cancer Research 12, 1972

LEUKEMOGENIC EFFECTS OF N-BUTYL-N-NITROSOUREA IN RATS*

Shigeyoshi ODASHIMA
*National Institute of Hygienic Sciences***

The leukemogenic effects of N-butyl-N-nitrosourea (BNU) was studied in a series of 3 animal experiments.

1) Female Donryu rats were given continuously 0.04, 0.02, and 0.01% BNU solution, 15 ml per day per rat, as their drinking water, until they were killed for autopsy. The higher concentrations of BNU resulted in a higher incidence of leukemia early in the experiment, 100% in those that received the 0.04% solution, and a lower dose resulted in more tumors in extrahematopoietic tissues in a later part of the experimental period.

2) A 0.04% BNU solution, 15 ml per day per rat, was given to female Sprague-Dawley rats for 5, 10, 15, or 20 weeks. Leukemia developed in 60 to 90% of the rats. The number of plaque-forming cells in the spleen against sheep red blood cell was at the zero level in all rats killed immediately after the end of BNU administration. This level continued until the end of the experiment in those rats that received BNU for more than 10 weeks.

3) A single application of BNU, 300 mg/kg body weight, to female Sprague-Dawley rats resulted in the development of leukemia in 20 to 30% of the animals.

4) Two types of leukemic cells, granulocytic and nongranulocytic, were observed. The majority of the animals with leukemia were characterized by enormous hepatosplenomegalia and by swelling of the adrenal gland and cysternal group of lymph nodes due to the metastatic lesions of leukemic cells.

A technique for the induction of leukemia by chemicals in adult rats has not yet been widely developed. Although several chemicals, such as 3-methylcholanthrene, 7,12-dimethylbenz[*a*]anthracene (DMBA) (*3*, *5*), 2-acetylaminophenanthrene (2-AAP) (*4*), aminopterine (*7*), *p*-nitroso (methylamino)azobenzene (*6*), ethyleneimine derivatives (*11*), N,N′-2,7-fluorenylenebisacetamide (2,7-FAA) (*8*), and N-ethyl-N-nitrosourea (ENU) (*1*), have been reported as leukemogenic, the incidence of leukemia induced was not high. Among these, a moderate yield of leukemias resulted from the following: 1) intravenous injections of pulse doses of DMBA to Long-Evans rats by Huggins and Sugiyama (*5*) and to female Donryu

* This work was carried out at the Sasaki Institute, Tokyo, and was supported by Grant DRG-96At from the Damon Runyon Memorial Fund for Cancer Research, Inc., New York, N.Y., U.S.A., and a Grant-in-Aid for Scientific Research from the Ministry of Education of Japan.
** 1-18-1 Kamiyoga, Setagaya-ku, Tokyo 158 (小田嶋成和).

rats by Fukunishi (*3*); 2) feeding of 0.02% 2-AAP to Holtzman rats by Hartmann *et al.* (*4*); 3) feeding of 0.025% 2,7-FAA to female Buffalo rats by Morris *et al.* (*8*); and 4) repeated intravenous injections of ENU to BD rats by Druckrey *et al.* (*1*). The incidence of leukemia was 36 to 56% except with Huggins and Sugiyama's experiment. These authors reported an incidence of 100% leukemia in rats that received 4 to 7 injections of pulse dose of DMBA.

According to Druckrey *et al.*, ENU was the only substance that showed a leukemogenic effect in their rats, among 65 N-nitroso derivatives tested (*1*). It produced leukemia in 9 of 16 rats that received intravenous injections of the chemical, 10 mg/kg body weight, for a total of 250 mg over 175 days. The authors also reported that subcutaneous injections of N-butyl-N-nitrosourea (BNU), the chemical employed in the present series of experiments, to rats resulted in only sarcomas at the injection site (*2*). There had been no other report in which the carcinogenicity of BNU was tested in experimental animals before the present author described its highly leukemogenic effect on female Donryu rats that received BNU in their drinking water (*9*, *10*). Thereafter, the leukemogenic effect of BNU was confirmed by Yokoro *et al.* (*12*) not only in rats but also in mice.

In the present paper, the results of a series of 3 different experiments are described: 1) continuous administration of 0.04, 0.02, and 0.01% solutions of BNU in the drinking water to female Donryu rats; 2) administration of a 0.04% BNU solution for 5, 10, 15, or 20 weeks to female Sprague-Dawley (S-D) rats; and 3) a single oral, subcutaneous, or intraperitoneal application of 300 mg/kg body weight of BNU in olive oil to female S-D rats.

The BNU used, mp 81 to 82°, was synthesized and supplied by Dr. Y. Sakurai, Division of Cancer Chemotherapy, Cancer Institute, Tokyo. It was kept refrigerated at 5° until it was used. In the first 2 experiments, the rats were separated into groups of 4 at 11 weeks of age and kept in hanging metal cages. Each day, 60 ml of freshly prepared solution of BNU in a distilled water, were placed in the drinking bottle glass in each cage. The bottle was completely covered with black vinyl tape to eliminate the effect of light.

Incidence of Leukemia

1. Effect of various concentrations of BNU in the drinking water on female Donryu rats

The localization and time of appearance of tumors in each rat, and the cumulative percentage of tumors in each group are given in Figs. 1 and 2. The average weight of the body, liver, and spleen, the average index of the liver and spleen in animals with and without leukemia, and the target organs for tumor development in each group are shown in Tables I and II.

In Group I (0.04% BNU solution), leukemia developed in 100%, and the animals were killed between the 19th and 24th experimental week, at an average period of 20 weeks. In Group II (0.02% BNU solution), 21 rats developed tumors and were killed for autopsy between the 25th and 29th week, at an average period of 27 weeks. Leukemia was found in 17 rats (81%) in the earlier part and extrahematopoietic tumors in 5 rats (24%) in the later part of the experimental

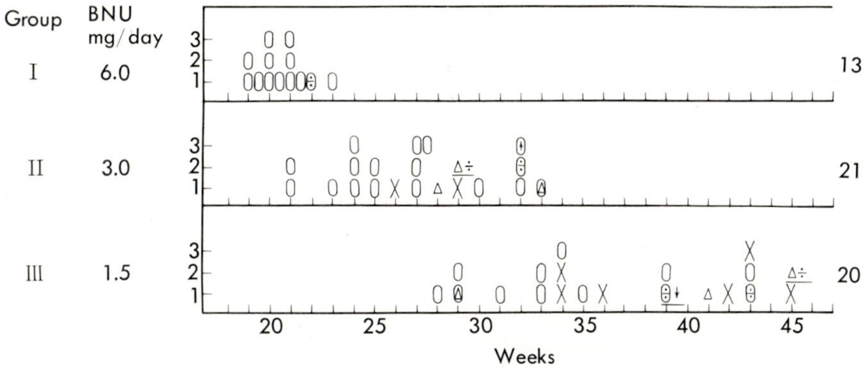

FIG. 1. Tumors in various organs and leukemias
0 leukemia ; ÷ esophagus ; ↑ small intestine ; ↓ mammary glands ; △ ear duct ; × no tumor.

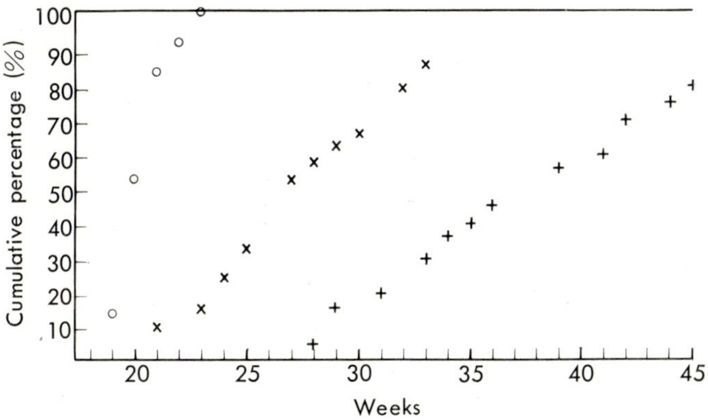

FIG. 2. Cumulative percentage of appearance of tumor in rats
○ 6.0 mg/day ; × 3.0 mg/day ; + 1.5 mg/day.

TABLE I. Average Weights of the Body, Liver, and Spleen and Indices of the Liver and Spleen

Daily dose (mg)	Nonleukemic			
	No. of rats	Body (g)	Liver (g)	Spleen (g)
1.5	8	158	6.3 (4.0)	0.4 (0.3)
3.0	5	144	6.5 (4.4)	0.7 (0.4)
6.0	0	—	— —	— —

Leukemic							
Aleukemic				Leukemic			
No. of rats	Body (g)	Liver (g)	Spleen (g)	No. of rats	Body (g)	Liver (g)	Spleen (g)
4	173	11.4 (6.5)	0.8 (0.4)	8	167	14.7 (8.9)	2.9 (1.5)
4	128	6.2 (4.8)	0.4 (0.3)	12	159	8.7 (5.5)	1.3 (0.7)
1	88	2.6 (2.9)	0.1 (0.1)	12	122	13.5(11.3)	0.8 (0.7)

Numbers in parentheses indicate indices. Liver or spleen weight/body weight ×100.

TABLE II. Localization of Tumors

Group	Daily dose (mg)	No. of rats	Leukemia and other tumors in various organs					
			Leukemia	Fore-stomach	Esophagus	Ear duct	Mammary gland	Small intestine
I	6.0	13	13	6	1	0	0	0
II	3.0	21	16	14	2	3	0	1
III	1.5	20	12	16	5	3	1	0

period. In Group III (0.01% BNU solution), 12 rats (60%) out of 20 developed leukemia between the 28th and 44th week, at the 33rd week on the average. Extrahematopoietic tumors developed in 6 rats (30%) in the later part of the experimental period.

The results of the first experiment showed that the higher concentration of BNU in the drinking water resulted in a higher incidence of leukemia early in the experiment, and the lower dose induced more tumors in extrahematopoietic tissues in the later part of the experiment.

2. Effect of various periods of treatment with a 0.04% solution of BNU in the drinking water on female Sprague-Dawley rats (Fig. 3, and Tables III and IV)

Four groups of female S-D rats, 11 weeks of age, were given 0.04% BNU solution continuously for 5, 10, 15, or 20 weeks. They were then kept on the basic diet alone until they were killed for autopsy.

Among 14 rats in Group I (5 weeks), 8 (57%) developed leukemia between the 26th and 47th week, at the 36th week on the average. Four out of these 8 leukemic rats simultaneously had mammary tumors. In Group II (10 weeks), leukemia was found in 12 (67%) out of 18 rats between the 16th and 42nd week,

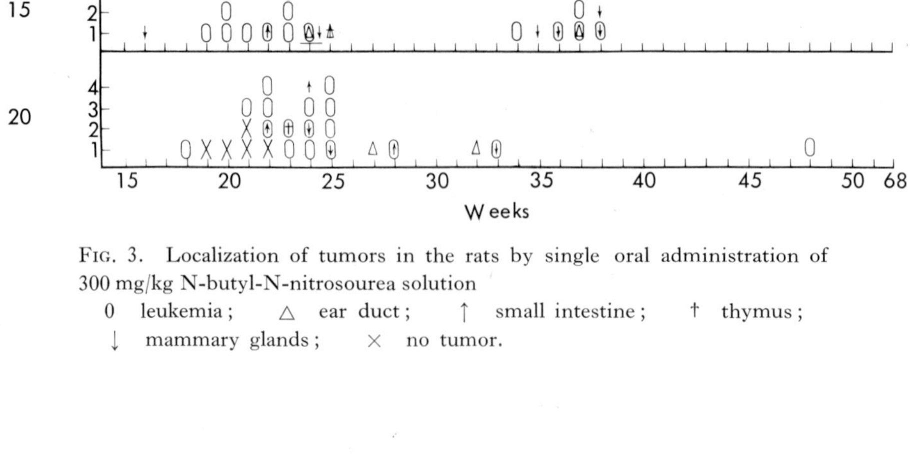

FIG. 3. Localization of tumors in the rats by single oral administration of 300 mg/kg N-butyl-N-nitrosourea solution
0 leukemia; △ ear duct; ↑ small intestine; † thymus;
↓ mammary glands; × no tumor.

Table III. Localization of Tumors in Rats Given 0.04% BNU Solution as Their Drinking Water for 5, 10, 15, or 20 Weeks

Group	Treatment (weeks)	No. of rats	Leukemia	Ear duct	Mammary gland	Small intestine	Others
I	5	14	8 (57)	0	6 (43)	0	4 (29)
II	10	18	12 (67)	3 (17)	4 (22)	0	2 (11)
III	15	20	17 (85)	3 (15)	6 (30)	1 (5)	3 (15)
IV	20	25	17 (68)	2 (8)	2 (8)	4 (16)	6 (24)

Numbers in parentheses indicate percents.

Table IV. Average Weights of the Body, Liver, and Spleen and Indices of the Liver and Spleen

Group	Treatment (weeks)	Nonleukemia				Leukemia			
		No. of rats	Body (g)	Liver (g)	Spleen (g)	No. of rats	Body (g)	Liver (g)	Spleen (g)
I	5	6	302	15.7 (5.1)	0.7 (0.2)	8	324	21.3 (6.8)	2.1 (0.8)
II	10	5	255	9.8 (3.8)	0.5 (0.2)	13	278	18.8 (6.8)	2.8 (1.0)
III	15	4	188	8.0 (4.2)	0.5 (0.3)	16	242	24.8(10.2)	2.2 (0.9)
IV	20	8	196	5.5 (2.8)	0.3 (0.2)	17	228	17.0 (7.5)	1.9 (0.8)

Numbers in parentheses are indices. Liver or spleen weight/body weight ×100.

at an average of 33 weeks. Among these 12 leukemia rats, 3 had mammary tumors also. In Group III (15 weeks), 17 rats (90%) died of leukemia between the 19th and 38th week, at the 24th week on the average. Among these 17 leukemic rats, 5 simultaneously had another tumor, 2 in the ear duct, 2 in the mammary gland, and 1 in the small intestine. In Group IV (20 weeks), leukemia developed in 17 (68%) out of 25 rats between the 18th and 48th week, at an average of 24 weeks. Among these 17, 6 simultaneously had tumors in other organs: 3 in the mammary gland, 3 in the small intestine, and 1 in the thymus.

It was confirmed in this second experiment that BNU caused a high incidence of leukemia in female S-D rats when it was given in their drinking water for more than 10 weeks. Although treatment for only 5 weeks led to development of leukemia in some rats, the incidence was low, 60%, and the induction period was very long, averaging 36 weeks. Extrahematopoietic tumors, specially mammary carcinomas, were found more frequently in S-D rats than in Donryu rats.

3. *Effect of a single application of BNU* (*Fig. 4 and Table V*)

The female S-D rats, at the age of 11 weeks, received 300 mg/kg body weight of BNU suspended in 1 ml of olive oil intraperitoneally, subcutaneously, or orally by means of a stomach tube. Thereafter they were maintained on the basic diet alone. In cases of oral administration, leukemia developed sporadically between the 20th and 66th week at which time all the survivors were killed for autopsy. Among 25 rats that survived longer than the 20th week after the single oral administration of BNU, 6 (24%) developed leukemia. Three of them had mammary tumors also.

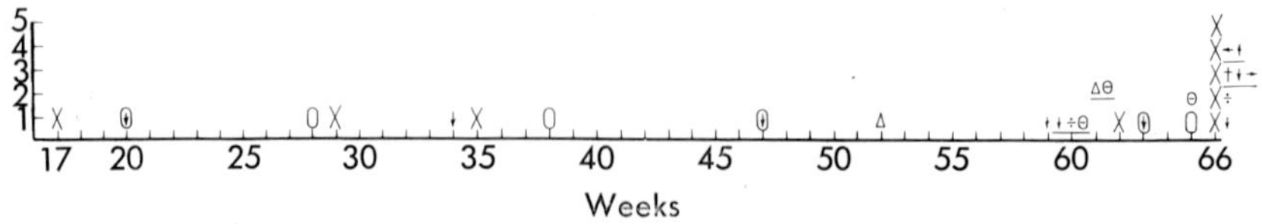

FIG. 4. Localization of tumors in the rats by single oral administration of 300 mg/kg N-butyl-N-nitrosourea solution

0 leukemia ; ↓ mammary glands ; ÷ adrenal ; → ovary ;
⊖ kidney ; △ uterus ; † liver ; ← stomach ;
↑ spleen ; × no tumor.

TABLE V. Localization of Tumors in Rats after a Single Oral Administration of 300 mg/kg BNU Solution

No. of rats	Leukemia	Mammary	Others	No tumor
25	6 (24%)	8 (32%)	11† (44%)	9 (36%)

† Kidney (12%), uterus and adrenal (8%), forestomach, spleen, liver and ovary (4%).

Although leukemia developed also in those rats that received BNU by the subcutaneous or intraperitoneal route, 2/7 and 3/9 of the rats, respectively, it was not possible to compare the target organs of BNU given by the different routes of application due to the small number of animals tested. Nevertheless, it was clearly confirmed in this third experiment that even a single dose was capable of producing leukemia in some animals.

Plaque-forming Cells in the Spleen

The number of plaque-forming cells (PFC) in the spleen against sheep red blood cells was studied in those rats that were killed immediately after the end of administration of 0.04% BNU solution for 5, 10, 15, or 20 weeks, and on every fifth week thereafter. The results are shown in Fig. 5.

Plaque-forming cells were almost nonexistent in all the rats that were killed immediately after the end of BNU administration. In the rats that received BNU for 5 weeks, the count recovered gradually thereafter, and it was about 60% of the control level at the end of the experiment, at the 25th week. In the other three groups however, the count remained continuously on the zero level until the end of the experiment.

Blood Cell Count

The animals that received 0.04% BNU solution lost approximately 15% of their body weight during the first experimental week and then maintained this level throughout the rest of the experimental period. The number of red and white blood cells in the circulating blood decreased gradually until around the 10th week, at which point they were about 50% of the normal level, and then the latter increased rather rapidly. In many cases, the white blood cell count recovered to

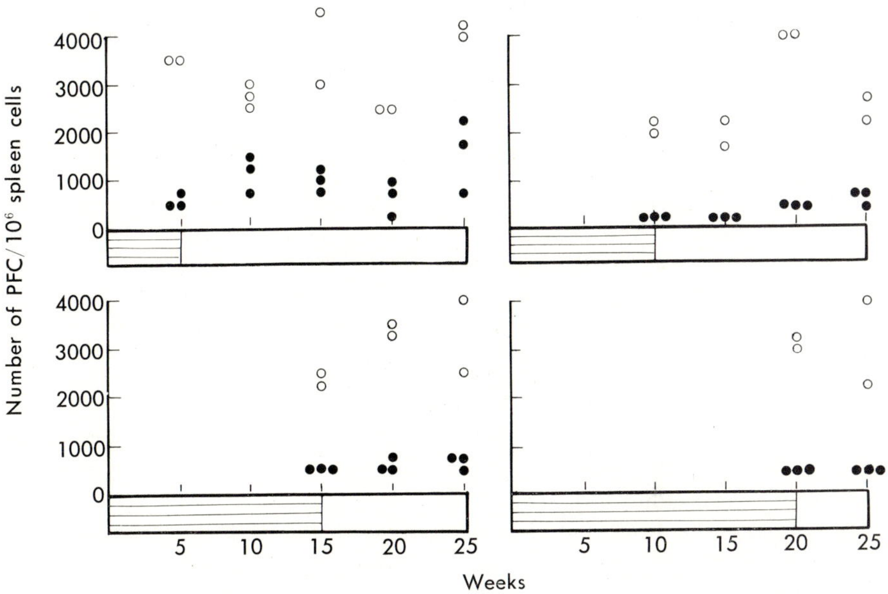

FIG. 5. Effect of N-butyl-N-nitrosourea administration on plaque-forming cell formation in Sprague-Dawley rats

○ control; ● treated; [hatched bar]; BNU administration.

the normal level by the 15th week. In some cases, leukemic cells began to appear in the peripheral blood from the 17th week. The white blood cell counts in leukemic animals varied greatly from case to case, ranging from the normal level to as high as 9×10^5 when they were examined at the time of autopsy. In the majority of cases, however, it was 2 to 5×10^4. Anemia was prominent in many cases.

Microscopic Findings

1. Leukemic cells

Two types of leukemic cells were found in the smear preparations of the peripheral blood, bone marrow, and ascitic fluid, stained with the Wright-Giemsa solution. The first type contained various amount of azurophilic granules in their cytoplasm and were positive in peroxidase reaction (Photo 1). The granules were larger than those in normal neutrophiles and smaller than those of eosino- and basophilic leucocytes. The number of granules was higher than that of normal neutrophiles in many cases. These granules were sometimes found even in mitotic cells. The nucleus, oval or kidney-shaped, consisted of a fine network of karyoplasm and several small nucleoli. These cells resembled promyelocytes, myelocytes, or metamyelocytes. The bone marrow and tumor nodules in some animals were characterized by greenish color (chloroleukemia).

The leukemic cells of the second type, nongranulocytic ones, had large, oval, bean-shaped, or lobulated nuclei which consisted of fine networks of karyoplasm and a few large nucleoli. The majority of these cells, particularly those that had an oval or round nucleus, had a narrow rim of very basophilic cytoplasm with a white halo (Photo 2). There were no azurophilic granules and neither the peroxidase nor the PAS reaction was positive. These cells resembled undifferentiated hemocytoblasts or sometimes erythroblasts.

2. *Histopathology in leukemic rats*

The leukemic rats were characterized by hepatosplenomegalia, as shown in Tables II, IV, and V, and by enlargement of the adrenal glands and cysternal lymph nodes due to metastatic proliferation of leukemic cells (Photo 3). Swelling of the systemic lymph nodes and thymus, however, was not seen in the majority of cases.

In the liver, leukemic cells appeared sporadically or in small groups in Glisson's capsules or in the hepatic sinusoids (Photo 4). Then, they proliferated widely and extensively in the sinusoids and central veins. The leukemic lesions were sometimes so extensive that atrophy and necrosis of hepatic cell cords were seen in many cases (Photo 5).

In the spleen, leukemic cells proliferated first in the venous sinuses of the red pulp and then infiltrated the white pulp. In some cases, the weight of the spleen was more than 1 g, and normal spleen architecture was seldom seen (Photo 6).

Invasion of leukemic cells was also commonly seen in the adrenal glands and kidneys (Photo 7), cysternal lymph nodes (Photo 3), and in the alveolar walls and peribronchial spaces of the lung (Photo 8).

In a few cases, leukemic cells were not detected in the circulating blood of rats that had leukemic lesions in the bone marrow, liver, spleen, and adrenal glands. These cases were diagnosed as aleukemic leukemia.

DISCUSSION

The results of these studies reveal 3 interesting facts. The first is that BNU showed a very strong leukemogenic effect on both Donryu and Sprague-Dawley rats when it was given to these animals continuously in their drinking water. The higher concentration of BNU in the drinking water and the longer period of administration resulted in a higher incidence of leukemia early in the experimental period, and the lower dose and shorter period of administration induced more tumors in extrahematopoietic tissues in the later part of the experimental period. Second, there was some strain specificity in the target organs of BNU carcinogenesis, *i.e.*, Donryu rats developed leukemia alone in the majority of cases while Sprague-Dawley rats developed both leukemia and mammary tumors simultaneously. Third, the immunosuppressive action of BNU was revealed. It was apparent that leukemic cells proliferated in and killed the host animals that had been in a highly immunosuppressive state so far as was indicated by the number of plaque-forming cells in the spleen against sheep red blood cells.

Although 2 types of leukemia, granulocytic and nongranulocytic, were observed in these studies, the histogenesis of these leukemias, including their target cells, was not studied. Since BNU caused a high incidence of leukemia in both Donryu and Sprague-Dawley rats in 20 weeks, it would be a useful tool in analyzing leukemogenesis, especially with respect to comparative studies on leukemogenic viruses.

Acknowledgments

The author wishes to thank Dr. Y. Sakurai of the Cancer Institute, Tokyo, for the synthesis and supply of N-butyl-N-nitrosourea, Dr. Y. Hashimoto and Miss Y. Oshima of the Tokyo Biochemical Research Institute, Tokyo, for performing the plaque-forming cell count, and Miss S. Yamazaki of the Sasaki Institute, Tokyo, for her technical assistance in the animal experiments.

REFERENCES

1. Druckrey, H. Organotrope carcinogene Wirkungen bei 65 verschiedenen N-Nitroso-Verbindungen an BD-Ratten. *Z. Krebsforsch.*, **69**, 103–201 (1967).
2. Druckrey, H., Preussmann, R., Ivankovic, S., So, B. T., Schmidt, C. H., and Bucheler, J. Zur Erzeugung subcutaner Sarkome an Ratten. Carcinogene Wirkung von Hydrazodicarbonsäure-bismethyl-nitrosamid, N-nitroso-N-*n*-butylharnstoff, N-Methyl-N-nitroso-N′-nitroguanidin, und N-Nitroso-imidazolidon. *Z. Krebsforsch.*, **68**, 87–102 (1966).
3. Fukunishi, R. Studies on tumor induction in rats with 7,12-dimethylbenz[*a*]-anthracene, with special references to the morphogenesis and fine-structural changes in the target organs. *Acta Pathol. Japon.*, **18**, 51–72 (1968).
4. Hartmann, H. A., Miller, E. C., Miller, J. A., and Morris, F. K. The leukemogenic action of 2-acetylaminophenanthrene. *Cancer Res.*, **19**, 210–216 (1959).
5. Huggins, C. B., and Sugiyama, T. Induction of leukemia in rat by pulse doses of 7,12-dimethylbenz[*a*]anthracene. *Proc. Natl. Acad. Sci. U.S.*, **55**, 74–81 (1966).
6. Ivanković, S. Übertragung einer Ratten Leukamie durch peripheres Blut. *Arzneimittelforsch.*, **14**, 836–837 (1964).
7. Iwahashi, Y., and Setsuda, T. Experimental studies on congenital bone marrow asthenia and leukemia. I. Haematological and cytological observations on the albino rats given continuously 4-amino-pterorylglutamic acid (in Japanese). *Acta Haematol. Japon.*, **20**, 393–405 (1957).
8. Morris, H. P., Wagner, B. P., Ray, F. E., Snell, K. C., and Stewart, H. L. Comparative studies of cancer and other lesions of rats fed N,N'-2,7-fluorenylene-bisacetamide or N-2-fluorenylacetamide. *Natl. Cancer Inst. Monograph*, **5**, 1–54 (1961).
9. Odashima, S. Development of leukemia in rats by oral administration of N-nitrosobutylurea in the drinking water. *GANN*, **60**, 237 (1969).
10. Odashima, S. Leukemogenesis of N-nitrosobutylurea in the rat. I. Effect of various concentrations in the drinking water to female Donryu rats. *GANN*, **61**, 239–244 (1970).
11. Walpole, A. I., Roberts, D. C., Rose, F. L., Hendry, J. A., and Homer, R. F. Cytotoxic agents. IV. The carcinogenic actions of some monofunctional ethyleneimine derivatives. *Brit. J. Pharm. Chemother.*, **9**, 306–323 (1954).
12. Yokoro, K., Imamura, N., Takizawa, S., Nishihara, H., and Nishihara, E. Leukemogenic and mammary tumorigenic effect of N-nitrosobutylurea in mice and rats. *GANN*, **61**, 295–296 (1970).

EXPLANATION OF PHOTOS

PHOTO 1. Leukemic cells in the peripheral blood; mononucleated cells with a light blue cytoplasm around a large, kidney-shaped or lobulated nucleus. A large number of azurophilic granules are seen in the cytoplasm. Taken from a rat that received 0.04% BNU solution for 10 weeks and was killed at the 22nd week. Wright-Giemsa stain.

PHOTO 2. Leukemic cells in the peripheral blood; mononucleated cells with a narrow rim of deep blue cytoplasm surrounding a large, round, kidney-shaped or slightly lobulated nucleus. From a rat that received 0.04% BNU for 15 weeks and was killed at the 21st week. Wright-Giemsa stain.

PHOTO 3. Leukemic invasion of cysternal lymph node and pancreas. From a rat given 0.04% BNU for 15 weeks and killed at the 21st week.

PHOTO 4. Invasion of leukemic cells in the liver. Leukemic cells are seen sporadically in the sinusoid and portal vein. From a rat that received 0.04% BNU for 5 weeks and was killed at the 30th week.

PHOTO 5. Leukemic lesions in the liver. Atrophy, disorder, and necrosis of hepatic cell cords due to intensive proliferation of leukemic cells. From the same rat shown in Photo 3.

PHOTO 6. Leukemic invasion of the spleen. Red and white pulp is replaced by leukemic cells. From the same rat shown in Photo 3.

PHOTO 7. Leukemic invasion of the kidney. Proliferation of leukemic cells in the interstitium of the kidney is seen. From a rat that received 0.04% BNU for 5 weeks and was killed at the 32nd week.

PHOTO 8. Leukemic lesions in the lung. Peribronchial and perivascular spaces as well as alveolar walls are invaded by leukemic cells. From the same rat shown in Photo 3.

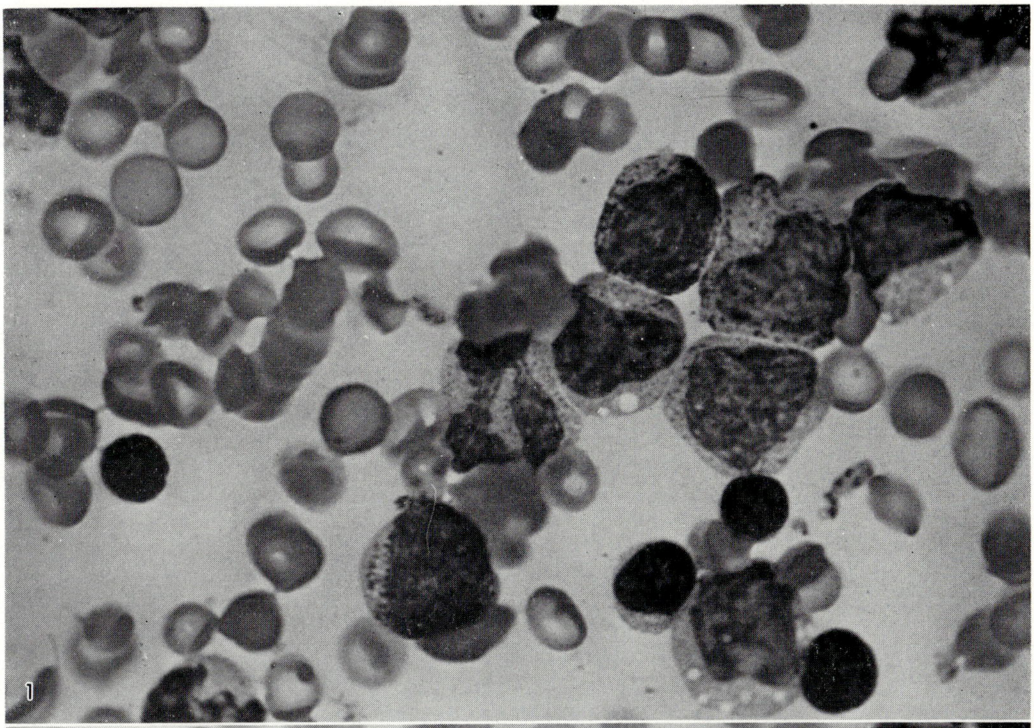

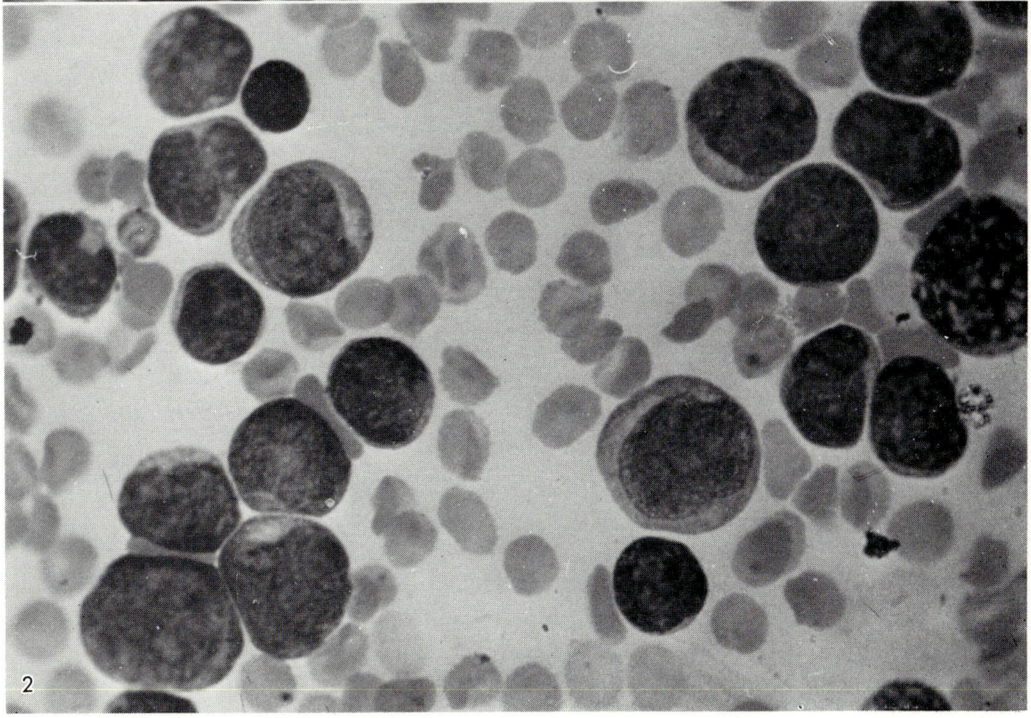

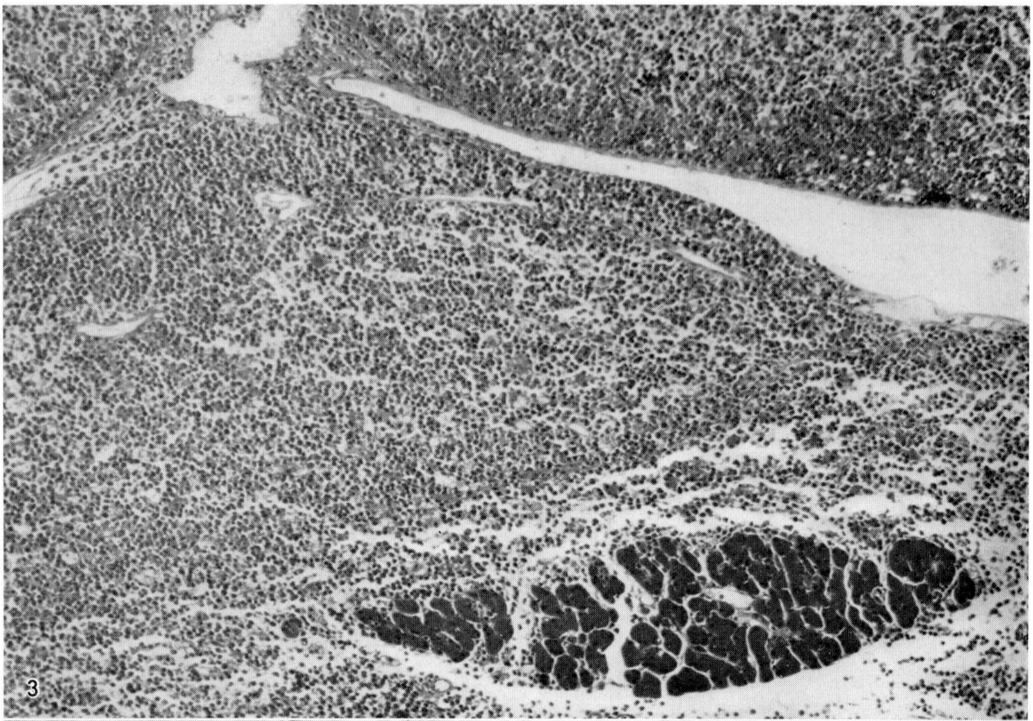
3

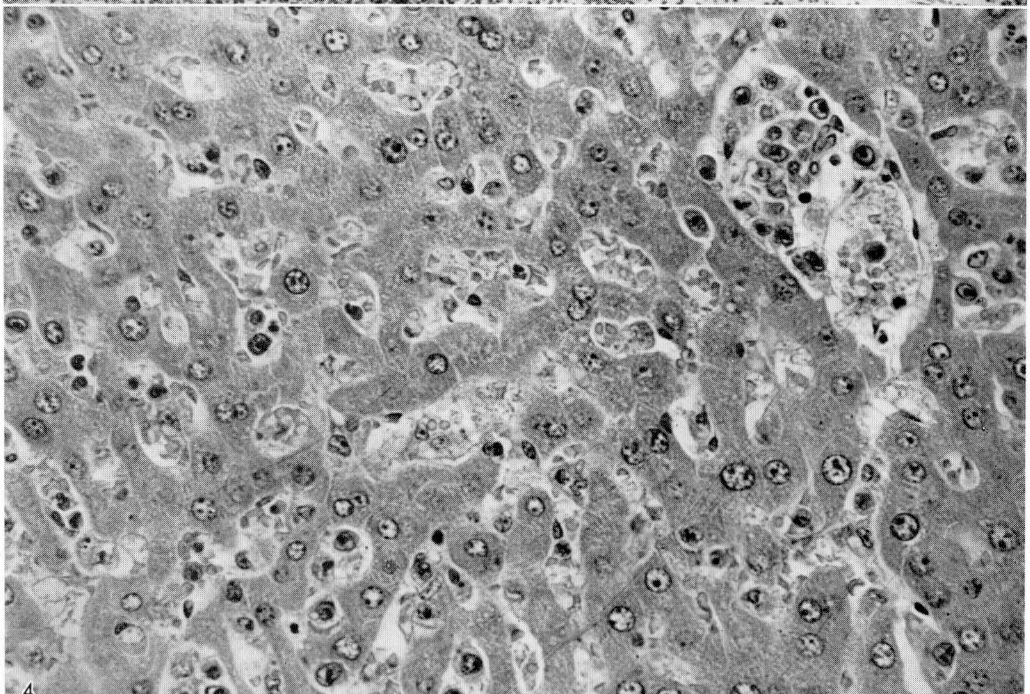
4

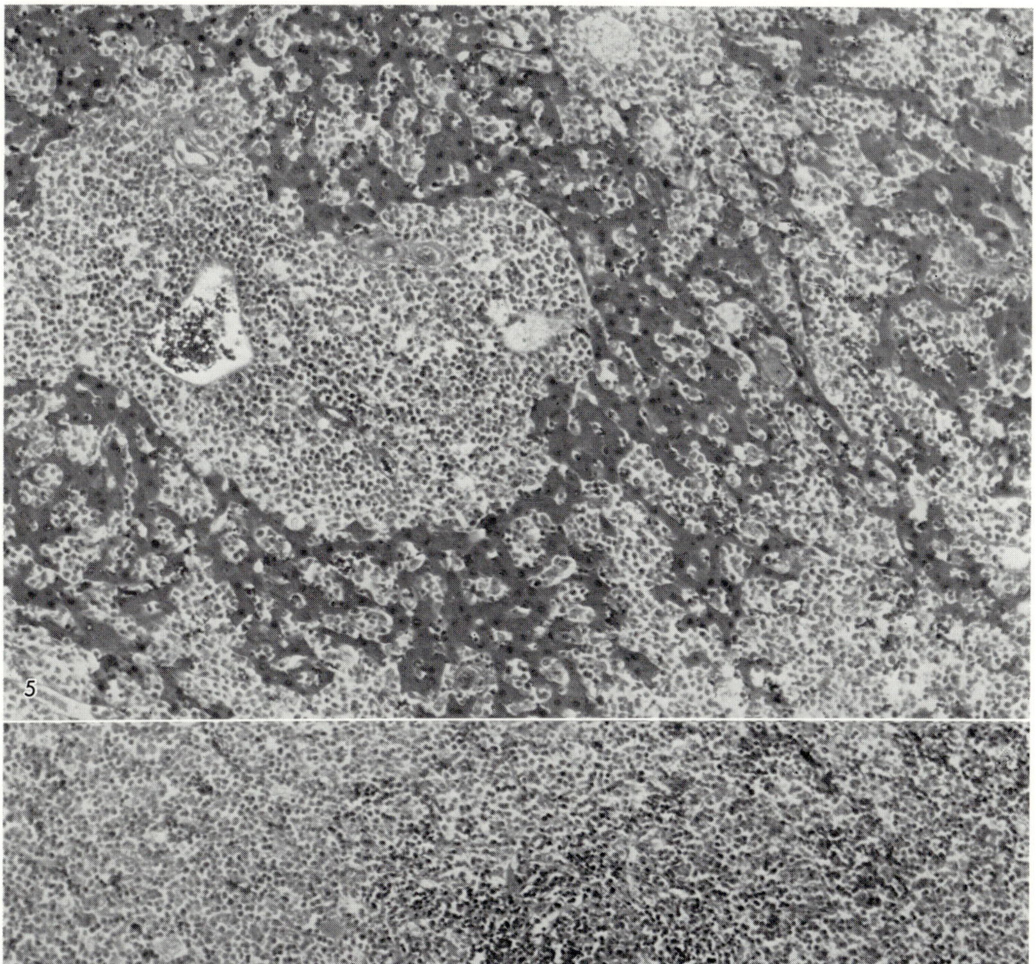
5

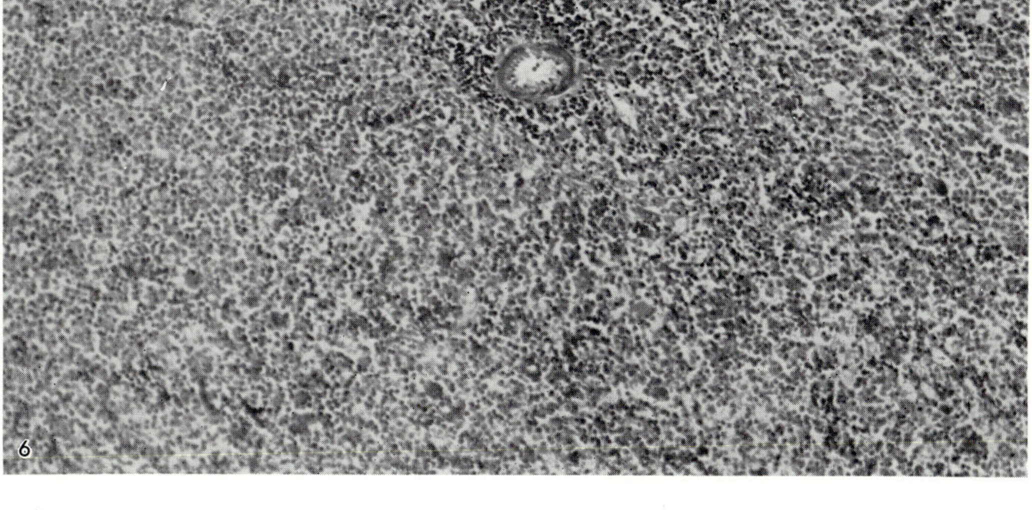
6

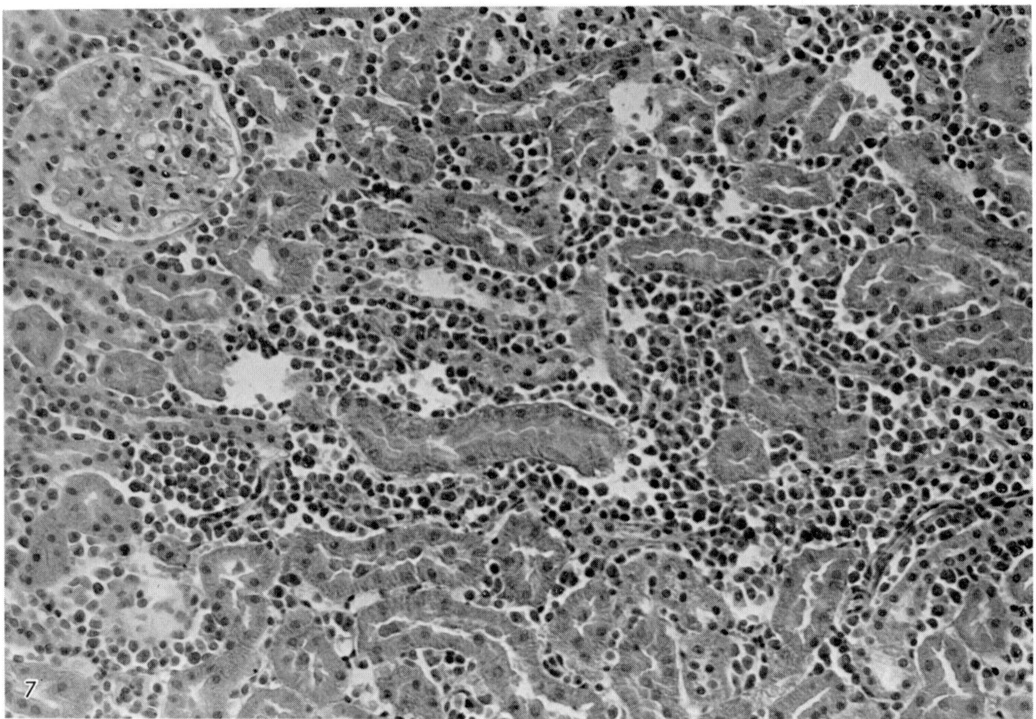
7

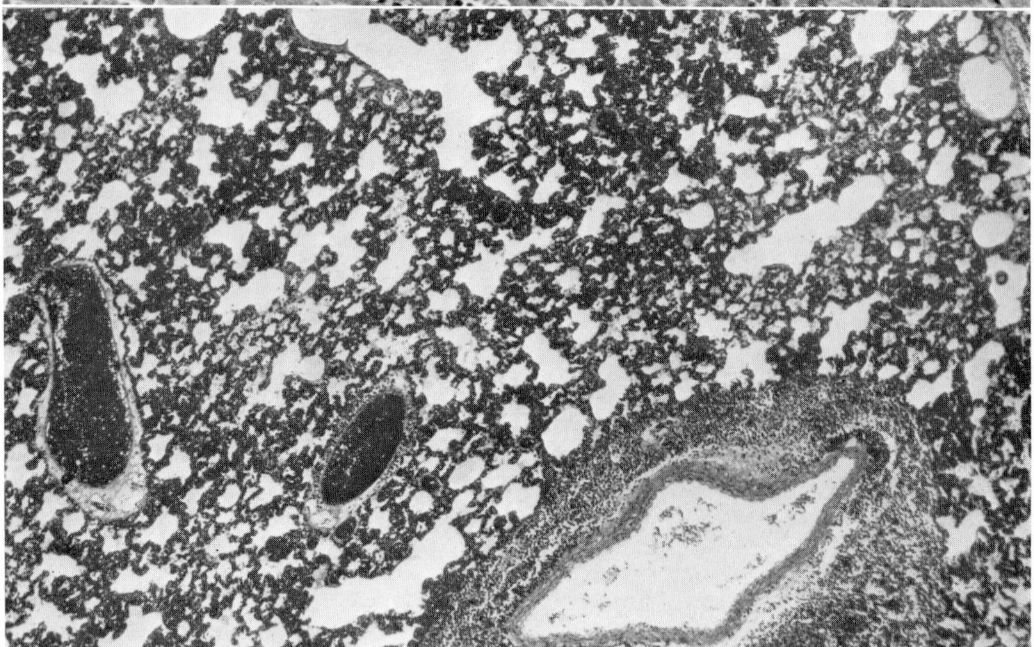
8

GANN Monograph on Cancer Research 12, 1972

MECHANISM OF LEUKEMOGENESIS BY 7,12-DIMETHYLBENZ[*a*] ANTHRACENE, WITH SPECIAL REFERENCE TO HOST FACTORS INFLUENCING ITS PATHOGENESIS*

Yasuaki NISHIZUKA and Hayase SHISA

*Laboratory of Experimental Pathology, Aichi Cancer Center Research Institute***

The results of recent experiments carried out to develop a basic understanding of chemical leukemogenesis in mice and rats are presented. The incidence, type, and pathology of leukemias evoked by 7,12-dimethylbenz[*a*]anthracene (DMBA) and by N-nitrosobutylurea (NBU) are analyzed in connection with the method of induction and the species and age of animals. It is demonstrated that leukemia of the lymphocytic cell series may be the prototype of mouse leukemias induced by chemical carcinogens, while those of the myelogenous cell series are predominant among rat leukemias. The role of the thymus as a determinant of the facility of leukemia development and of the morphological character of mouse leukemia is emphasized in experiments with mice under different conditions. In the rat, specificity of leukemia with trisomy of the longest telocentric chromosome (C-1 trisomy), evoked only in Long-Evans rats by DMBA, is also stressed and discussed.

The induction of leukemia by chemical carcinogens has been studied extensively in many laboratories (*2*). It is known that neonatal and suckling mice are very susceptible to leukemia induction by various types of chemical carcinogens (*20*). Recent reports by Huggins and Sugiyama (*7*), Odashima (*19*), and others (*3*, *31*) have described useful methods of leukemogenesis in rats. The present report will present a survey of our recent data on the highly sensitive leukemogenic responses in mice and rats which, as newborns or adults, were administered 7,12-dimethylbenz[*a*]anthracene (DMBA) under various conditions. Recent experiments on leukemia induction by N-nitrosobutylurea (NBU) will also be described briefly. The main aim of our study is to clarify the pathogenesis of chemical murine leukemogenesis with special reference to comprehensive analysis of the host factors that appear to be responsible for determining the age of leukemia occurrence and the type of leukemia thus evoked.

* This work was supported in part by a Grant-in-Aid for Scientific Research from the Ministry of Education of Japan.

** Kanokoden 81, Tashiro-cho, Chikusa-ku, Nagoya 464 (西塚泰章, 志佐　湍).

Experimental Procedures

The results described here cover experiments with 1) inbred strains of C57BL/6J, A/Jax, 129/J, AKR/Ms, SL/Ms, and C3Hf/He mice, and noninbred Swiss/Ms mice; and 2) inbred strains of ACI/Ms and Wistar/Ms rats and non-inbred Long-Evans and Donryu rats. All the animals were raised in our laboratory. The methods of leukemia induction have been fully described previous publications (*7*, *12*, *21*). DMBA (Eastman Organic Chemicals, Rochester, N.Y.) was used in the form of a lipid emulsion (0.5%) or aqueous gelatin suspension (1.0%). A single subcutaneous injection of a relatively low dose of DMBA (50 μg/g body weight) given at 0 to 3, 25 to 35, or 70 days of age was the standard method for leukemia induction in mice (*21*, *24*). Intravenous injections of multiple pulse doses of DMBA (20–30 mg/kg body weight), starting at the age of 25 to 30 days, were employed for rat leukemia induction (*7*, *12*). Mice and rats were given a 0.04% solution of NBU (supplied by Dr. S. Odashima) continuously as their drinking water from the age of 30 to 40 days (*19*). Procedures for care of animals and checking for tumor development and techniques for cytogenetical histological observations have been described in previous papers (*13*, *14*).

DMBA-induced Leukemias in Mice

1. Induction of leukemias in different strains and ages of mice

Lymphocytic and lymphoblastic leukemias which appear, at the histological level at least, to originate in the thymus can be induced with high incidence in mice given a single injection of DMBA shortly after birth (*20*). As seen in Table I, there is a remarkable strain difference in leukemogenic response, however (*21*). Swiss mice are most susceptible, followed by 129/J and C57BL mice, and A/Jax

TABLE I. Incidence of Leukemia in Various Strains of Mice after Single Subcutaneous Injection of DMBA at Birth

Strain	Incidence of leukemia			
	Spontaneous leukemic mice (at age 12 mos.)	Total mice (%)	DMBA-induced leukemic mice (at age 6 mos.)	Total mice (%)
Swiss/Ms	3/201	(1.4)	76/111	(82.9)
C57BL/6J	0/112	(0.0)	10/48	(20.8)
129/J	1/101	(0.9)	13/42	(30.9)
A/Jax	3/237	(1.3)	4/29	(13.8)
AKR/Ms	81/99 (1)†	(81.1)	38/48	(79.2)
SL	57/87 (0)†	(67.9)	17/30	(56.6)

Mice were given 60 μg of DMBA within 24 hr after birth; mice at 3 days of age were given 100 μg of DMBA.

† Number of mice with leukemia at 6 months of age.

mice are the least susceptible. Newborn AKR and SL mice of high-leukemia strains also show a more rapid occurrence of thymic leukemia after injection of DMBA. It seems that no positive relation between the DMBA sensitivity and the susceptibility to Gross virus can be recognized.

It is clear from Table II that cortisone treatment preceding DMBA exposure has an enhancing effect on leukemia development in susceptible Swiss mice. The leukemogenic response of the cortisone-pretreated C57BL and A/Jax mice could be ranked at almost the same level as that of Swiss mice. This may indicate that the susceptibility of each strain to DMBA leukemogenesis can be modified by exogeneous host-conditioning factors (*18*, *23*). An explanation of the potentiation introduced may be provided by the fact that cortisone causes severe thymic involution which is followed by rapid regeneration with a concomitant repopulation by immature lymphocytes (*9*). It has been proposed also that the population of immature lymphocytes in the thymus may be correlated with the susceptibility to viral leukemogenesis (*1*).

A previous report indicated that mice receiving DMBA injections as newborns show a higher incidence of leukemia development in a shorter time than

TABLE II. Acceleration of DMBA-Leukemia Development by Cortisone Pretreatment of Neonatal Mice

Strain	Cortisone treatment† (mg)	Incidence of leukemia: Leukemic mice	Incidence of leukemia: Total mice (%)	Latent period (days)
Swiss/Ms	—	29/36	(80.5)	107
	0.2	29/33	(87.8)	84
C57BL/6J	—	7/22	(31.8)	137
	0.15	24/29	(82.9)	126
A/Jax	—	2/13	(15.3)	181
	0.2	11/18	(61.1)	175

† Cortisone acetate was given i.p. within 24 hr after birth and a DMBA injection (100 μg) was given s.c. at 3 days of age.

TABLE III. Incidence and Type of Leukemia Induced by DMBA Lipid Emulsion Given to Newborn and Adult Swiss Mice

Treatment	Incidence of leukemias: Leukemic/total (%)	Incidence of leukemias: Latent period (days)	No. of mice with: Thymic leuk.	No. of mice with: Nonthymic leuk.
DMBA (100 μg) at 3 days of age	29/35 (82.9)	107	28	1
DMBA (1 mg) at 35 days of age	18/22 (81.8)	125	9	9
DMBA (1 mg) at 70 days of age	23/28 (82.1)	102	6	17
Cortisone (3.5 mg) at 32 days of age +DMBA (1 mg) at 35 days of age	23/28 (82.1)	105	21	2
DMBA (1 mg) at 3 days after delivery (70 days average)	21/24 (87.5)	134	15	6

would be expected in mice receiving injections as adults (*20*). Our results demonstrated however, that subcutaneous injection of DMBA when given in the form of a lipid emulsion yields an equally high incidence of leukemias in both newborns and adults (Table III). It is obvious, therefore, that target cells sensitive to DMBA exist in the hematopoietic tissues of host animals at all ages. However, differences in the pathology of leukemias thus evoked can be noticed among the age groups examined; thymic lymphocytic leukemias are most frequent when the chemical is given to neonatal mice, whereas undifferentiated cell leukemias without thymus involvement are common when DMBA is injected into adult mice. Table III illustrates also that frequent occurrence of thymic lymphocytic leukemias is observed in adult mice injected with DMBA either in the post partum period or after a single injection of cortisone acetate. Cytological analysis of the thymuses in these 2 groups of animals revealed a prompt decrease in their weights due to marked depletion of the lymphocyte population, which was followed by a rapid increase in weights due to lymphocyte proliferation. It is probable that the status of cell kinetics in the thymus after cortisone treatment or in the post partum period is comparable to that of the thymus in the neonatal stage. So far as chemical leukemogenesis is concerned, the procedures employed here could be referred to as " neonatalization " of the thymus which, in turn, might be a major factor determining the type of leukemia in adult mice (*24*).

2. *Leukemia induction in thymectomized mice*

The thymus is of critical importance in determining susceptibility to lymphocytic leukemia in spontaneous murine leukemogenesis of viral etiology (*4*). In AKR mice, the development of leukemia usually commences at 6 months of age. Thymectomy at varying ages, even when performed at an age shortly before the clinical appearance of leukemia, can prevent the occurrence of leukemia (*15*), and thymus grafting is capable of accelerating and restoring susceptibility to leukemia development (*16*, *17*). Similar roles of the thymus are also elucidated in

TABLE IV. Role of Thymuses in DMBA-Leukemia Development in Swiss Mice (A)

Treatment			Incidence of leukemias		
DMBA injection (age in days)	Thymectomy (age in days)	Thymus grafting†	Leukemic/ total (%)	Latent period (days)	No. of mice with enlarged grafted thymus
—	20	—	5/24 (20.8)	245	0
—	35	—	15/53 (28.3)	142	0
—	35	1-day-old thymuses	10/34 (29.4)	195	7
—	35	Autochthonous thymuses	4/22 (18.2)	183	4
—	60	—	2/28 (16.6)	125	0

† Grafting of thymuses was performed at 35 days of age, immediately after removal of *in situ* thymuses.

TABLE V. Role of Thymuses in DMBA-Leukemia Development in Swiss Mice (B)

Treatment		Incidence of leukemias		No. of mice with enlarged grafted thymus
At 3 days of age	At 35 days of age	Leukemic/total (%)	Latent period (days)	
Tx (thymectomy) +DMBA[a]	—	7/22 (31.8)	157	—
Tx+DMBA+ thymus graft[b1]	—	4/13 (30.9)	176	1
—	Tx+DMBA[a]	5/12 (41.7)	125	—
—	Tx+DMBA+ thymus graft[b2]	13/19 (68.4)	132	3
Tx	DMBA[a]	32/53 (60.4)	116	—
Tx	DMBA+ thymus graft[b1]	11/17 (64.7)	111	6

[a] Spleen (1 to 5×10^6) cells from adult Swiss mice were inoculated (i.p.) 7 days after DMBA injection. Neonatal (—[b1]) and young adult (—[b2]) thymuses were grafted (s.c.) 4 days after DMBA injection.

X-ray leukemogenesis (*10*). Hence, the effects of thymectomy in DMBA-leukemogenesis is of great importance and should be studied extensively. Table IV shows clearly that the incidence of leukemia in Swiss mice thymectomized after DMBA injection is markedly reduced and falls into the range of 15 to 30% in all the groups examined. The inhibitory effect of thymectomy is not reversed by reimplantation of autochthonous or isologous intact neonatal thymuses. Inoculation of spleen cells into thymectomized mice does not augment DMBA leukemogenesis. Table V shows that leukemias develop in about 30% of thymectomized mice even when they underwent thymus grafting 7 days after DMBA exposure. This may suggest that the leukemogenic action of DMBA is of short duration, and that neoplastic transformation of target cells may take place shortly after injection. A chronological study of the histology of thymuses of DMBA-treated mice revealed the presence of small foci or aggregates of leukemic cells, first detected in the deeper zones of the thymus cortex 35 days after DMBA exposure (unpublished data). However, transplantation assays have not so far succeeded in demonstrating that 35- to 42-day-old thymuses of neonatally DMBA-treated mice contain a sufficient number of autonomous leukemic cells to produce transplantable tumors in new intact or thymectomized hosts (*22*). Table V illustrates further studies indicating that DMBA is able to induce leukemias in 30 to 70% of thymectomized hosts and that thymuses grafted either in the neonatal stage or in adult mice are unable to potentiate or accelerate the occurrence of leukemias. It is possible to hypothesize that, although the thymus contains the cells probably most susceptible to DMBA leukemogenesis, other hematopoietic tissues harbor target cells. Hence, the possibility remains to be studied that in thymus-bearing mice the cells outside the thymus can migrate into the thymus after neoplastic transformation and form a tumor, since the thymus provides the most favorable site for proliferation of leukemic cells. This assumption may relate to our results

TABLE VI. Incidence and Type of Leukemias Induced by NBU in Normal and Thymectomized Mice of Various Strains

Strain	Oral administration†		Thymectomy at 32 days of age	Incidence of leukemia		No. of mice with	
	Duration (days)	Total dose (mg)		Leukemic/total (%)	Latent period (days)	Thymic leuk.	Non-thymic leuk.
Swiss/Ms	62	57–72	−	20/20 (100.0)	73	16	4
			+	7/7 (100.0)	97	0	7
C57BL/6J	70	38–54	−	18/19 (94.7)	103	15	3
			+	9/11 (81.8)	103	0	9
$C3H_f$/He	62	39–48	−	10/11 (90.9)	103	9	1
AKR/Ms	70	37–50	−	18/18 (100.0)	90	18	0
			+	5/5 (100.0)	103	0	5

† Administration of NBU (0.4 mg/ml) was started at the age of 35 to 40 days.

indicating that the frequency of chromosomal aberrations evoked by DMBA exposure in cells of the hematopoietic organs appears to be correlated to the incidence of DMBA-leukemias. The cells of the bone marrow were most susceptible to chromosomal aberrations and cells of the thymus were less susceptible than those of the bone marrow (*11*).

Table VI shows preliminary data on leukemia induction by oral administration of NBU. It is clear that NBU is the most potent leukemogenic agent since it can evoke leukemias in almost 100% of both intact and thymectomized mice of all strains examined. The gross and microscopic pathology thus induced is the same as that of DMBA-induced leukemia. Hence, it seems likely that the target cells of leukemogenic chemicals are distributed inside and outside the thymus.

3. *Induction of leukemias by pulse doses of DMBA injections*

Intravenous injections of pulse doses of DMBA result in a higher incidence of leukemias in adult Swiss mice (Table VII). However, a distinct difference in

TABLE VII. Incidence and Type of Leukemia Evoked by Multiple Pulse Doses of DMBA in Swiss Mice

Treatment		Incidence of leukemias		No. of mice with	
Pulse doses	Duration of injection (days)	Leukemic/total[a] (%)	Latent period (days)[b]	Thymic leuk.	Non-thymic leuk.
3–4	25–50	11/20 (55.0)	108	9	2
6	25–65	9/10 (90.0)	57	0	9

[a] Mice surviving more than 7 days after the last injection of DMBA.
[b] Days after the first injection of DMBA.

leukemogenic response can be seen between the group receiving 3 to 4 successive injections at 7-day intervals and the group receiving 6 injections at the same interval. Namely, thymic lymphocytic leukemias are frequently induced in the former group, whereas, in the latter leukemias were induced rapidly and proved to be stem-cell leukemias without any thymic involvement. Histological examination demonstrated that such a prolonged series of injections of pulse doses of DMBA resulted in complete loss of lymphocytes from the thymus cortex and produced severe atrophic thymuses.

4. *Pathology of leukemias induced by DMBA*

Classification of chemical-induced leukemias into 2 categories, thymic and nonthymic, is utilized in the present report (*21*, *24*). Typical thymic leukemia is the most prevalent type and develops in DMBA- and NBU-treated thymus-bearing mice. It is characterized by initial enlargement of the thymus and subsequent involvement of the lymph nodes, spleen, and liver. The cellular structure is monotonously uniform and is composed of immature lymphocytes or lymphoblasts. The " starry sky " pattern is also common. The histological and electronmicroscopic patterns are similar to those of Gross virus-induced and X-rayinduced leukemias. Nonthymic leukemias are of 3 types: myeloid, undifferentiated cell, and stem-cell leukemias. It is clear that myeloid leukemia is rare among chemical leukemias in mice. Undifferentiated cell leukemia usually appears earlier than lymphocytic leukemia and shows a moderate or marked enlargement of the lymph nodes and spleen without thymic involvement. Histologically, leukemic cells are generally large, polygonal, well-defined forms possessing ample cytoplasm that surrounds an oval, sharply outlined nucleus in which chromatin is abundant and evenly distributed. These cells have a tendency to aggregate and to show nodular infiltration. Our studies demonstrate that this type is found frequently in intact adult or thymectomized mice that become the recipients of chemical carcinogens (*22*, *24*). A striking difference in histological patterns is observed between leukemias developing in thymectomized hosts and those occurring in thymectomized hosts with thymus grafts. The large leukemic cells in thymectomized hosts appear to be of the undifferentiated cell type. In the hosts with thymus grafts, leukemic cells are usually typical lymphoblasts. In addition, remarkable infiltration of the grafted thymuses by these leukemic cells is frequently observed (Tables IV and V). Although thymus grafting does not augment the incidence of leukemia in thymectomized hosts, it is likely that thymus grafting gives rise to the cytological shift toward lymphocytic maturation of leukemic cells. Namely, it can be postulated that the determination of the phenotype of leukemia as " lymphocytic leukemia " is strongly influenced by the presence of the thymus. However, we do not know whether this is mediated by a systemic humoral action of the thymus or by local or environmental properties of the thymic tissues.

Stem-cell leukemia, developing only in mice receiving large doses of pulse injections of DMBA, is accompanied by moderate splenomegaly and lymphadenopathy without thymus involvement. The cellular structure may suggest a somewhat myeloid nature. Probably the development of this leukemia is not related to any thymus functions.

Chemically Induced Leukemias in Rats

1. Induction of leukemias in rats by DMBA and NBU

In Long-Evans rats, leukemias can be easily induced by intravenous injections of pulse doses of DMBA (*7*). The toxicity of DMBA may differ from strain to strain, Donryu rats being too sensitive to survive for a period long enough for leukemia development. As reported by Odashima (*19*), oral administration of NBU can regularly evoke leukemia in all the strains of rats examined (Table VIII). Repeated attempts to find a simple method of leukemia induction by subcutaneous or intraperitoneal injection of DMBA and NBU, single or multiple, at varying intervals, have been unsuccessful to date in neonatal and suckling rats.

2. Pathology of leukemias induced by DMBA and NBU

The rat leukemias thus induced differ in their pathology from the chemically induced mouse leukemias (Table VIII). Thymic lymphocytic leukemia was less frequent even when the rats were pretreated with cortisone acetate (unpublished data). The predominant type of leukemia in rats was stem-cell leukemia which has a predilection for growth in the liver, usually associated with erythroblastosis. Erythroblastic leukemias were evoked frequently also. These 2 types usually are accompanied by huge hepatomegaly and are referred to as " hepatic type " (*7, 27*) in gross appearance. Nodular or diffuse enlargement of the spleen is observed not infrequently in hepatic leukemia. Chloroleukemia was also observed in rats. Mammary tumors developed occasionally at a rather late stage in NBU-treated rats, especially in Wistar rats (Table VIII).

One distinct characteristic of the rat leukemias induced by DMBA was the presence of a high percentage of consistent chromosome abnormality, trisomy of the longest telocentric chromosome, *i.e.*, C-1 trisomy (*12, 27*). The cells with C-1 trisomy are large, mononuclear, and erythroblastic showing maturation arrest at the stage of polychromatic normoblast (*28*). Our cytogenetic analysis of leukemic rats clearly demonstrated that, although leukemic cells are found to be of multiple

TABLE VIII. Incidence and Type of Leukemias Induced by NBU in Rats of Various Strains

Strain	Oral administration[a]		No. of rats	Incidence of leukemia			Macroscopic type of leukemia			Mammary tumors
	Duration (days)	Total dose (mg)		No.	%	Latent period (days)	Thymic	Hepatic	Myeloid	
Long-Evans	92–94	266–335	26	21	80.7	130	4	17	0	6/12[b]
(Don×L-E) F_1	95–98	310–450	26	21	80.7	143	1	20	0	4/13
Donryu	91–94	301–390	30	27	90.0	138	0	24	3	3/16
ACI/Ms	91–95	289–358	14	11	78.5	138	0	9	2	3/10
Wistar/Ms	92–94	320–348	13	7	53.8	176	0	6	1	8/9

[a] Administration of NBU (0.4 mg/ml) was begun at the age of 30 to 40 days.
[b] Number of female rats.

clonal origin, predominant growth of cells with C-1 trisomy may occur, especially in severely anemic hosts. C-1 trisomy cells were present in 49 rats (53%) as stemline of leukemic cells out of total of 93 leukemic rats examined (*13*). It was of interest that the susceptibility of chromosomes to induction of aberrations by DMBA was proportional to the length of the chromatid, and that the largest telocentric chromosome (C-1) had the highest susceptibility to DMBA in acute stages (*14*). Further, it was also reported by Sugiyama (*25*) that aberrations involving the C-1 chromosome appear in a non-random manner and occur more frequently in anemic hosts or hosts given erythropoietin shortly before injection of DMBA. In addition, it was demonstrated that 7,8,12- and 6,8,12-trimethylbenz[*a*]anthracene yielded leukemias with the same chromosomal abnormality (*26*). In contrast, our extensive studies on leukemias induced by NBU in Long-Evans and other rats have failed to demonstrate the presence of C-1 trisomic leukemia (unpublished data). However, it seems likely that chromosomal abnormalities without any regularity may occur frequently in hepatic type leukemias with nodular splenic enlargement. From these studies, it appears that C-1 trisomic change in Long-Evans rats may be rather specific for polycyclic hydrocarbon carcinogens when they are given in pulse doses.

COMMENTS AND CONCLUSIONS

Based on the present studies on chemical leukemogenesis in mice and rats, the following conclusions can be drawn.

1) The most effective method of leukemia induction by DMBA differs for the 2 species, but when NBU is used the same method is most desirable in both species.

2) The pathology of leukemias evoked by the chemicals is also different in mice and rats. In mice, lymphocytic leukemias involving the thymus predominate, whereas in rats stem-cell or erythroblastic leukemias with huge hepatomegaly are predominant. It seems significant that blood cells of the lymphatic series are very sensitive in mice, while those of the myelogenous series are more sensitive in rats.

3) Considering the many studies on the leukemogenic response of mice to Gross virus and X-ray irradiation, it is significant that target cells that are highly sensitive in their leukemogenic response to chemical agents may be distributed widely both inside and outside the thymus. Further, the presence or absence of the thymus and its functional situation have a profound influence on both the macroscopic and microscopic patterns of chemically induced leukemias in the mouse.

4) In the rat, leukemias accompanied by a specific chromosomal abnormality (C-1 trisomy) can be consistently evoked only in the system where Long-Evans rats were exposed to pulse doses of DMBA. This system may provide a useful tool for clarifying the relationship between chromosomal or gene changes and neoplastic change in cells in chemical tumorigenesis.

5) The demonstration of a possible leukemogenic virus in cell-free filtrates prepared from chemically induced mouse leukemias has been described by re-

searches from several laboratories (*5*, *8*, *29*). On the other hand, similar experiments in our laboratory resulted in essentially negative data (*30*). Our attempts to transfer cell-free filtrates from thymic leukemias induced by DMBA in Swiss mice and evoked by NBU in Long-Evans rats have failed so far (*21*, unpublished data). However, more extensive studies along this line on chemically induced leukemias, especially on rat leukemias, may be needed to clarify the mechanism of chemical tumorigenesis connected with the oncogene theory of RNA tumor viruses (*6*).

REFERENCES

1. Axelrad, A. A., and Van Der Gaag, H. C. Susceptibility to lymphoma induction by Gross'passage A virus in C3Hf/Bi mice of different ages: Relation to thymic cell multiplication and differentiation. *J. Natl. Cancer Inst.*, **28**, 1065–1093 (1962).
2. Bergs, V. V. Chemical and hormonal induced leukemia. *In* "Experimental Leukemia," ed. by M. A. Rich, Appleton-Century-Crofts, New York, pp. 159–172 (1968).
3. Fukunishi, R. Studies on tumor induction in rats with 7,12-dimethylbenz[*a*]-anthracene, with special reference to the morphogenesis and fine-structural changes in the target organs. *Acta Pathol. Japon.*, **18**, 51–72 (1968).
4. Gross, L. Mouse leukemia. *In* "Oncogenic Viruses," Pergamon Press, Oxford, pp. 286–469 (1970).
5. Haran-Ghera, N. Leukemogenic filtrable agent from chemically induced lymphoid leukemia in C57BL mice. *Proc. Soc. Exp. Biol. Med.*, **124**, 697–699 (1967).
6. Huebner, R. J., and Todaro, G. J. Oncogenes of RNA tumor viruses as determinants of cancer. *Proc. Natl. Acad. Sci. U.S.*, **64**, 1087–1094 (1969).
7. Huggins, C. B., and Sugiyama, T. Induction of leukemia in rat by pulse doses of 7, 12-dimethylbenz[*a*]anthracene. *Proc. Natl. Acad. Sci. U.S.*, **55**, 74–81 (1966).
8. Irino, S., Ota, Z., Sezaki, T., Suzaki, M., and Hiraki, K. Cell-free transmission of 20-methylcholanthrene-induced RF mouse leukemia and electron microscopic demonstration of virus particles in its leukemic tissue. *GANN*, **54**, 225–237 (1963).
9. Ito, T., and Hoshino, T. Histological changes of the mouse thymus during involution and regeneration following administration of hydrocortisone. *Z. Zellforsch.*, **56**, 445–464 (1962).
10. Kaplan, H. S., Brown, M. B., and Paull, J. Influence of postirradiation thymectomy and of thymic implants on lymphoid tumor incidence in C57BL mice. *Cancer Res.*, **13**, 677–680 (1953).
11. Kurita, Y., Shisa, H., Matsuyama, M., Nishizuka, Y., Tsuruta, R., and Yoshida, T. H. Carcinogen-induced chromosome aberrations in hematopoietic cells of mice. *GANN*, **60**, 91–95 (1969).
12. Kurita, Y., Sugiyama, T., and Nishizuka, Y. Cytogenetic studies on rat leukemia induced by pulse doses of 7,12-dimethylbenz[*a*]anthracene. *Cancer Res.*, **28**, 1738–1752 (1968).
13. Kurita, Y., Sugiyama, T., and Nishizuka, Y. Cytogenetic analysis of cell populations in rat leukemia induced by pulse doses of 7,12-dimethylbenz[*a*]anthracene. *GANN*, **60**, 529–535 (1969).
14. Kurita, Y., Sugiyama, T., and Nishizuka, Y. Chromosome aberrations induced in rat bone marrow cells by 7,12-dimethylbenz[*a*]anthracene. *J. Natl. Cancer Inst.*, **43**, 635–641 (1969).

15. Nakakuki, K., Shisa, H., and Nishizuka, Y. Prevention of AKR leukemogenesis by thymectomy at varying ages. *Acta Haematol.*, **38**, 317–323 (1967).
16. Nishizuka, Y. Viral and chemical leukemogenesis and host conditioning. *Acta Pathol. Japon.*, **18**, 357–361 (1968).
17. Nishizuka, Y., and Nakakuki, K. Acceleration of leukemogenesis in AKR mice by grafts, cell suspensions, and cell-free centrifugates of thymuses from preleukemic AKR donors. *Int. J. Cancer*, **3**, 203–210 (1968).
18. Nishizuka, Y., and Shisa, H. Enhancement of 7,12-dimethylbenz[*a*]anthracene leukemogenesis in mice by neonatal injection of cortisone acetate. *Brit. J. Cancer*, **32**, 290–295 (1968).
19. Odashima, S. Leukemogenesis of N-Nitrosobutylurea in the rat. I. Effect of various concentrations in the drinking water to female Donryu rats. *GANN*, **61**, 245–253 (1970).
20. Pietra, G., Spencer, K., and Shubik, P. Response of newly born mice to a chemical carcinogen. *Nature*, **183**, 1689 (1959).
21. Shisa, H. Studies on the mechanism of 7,12-dimethylbenz[*a*]anthracene leukemogenesis in mice. I. Strain difference in susceptibility of DMBA leukemogenesis. *Mie Med. J.*, **19**, 89–99 (1969).
22. Shisa, H. Studies on the mechanism of 7,12-dimethylbenz[*a*]anthracene leukemogenesis in mice. II. The role of thymus in DMBA leukemogenesis. *Mie Med. J.*, **19**, 101–109 (1969).
23. Shisa, H. Studies on the mechanism of 7, 12-dimethylbenz[*a*]anthracene leukemogenesis in mice. III. Acceleration of DMBA leukemogenesis in mice by pretreatment of cortisone acetate. *Mie Med. J.*, **19**, 111–121 (1969).
24. Shisa, H., and Nishizuka, Y. Determining role of age and thymus in pathology of 7,12-DMBA-induced leukemia in mice. *GANN*, **62**, 407–412 (1971).
25. Sugiyama, T. Specific genome change in hydrocarbon-induced rat leukemia. *Abstr. Papers, Xth Int. Cancer Congress*, 64 (1970).
26. Sugiyama, T., and Brillantes, F. P. Cytogenetic studies of leukemia induced by 6,8,12- and 7,8,12-trimethylbenz[*a*]anthracene. *J. Exp. Med.*, **131**, 331–341 (1970).
27. Sugiyama, T., Kurita, Y., and Nishizuka, Y. Chromosome abnormality in rat leukemia induced by 7,12-dimethylbenz[*a*]anthracene. *Science*, **158**, 1058–1059 (1967).
28. Sugiyama, T., Kurita, Y., and Nishizuka, Y. Biologic studies on 7,12-dimethylbenz[*a*]anthracene-induced rat leukemia with special reference to the specific chromosomal abnormalities. *Cancer Res.*, **29**, 1117–1124 (1969).
29. Toth, B. Development of malignant lymphomas by cell-free filtrates prepared from a chemically induced mouse lymphoma. *Proc. Soc. Exp. Biol. Med.*, **112**, 873–875 (1963).
30. Toth, B., and Shubik, P. Studies with malignant lymphomas: Possible interaction problems between chemical and viral-inducing agents. *Natl. Cancer Inst. Monograph*, **22**, 313–328 (1966).
31. Yokoro, K., Imamura, N., Takizawa, S., Nishihara, H., and Nishihara, E. Leukemogenic and mammary tumorigenic effects of N-Nitrosobutylurea in mice and rats. *GANN*, **61**, 287–289 (1970).

COMMENTS

SYNCARCINOGENIC ROLE OF ONCOGENIC VIRUS

Waro NAKAHARA
*National Cancer Center Research Institute**

The concept of syncarcinogenesis, as it is now understood, means the eventual production of cancer through the summation of many small but apparently permanent alterations in the genetic material of the cell, the alterations summarized being induced by more than one, possibly numerous, carcinogenic agents (*2*). The carcinogenic agents involved may be chemical, physical, or biological. To say this much is tantamount to including oncogenic viruses among the agents, the carcinogenic effects of which may summate with those of other carcinogenic agents.

There are in the literature reports of many experimental results that support, directly or indirectly, viral and chemical syncarcinogenesis. One of the most pertinent examples may be the observation of Mackenzie and Rous (*1*), showing that benign warts induced by percutaneous applications of tar on rabbit ear rapidly turn into malignant eptheliomas when the virus of Shope papilloma is injected intravenously. I point out this observation now, in particular, because its real significance does not seem to have been fully appreciated. Here we have Shope virus, which, by itself, seldom produces anything but benign papillomas. Tar painting on the rabbit ear (performed in Yamagiwa and Ichikawa's classic experiments) produces epithelioma only with great difficulty and after a long period of repeated applications. These 2 materials, a virus and a chemical substance, each weakly carcinogenic, precipitously induce malignant tumors when applied one after the other. Clearly, this may be a case of the summation of the effects of viral and chemical carcinogens.

The production of tumors of the lymphoma-leukemia complex in rodents by exposure to radiant energy, and the occurrence of the leukemia virus (type C particles) in the tumors produced is now too well documented to require any comment. These cases may well be examples of radiation-virus syncarcinogenesis. The possibility of the leukemia virus originally present in the animal body in a latent form having been " activated " by irradiation, however, cannot be entirely excluded.

A virus could produce malignant tumors apparently without the aid of helping cofactors, as demonstrated by massive injections of certain adenoviruses.

Potentially oncogenic viruses may remain latent without ever showing their oncogenic properties. Such viruses may be activated, or induced to mature into an actively oncogenic form, by influences external to the viruses.

The present discussion is based on the idea of regarding oncogenic viruses simply as another class of carcinogenic agents. From this point of view, the role of

* Tsukiji 5-1-1, Chuo-ku, Tokyo 104 (中原和郎).

an oncogenic virus in the causation of malignant growths may be considered on an equal footing with chemical carcinogens and carcinogenic radiant energy. It would perhaps be profitable for the study of viral carcinogenesis to take into account the concept of the summation of syncarcinogenic effects.

REFERENCES

1. Mackenzie, I., and Rous, P. The experimental disclosure of latent neoplastic changes in tarred skin. *J. Exp. Med.*, **73**, 391–415 (1941).
2. Nakahara, W. Critique of carcinogenic mechanism. *Progr. Exp. Tumor Res.*, **2**, 158–202 (1961); Summation synkarzinogener Wirkungen. *Med. Klinik*, **61**, 661–64 (1966).

GANN Monograph on Cancer Research 12, 1972

A FEW COMMENTS

Hisao Uetake
*Institute for Virus Research, Kyoto University**

I would like to make a few comments on virus-cell interactions and the viral etiology of human tumors from the virological and immunological viewpoints.

1) It is now generally accepted that usually the tumor cell carries tumor-specific transplantation antigen(s) (TSTA) on its surface, which is virus-specific in virus-induced tumors and strain-specific in chemically induced tumors. In this regard, what I would like to point out is that the appearance of change(s) in the cell surface structure is a fairly common phenomenon in virus-infected cells and is not confined to virus-induced tumor cells. In my opinion, this type of antigenic change is important in that it evokes cell-mediated immunity in the host not only against tumor cells but also against virus-infected cells.

2) The appearance of TSTA in tumor cells is suggestive of its important role in carcinogenesis but nothing is known as yet about their direct relationships. Human adenovirus-induced hamster or mouse tumor cells carry TSTA, and the virus-infected human cells which are destined to death also synthesize TSTA. Both types of cells with TSTA are subjected to host immunological surveillance. However, human adenoid tissue cells in which adenovirus resides in a dormant state do not seem to carry TSTA, because they are not rejected by the host immune mechanisms. If they carried TSTA, they would be rejected. They have no TSTA, and they are not cancer cells.

The same holds true for SV40; SV40-induced hamster or mouse tumor cells carry specific TSTA, and the virus-infected African green monkey cells which are going to die also synthesize the same TSTA. On the other hand, however, SV40 is known to be carried in a latent state in monkeys, and in this case virus-carrying cells may not show TSTA so they are not rejected by immune response, since if they showed TSTA, they would be rejected. They have no TSTA and they are not cancer cells.

Herpes simplex virus (HSV) is thought to be harbored in cells as a provirus. These virus-carrying cells are not rejected by the host immune mechanism. Hence, the HSV genome persists throughout the life of the host. Here again, though it is not definitely proved, the cells that harbor HSV genome do not seem to show TSTA or the like, and they are not cancer cells. On the contrary, cells freshly infected with HSV which are destined to destruction show new antigen(s) on their surfaces and these cells are eliminated.

Recent investigations suggest that cytomegalovirus is carried in a latent form and is activated by hormones, immunosuppressive agents, and/or pregnancy. If so, cells harboring the virus genome might not show any virus-specific

* Kawara-machi, Shogoin, Sakyo-ku, Kyoto 606 (植竹久雄).

structure on their surface, since they are exempt from immunological rejection.

In connection with Rous sarcoma virus (RSV), it has recently been clarified that cells of some chicken lines may carry a genetic factor designated as " chick cell-associated helper factor (chf or f)," which provides an envelope component(s) to defective RSV, resulting in reproduction of infective RSV. This genetic entity seems to be a defective genome of Rous-associated virus (RAV). It indicates that RAV is not oncogenic but may be integrated into host cells.

The above examples imply that the incorporation or integration of the viral genome into the host cell is not confined to oncogenic viruses but also occurs in nononcogenic viruses and that in any case structural change(s) on the cell surface does not seem necessary in order for viral genome-carrying cells to persist in the host organism. In turn it implies that the presence of viral genome does not always lead to alteration in the cell surface structure even in the host-virus combinations in which cell surface changes appear in cytocidal infections, and such cells are not tumor cells.

3) In this symposium Dr. Toyoshima reported the isolation of unique temperature-sensitive mutants from Rous sarcoma virus B77. This type of mutant-infected cell undergoes focus formation when kept at a permissive temperature, but when shifted to a nonpermissive temperature they lose their focus-forming ability quickly and reversibly. These findings seem to be very important in the sense that this type of mutant RSV may be of great help in elucidating the mechanism of transformation by RSV, possibly in connection with changes in cellular surface structures.

4) Are human cancers virus-induced? If so, are they transmitted vertically, as suggested by Huebner and Todaro?

I and K. E. Hellströms recently reported that in human neoplasms the cell-mediated immunity, its blocking by patient sera, and immunological cross-reactions in neuroblastomas, malignant malanomas, breast carcinomas, endometrial carcinomas, colon carcinomas, seminomas, ovarian carcinomas, and sarcomas, respectively, but no cross-reactions between tumors of different types. The presence of cross-reactions among a certain type of carcinomas seems favorable for viral etiology, since virus-induced tumors show virus-specific TSTAs, while chemically or physically induced tumors show individual tumor-specific TSTAs. However, if such a hypothetical virus were transmitted vertically, the host would become tolerant of the said virus-induced TSTA and thus unable to produce blocking antibodies against the TSTA, as observed in animal tumor viruses. Thus, these are not compatible with the Hellströms' findings cited above. What would be the explanation? Are they not induced by viruses? If virus-induced, are they not transmitted vertically?

5) Group-specific (gs) antigen is a kind of viral antigen. In virus infections, it is a general rule that there is no expression of late function genes without expression of early function genes. And the synthesis of viral antigens is one of the late functions. TSTA synthesis is one of the early functions, whereas gs synthesis seems to be one of the late functions. Hence, it should be reasonable to presume that gs synthesis always follows TSTA synthesis. If so, gs antigen-positive cells must carry TSTA, too. This can be tested experimentally.

6) Generally speaking, based on experimental tumor research, the oncogenic activity of leukemia viruses is species specific whereas that of sarcoma viruses and DNA tumor viruses is not species specific, inducing tumors in different species of animals. And sometimes DNA tumor viruses can induce tumors only in animals that are not their natural hosts, and in natural hosts they multiply and kill the cells. Accordingly, if human tumors were induced by DNA viruses, we would have to take into consideration the possibility that they would be induced by animal viruses of which the natural hosts are not humans. On the contrary, in regard to human leukemias, if they were of viral nature, it is likely that they would be induced by a human-specific virus or viruses, and human sarcoma may stand in between.

A GENERAL DISCUSSION OF EXPERIMENTAL LEUKEMOGENESIS

Susumu WATANABE
*National Cancer Center Research Institute**

Personally, I think that research on experimental leukemia should contribute to the clarification of the mechanism of human leukemogenesis.

Leukemia in experimental animals has been most extensively studied using mice. Also, the greater part of experimental and spontaneous leukemias of mice belong to the lymphoid type (including the thymus type). This type of leukemia, initially developing from the lymphoid tissue and thymus, has the character of a lymphosarcoma, which at the terminal stage disseminates into the blood-stream. Thus, this type of leukemia in mice shows the characteristics of a malignant growth in the narrower sense. Furthermore, the process of leukemic changes in mice manifests itself in acute form. We have not encountered a leukemic process in mice of the chronic type which is compatible with those in human cases. Also, with the rat, we have only cases of the acute type, although sometimes leukemia of the myeloid type has also been observed.

In contrast to these observations based on leukemic cases in experimental animals, both the myeloid and lymphoid types of leukemia have been observed among humans, and in particular we have many more cases of the myeloid type here in this country. Furthermore, among cases of human leukemia, we have separated 2 distinct groups, *i.e.*, acute and chronic. Although the chronic type may sometimes terminate with an acute crisis, the acute type does not transform itself into the chronic type. In this country most cases of chronic leukemia belong to the myeloid type, and we rarely encounter chronic lymphoid leukemia, which is frequently observed in Western countries.

When we examine the cases of acute leukemia, we are able to include this type of leukemic process among malignancies on the condition that this process shows the irreversible growth of immature hematopoietic cells. However, such immature cells do not show the definite destructive invading growth pattern that is usually observed in the case of other malignancies, and these cells seem merely to be filling the intercellular spaces. While this type of proliferation of leukemic cells is not sufficient to bring about the termination of the individual life by itself, massive hemorrhage and bacterial or fungus infection may contribute to the death.

When Virchow (1847) first defined leukemia, he dealt only with chronic myeloid leukemia, and acute leukemia was first described by Epstein (1880) some 30 years later. Up to the beginning of this century acute leukemia had been viewed in the sense of an infective or reactive process; Sternberg, in particular, understood it as a septic process. Nageli criticized this opinion and applied the

* Tsukiji 5-1-1, Chuo-ku, Tokyo 104 (渡辺　漸).

concept of neoplastic growth to the leukemic process, and this view has been supported by Apiz, Rohr, and Moeschlin. My co-workers and I published our opinion in 1941, supporting the neoplastic theory of human leukemia; however, at that time, this theory had not yet won unanimous approval.

At the present time, viewing leukemia as a whole, including both the myeloid and lymphoid types, we assume this process to be neoplastic growth. However, I wonder whether or not chronic leukemia, especially chronic myeloid leukemia, belongs in the category of true neoplastic growth. Damshek (1964) presented the new concept that chronic lymphoid leukemia is an immune incompetent disorder. My own opinion is that chronic myeloid leukemia may also include such a process. In other words, I suspect that acute and chronic leukemias should not be treated as belonging to the same category.

Among leukemic cases of atomic bomb survivors in Hiroshima, we have noticed a definite increase of the chronic myeloid type. Furthermore, we have presented our opinion that the chronic myeloid leukemia among the atomic bomb survivors developed from generalized hyperplasia of the bone marrow following repeated physiological restorations of bone marrow activity, while the acute myeloid leukemia among the atomic bomb survivors developed from local circumscribed foci, as has been observed in cases of other malignancies.

I am now of the opinion that in the cases of chronic myeloid leukemia among atomic bomb survivors the total body irradiation might have contributed not only to generalized hematopoietic hyperactivity following the injuries but also to the deterioration of immune mechanisms in general.

On the basis of the concepts stated above, I think it is reasonable to separate acute and chronic leukemia and to assume the existence of two different categories of leukemia. Acute leukemia will be effected when predominantly localized injuries are sustained by the hematopoietic tissues, and chronic leukemia will develop when there exists a moderate to serious modification of the generalized immune response accompanied by slight, but more generalized damage to the hematopoietic tissues.

Therefore, investigations on experimental leukemia which simulate human acute leukemia will be evaluated in order to clarify the mechanisms of acute leukemia only. We need to produce the chronic type of leukemia among experimental animals in order to clarify the mechanism of the development of human leukemia as a whole. Furthermore, we find many discrepancies between the findings based on human and experimental acute leukemia.

For the purpose of pushing leukemia research further, we must discriminate between the diverse findings on human and experimental leukemia. Through precise recognition and analysis of these findings, our hopes will be realized in the near future.

A COMMENT BY AN OLD PATHOLOGIST

Tomizo YOSHIDA
*Cancer Institute**

There is a traditional concept of cancerization of the cell which many pathologists still harbor in the depths of their minds. In order to outline this concept I would like to use 2 simple drawings, Figs. 1 and 2.

The black point in the nucleus of the cell (Fig. 1) indicates a functional center which is postulated to regulate the mitotic division of a cell. According to Rudolf Virchow (1821–1902), the cell is provided with such a center which will respond only to an appropriate stimulation from outside the cell, resulting in cell division. The center remains silent and inactive as long as proper stimulation is absent.

On the other hand, when this external stimulation of cell division is repeated at an unusual frequency and lasts for a certain long period of time, a change can occur in the center such that the center begins to operate autonomously and cell division continues without any external stimulation. This change of the center is regarded as stable and irreversible. This is an explanation, based on Virchow's stimulation theory, of how the cancerization of a normal cell takes place.

It is obvious that the origination of a cancer cell in this way implies the origination of a new type (species) of cell, or " a new cell race " (eine neue Zellrasse) as it was once called by Gustav Hauser (1903) of Germany. Consequently, the development (growth) of a " malignant tumor " which is actually the result of multiplication (numerical increase) of this new cell race excludes the possibility of a process by which surrounding normal cells are added to established tumors as their constituents one after another through cancerization on their own side. This is an important aspect of the traditional concept, for it strictly excludes the additional or

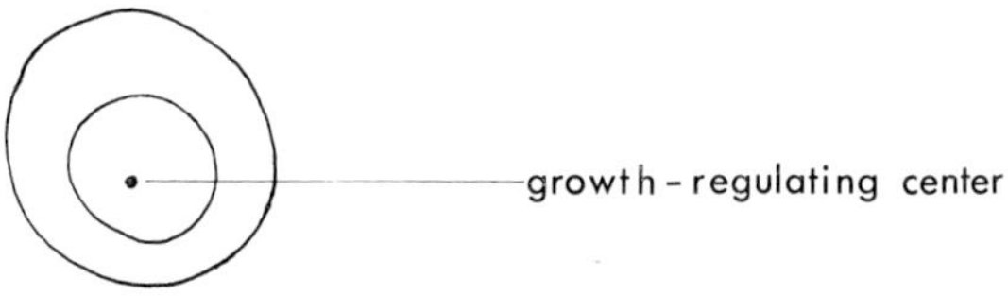

FIG. 1

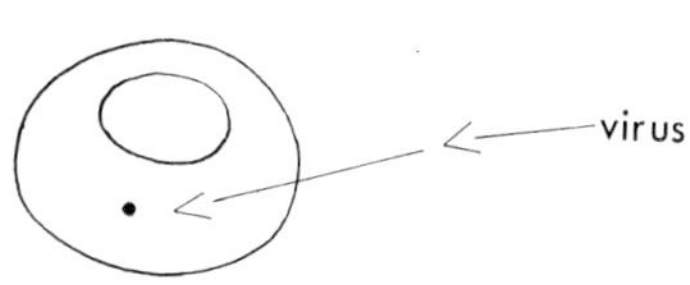

FIG. 2

* Kami-Ikebukuro 1-37-1, Toshima-ku, Tokyo 170 (吉田富三).

appositional growth of malignant tumor. Under certain carcinogeneous conditions of a tissue, there may originate a great number of cancer cells. However, this does not immediately mean the additional growth of any established tumor; rather, it means multicentric development of different tumors, each of which is initiated by a separate original cancer cell.

On the contrary, in the case of virus tumors, the virus enters the cell body from outside, as indicated in Fig. 2. Following the invasion by the virus, cell division takes place as the result of a reaction of the cell to the activity of the virus. In this relation, a virus tumor must differ from traditional cancerization in at least the following 2 points.

1) Tumor cells infected with a virus cannot be regarded as a new type of cell since their pathological proliferation is the result of their reaction with the virus and consequently the change is reversible.

2) In the growth of virus tumors the additive type of growth is inevitably involved, since the same kind of virus or those released from virus tumor cells should cause exactly the same kind of reactive growth in the surrounding normal cells, one after another.

As stated above, the exclusion of additional growth of a tumor is the fundamental point of traditional discussions of neoplastic growth, but when multiple cancer cells originating in the area of the tissue under certain carcinogeneous circumstances are all alike in nature and indistinguishable from each other, then this becomes a weak point in the traditional concept. This has been a great concern to me for a long time. However, comparative research by our study group on malignant growth using ascites hepatomas of the rat revealed materials which support the traditional concept. It was demonstrated that every one of the hepatoma nodules induced in the rat liver by azo-dye feeding was constituted of tumor cells which were more or less, and sometimes to a great extent, different from those constituting another hepatoma. This difference was noted not only between hepatomas induced in separate animals but even between hepatomas induced in one and the same liver of the same animal. These findings would provide a basis for the assumption that the development of each hepatoma nodule could be traced to a single initial hepatoma cell which is different from the initial cell of another tumor, that is, every tumor is constituted exclusively of descendant cells of a single ancestor hepatoma cell, although conglomeration of many tumors which are growing in their own way may sometimes give rise to a large tumor mass of mosaic constitution of different tumors. It seems to me that this result is quite favorable to the traditional theory.

On the other hand, there is some talk about integration of the virus genome into the host chromosome or host genome. When the growth of a virus tumor is due to such a biological or biochemical change in the host genome caused by the integration of a virus genome, it could be regarded as a stable and irreversible change, and, if so, the situation will be the same, in principle, as that of the traditional theory. In other words, tumor cells of virus tumors could be regarded as a new type of cell like the cancer cells described by the traditional theory. I would like to hear comments from specialists on virus tumors as to whether or not such a concept is correct.

Virchow's hypothesis of a growth-regulating center is apparently a product of his anatomical thinking (anatomischer Gedanke), which goes back to Morgagni's idea of " the seat of disease " (1761). Virchow pursued the seat of disease from macroscopic organs and tissues down to the microscopic cell level and established " cellular pathology " as a guiding principle for pursuing the pathogenesis of general diseases. As to the cancerization of a normal cell, it is in fact a disease of the cell itself, apart from any general disease of the body. Therefore, in order to pursue the anatomical mode of thinking to the last, the seat of this disease of the cell must be found inside the cell. It seems quite natural that this train of thought leads to the assumption of a central organization within the cell which regulates cell division. This is in fact a working hypothesis and is subject to scientific proof. In this relation, I wonder whether the " integration of a virus genome into the host genome " could be deemed as a scientific proof, or an approach to the proof, of this hypothesis?

At any rate, in the traditional concept of carcinogenesis the focus of discussion is found in the " centrum " of origination as well as in the further development of the tumor. Actually, in the case of malignant epithelial growths (carcinomas), a localized center of the growth can be demonstrated under the microscope, and examination of the earliest stage of circumscribed tumor formation leads to the assumption of an initial cancer cell, although this is beyond direct observation.

In contrast, in the case of nonepithelial neoplasms (sarcomas), the demonstration of a focus of the growth in any stage of its development is quite difficult. Above all, exclusion of the additional growth in the early stage of sarcoma development, not only in human cases but also in experimental induction of sarcomas in animals, is extremely difficult, and this condition is most prominent in the development of leukemias.

About 30 to 40 years ago, it was a topic of earnest discussion among pathologists in Japan whether leukemia in general should be included in the category of " true " (according to the traditional concept) neoplasm (neoplastic growth). Dr. O. Kimura, professor of pathology at Tohoku University at that time, was against its inclusion among true neoplasms. He pointed out that the formation of a tumor, that is, a focus of the growth, is lacking in the growth of leukemia. The record of this discussion has, regrettably, not been left, but I think that this may remain a point of discussion in tumor pathology.

It is a question harbored in my mind since a long time ago whether some fundamental difference does not exist between epithelial and nonepithelial neoplasms, although they are discussed at the present time on an equal footing under the collective term of " malignant growths."